pathology

pathology

The National Medical Series for Independent Study

pathology

EDITORS

Virginia A. LiVolsi, M.D.

Professor of Pathology
University of Pennsylvania School
of Medicine
Director of Surgical Pathology
Hospital of the University
of Pennsylvania
Philadelphia, Pennsylvania

Maria J. Merino, M.D.

Associate Chief of Surgical Pathology
and Postmortem
National Cancer Institute
National Institutes of Health
Bethesda, Maryland

Ronald D. Neumann, M.D.

Assistant Chief, Department of
Nuclear Medicine
National Institutes of Health
Bethesda, Maryland

ASSOCIATE EDITOR

Paul H. Duray, M.D.

Assistant Professor of Pathology
Yale University School of Medicine
Attending Surgical Pathologist
Director of Autopsy Pathology
Yale-New Haven Hospital
New Haven, Connecticut

A WILEY MEDICAL PUBLICATION
JOHN WILEY & SONS
New York • Chichester • Brisbane • Toronto • Singapore

Harwal Publishing Company, Media, Pa.

Library of Congress Cataloging in Publication Data
Main entry under title:

Pathology.

(The National medical series for independent study)
(A Wiley Medical publication)
Includes index.
1. Anatomy, Pathological—Outlines, syllabi, etc.
I. LiVolsi, Virginia A. II. Merino, Maria J.
III. Neumann, Ronald Daniel. IV. Series. [DNLM:
1. Pathology—Examination questions. QZ 18 P2965]
RB32.P37 1983   616.07   83-18608
ISBN 0-471-09623-7

©1984 by Harwal Publishing Company, Media, Pennsylvania

10 9 8 7

Contents

v

Preface

Pathology is fundamentally a review of anatomic pathology; it is not intended to be a primary textbook of pathology. Much of the information is based on current teachings and the discussions covered in the major pathology textbooks. As in all fields of medicine, controversies in pathology exist. Rather than adhere to any single reference, we have gathered material from many sources, including our own publications and lecture notes.

Pathology encompasses all of medicine. The amount of material to be learned is awesome, yet the time devoted to pathology courses has decreased in many medical schools. If this book helps the student learn the essentials of anatomic pathology, it will have served its intended purpose.

Ronald D. Neumann

Acknowledgments

The editors wish to extend their gratitude to Pamela Hinman for her preparation and typing of this manuscript and to Robert Specht for his preparation of the photographs.

Publisher's Note

The objective of the *National Medical Series* is to present an extraordinarily large amount of information in an easily retrievable form. The outline format was selected for this purpose of reducing to the essentials the medical information needed by today's student and practitioner.

While the concept of an outline format was well received by the authors and publisher, the difficulties inherent in working with this style were not initially apparent. That the series has been published and received enthusiastically is a tribute to the authors who worked long and diligently to produce books that are stylistically consistent and comprehensive in content.

The task of producing the *National Medical Series* required more than the efforts of the authors, however, and the missing elements have been supplied by highly competent and dedicated developmental editors and support staff. Editors, compositors, proofreaders, and layout and design staff have all polished the outline to a fine form. It is with deep appreciation that I thank all who have participated, in particular, the staff at Harwal—Debra L. Dreger, Jane Edwards, Gloria Hamilton, Jeanine Kosteski, Wieslawa B. Langenfeld, Keith LaSala, June A. Sangiorgio, Mary Ann C. Sheldon, and Jane Velker.

The Publisher

Introduction

Pathology is one of seven basic science review books in a series entitled *The National Medical Series for Independent Study*. This series has been designed to provide students and house officers, as well as physicians, with a concise but comprehensive instrument for self-evaluation and review within the basic sciences. Although *Pathology* would be most useful for students preparing for the National Board of Medical Examiners examinations (Part I, FLEX, and FMGEMS), it should also be useful for students studying for course examinations. These books are not intended to replace the standard basic science texts but, rather, to complement them.

The books in this series present the core content of each basic science area, using an outline format and featuring a total of 300 study questions. The questions are distributed throughout the book at the end of each chapter and in a pretest and post-test. In addition, each question is accompanied by the correct answer, a paragraph-length explanation of the correct answer, and specific reference to the outline points under which the information necessary to answer the question can be found.

We have chosen an outline format to allow maximal ease in retrieving information, assuming that the time available to the reader is limited. Considerable editorial time has been spent to ensure that the information required by all medical school curricula has been included and that each question parallels the format of the questions on the National Board examinations. We feel that the combination of the outline format and board-type study questions provides a unique teaching device.

We hope you will find this series interesting, relevant, and challenging. The authors, as well as the John Wiley and Harwal staffs, welcome your comments and suggestions.

Pretest

QUESTIONS

Directions: Each question below contains five suggested answers. Choose the **one best** response to each question.

1. The most common type of malignancy that is found in a pleural effusion cytology in a man without a known primary cancer is

(A) lymphoma
(B) mesothelioma
(C) carcinoma of the colon
(D) carcinoma of the lung
(E) carcinoma of the pancreas

2. The term used to describe the unidirectional migration of leukocytes toward a target is

(A) diapedesis
(B) chemotaxis
(C) meiosis
(D) endocytosis
(E) margination

3. Permanent myocardial damage due to irreversible myocardial ischemia is identified best by which of the following terms?

(A) Myocardial infarction
(B) Angina pectoris
(C) Ischemic heart disease
(D) Paroxysmal nocturnal dyspnea
(E) Ventricular aneurysm

4. The most serious common complication of lower extremity thrombophlebitis is

(A) cerebral infarction
(B) kidney infarction
(C) myocardial infarction
(D) pulmonary infarction
(E) intestinal infarction

5. Glomus tumors or glomangiomas originate in structures that are responsible for which of the following functions?

(A) Blood pressure regulation
(B) Temperature regulation
(C) Taste sensation
(D) Tactile sensation
(E) Temperature sensation

6. The hereditary form of multiple aneurysmal telangiectasias is called

(A) Mönckeberg's disease
(B) Takayasu's disease
(C) Buerger's disease
(D) Lindau-von Hippel disease
(E) Osler-Rendu-Weber disease

7. What is the term given to the group of lung diseases that result from the chronic inhalation of particulate or gaseous agents as a result of occupational exposure?

(A) Granulomatous disease
(B) Pneumoconiosis
(C) Mycobacteriosis
(D) Pseudolymphoma
(E) Bronchiectasis

8. Which of the carcinomas listed below grows as well-differentiated cells that line the respiratory air spaces without invading the stroma of the lung?

(A) Squamous cell
(B) Anaplastic
(C) Large cell
(D) Small cell
(E) Bronchioalveolar

1

9. What is the most common cause of chronic obstructive pulmonary disease in the United States?

(A) Pneumoconiosis

(B) Pneumonia

(C) Interstitial lung diseases

(D) Emphysema

(E) Cystic fibrosis

10. A 58-year-old man was hospitalized for evaluation of intermittent upper abdominal pain. His history disclosed a 15-lb weight loss over the preceding months. Physical examination revealed upper abdominal tenderness, but neither masses nor ascites were present. The diagnostic approach and preliminary diagnosis would include

(A) oral cholecystogram: chronic cholecystitis with cholelithiasis

(B) measurement of serum bilirubin: chronic cholecystitis with cholelithiasis

(C) endoscopy: carcinoma of the ampulla of Vater

(D) celiotomy: carcinoma of the head of the pancreas

(E) computed axial tomography scan: carcinoma of the body of the pancreas

11. Of the tumors of the liver listed below, which is the most common?

(A) Hepatocellular carcinoma

(B) Angiosarcoma

(C) Cholangiocarcinoma

(D) Hamartoma

(E) Hemangioma

12. Which of the following liver tumors has been most frequently associated with the use of oral contraceptives?

(A) Bile duct adenoma

(B) Hepatocellular adenoma

(C) Nodular hyperplasia

(D) Hepatoma

(E) Cholangiocarcinoma

13. Malacoplakia of the renal pelvis occurs following infection by which of the following organisms?

(A) *Mycoplasma pneumoniae*

(B) *Cryptococcus neoformans*

(C) *Escherichia coli*

(D) *Streptococcus viridans*

(E) *Staphylococcus aureus*

14. A kidney biopsy specimen that shows subendothelial granular electron-dense deposits is characteristic of which of the following disease states?

(A) Rapidly progressive glomerulonephritis

(B) Poststreptococcal glomerulonephritis

(C) Membranous glomerulonephritis

(D) Systemic lupus erythematosus

(E) Goodpasture's syndrome

15. The best 5-year survival rate is found in patients with which of the following tumors?

(A) Choriocarcinoma

(B) Seminoma

(C) Embryonal cell carcinoma

(D) Teratoma

(E) Yolk sac tumor

16. The most common type of testicular germ cell tumor is termed

(A) seminoma

(B) embryonal cell tumor

(C) yolk sac tumor

(D) choriocarcinoma

(E) teratoma

17. Which of the following conditions probably is the most common cause of recurrent urinary tract infections in males?

(A) Immune deficiency disease

(B) Malacoplakia

(C) Chronic prostatitis

(D) Kidney stones

(E) Syphilis

18. Which of the following is the most common type of breast carcinoma?

(A) Intraductal
(B) Medullary
(C) Papillary
(D) Mucinous
(E) Infiltrating ductal

19. A 16-month-old boy presents with a right-sided abdominal mass, which examination discloses to be associated with the liver. X-rays show a partially calcified tumor occupying most of the right abdomen. The correct diagnosis is

(A) Wilms' tumor
(B) hepatoblastoma
(C) pancreatoblastoma
(D) neuroblastoma
(E) islet cell carcinoma

20. A 38-year-old man is injured in a head-on automobile collision. When he is brought to the emergency room, he is in shock, is unconscious, and requires mechanical respiratory assistance. Despite heroic efforts, he dies. Neuropathologic examination most likely will disclose

(A) ruptured basilar artery aneurysm
(B) Duret's hemorrhage
(C) severed medulla oblongata
(D) cerebral infarct
(E) arteriovenous malformation

21. An 8-year-old girl has a 3-month history of intermittent right lower quadrant pain. Two previous visits to the emergency room ruled out acute appendicitis. At this visit, a mass is palpated in the lower abdomen. The differential diagnosis includes each of the following conditions EXCEPT

(A) periappendiceal abscess
(B) Burkitt's lymphoma
(C) Crohn's disease
(D) ovarian cyst
(E) Hodgkin's disease

22. Acute leukemia is found with higher than expected frequency in each of the following conditions EXCEPT

(A) mongolism
(B) Fanconi's anemia
(C) Wiskott-Aldrich syndrome
(D) sideroblastic anemia
(E) sickle cell disease

23. Megaloblastic anemia results from each of the following EXCEPT

(A) *Diphyllobothrium latum* infection
(B) intestinal bypass surgery
(C) gastric atrophy
(D) oral contraceptive use
(E) chronic pancreatitis

24. What is the most common fungal infection of the oral mucosa occurring in young children and in immunocompromised adults?

(A) Actinomycosis
(B) Histoplasmosis
(C) Moniliasis
(D) Mucormycosis
(E) Nocardiosis

25. The most common benign bone tumor affecting individuals under the age of 21 years is

(A) chondromyxoid fibroma
(B) osteochondroma
(C) giant cell tumor
(D) aneurysmal bone cyst
(E) osteogenic sarcoma

Directions: Each question below contains four suggested answers of which **one or more** is correct. Choose the answer

A if **1, 2, and 3** are correct
B if **1 and 3** are correct
C if **2 and 4** are correct
D if **4** is correct
E if **1, 2, 3, and 4** are correct

26. Host inflammatory response includes which of the following functions?

(1) Isolation of infected tissues
(2) Inactivation of causative agents
(3) Neutralization of toxins
(4) Removal of devitalized tissue debris

27. Autopsy shows which of the following findings in the heart of a patient with long-standing hypertension?

(1) Left ventricular hypertrophy
(2) Papillary muscle hypertrophy
(3) Decreased left ventricle volume
(4) Endocardial fibrous thickening

28. Adult respiratory distress syndrome (ARDS) shows which of the following anatomic signs?

(1) Pulmonary edema
(2) Hyaline membrane formation
(3) Proliferation of type II pneumonocytes
(4) Alveolar wall damage

29. The various forms of viral hepatitis are transmitted by which of the following routes?

(1) Fecal-oral contamination
(2) Injection of antihemophilic factor
(3) Ingestion of contaminated raw shellfish
(4) Use of contaminated hypodermic needles

30. Chronic congestive heart failure produces which of the following hepatic morphologic changes?

(1) Biliary duct proliferation
(2) Formation of Mallory's bodies
(3) Lymphocytic infiltration of the triads
(4) Central lobular congestion and necrosis

31. Amyloid deposition is a part of the histopathologic process in which of the following diseases?

(1) Plasmacytoma
(2) Medullary carcinoma of the thyroid
(3) Chronic infection of the kidney
(4) Kimmelstiel-Wilson lesion

32. Acute orchitis refers to an acute inflammation of the testicular parenchyma. True statements concerning this condition include

(1) it is a common complication of mumps
(2) it results in a relatively high incidence of testicular cancer
(3) it is more frequent in patients with cryptorchidism
(4) it may result from epididymal infection

33. True statements concerning squamous cell carcinoma of the cervix include which of the following?

(1) It can be detected by cytologic screening tests
(2) It has an incidence equal to that of endometrial carcinoma
(3) It begins in the junction between the cervix and endocervix
(4) It is treated by hysterectomy and radiation therapy

34. Complications of gonorrheal infections in women that can cause sterility include

(1) permanent damage of the tubular epithelium
(2) extensive peritoneal and tubo-ovarian adhesions
(3) chronic salpingitis
(4) cervical stenosis

35. The epidemiology of squamous cell carcinoma of the cervix includes

(1) a low socioeconomic status
(2) a history of multiple sex partners
(3) early age at first coitus
(4) multiparity

36. Factors that carry an increased risk for the development of breast carcinoma include

(1) nulliparity
(2) fibrocystic disease
(3) family history of breast cancer
(4) amastia

37. Characteristics of laryngeal papillomatosis include

(1) occurrence at any age
(2) viral etiology
(3) positive response to surgical treatment
(4) malignant transformation

38. Conditions that predispose to the development of osteosarcoma include

(1) Paget's disease of the bone
(2) trauma to the bone
(3) previous radiation therapy involving bone
(4) multiple enchondromatoses

39. True statements concerning tuberculosis of the bone include

(1) it affects both children and adults
(2) vertebrae and the long bones are most commonly affected
(3) it often occurs via hematogenous spread of the organism
(4) bone can be the primary focus of infection

40. A patient complains that his hat size is increasing frequently; he walks bowlegged due to tibial deformities. Bone biopsy shows which of the following findings?

(1) Increased rate of calcification
(2) Mosaic pattern of bone
(3) Marked medullary fibrosis
(4) Increased number of osteoclasts

41. The main forms of leprosy include which of the following?

(1) Lepromatous
(2) Granulomatoid
(3) Tuberculoid
(4) Lupoid

Directions: The groups of questions below consist of lettered choices followed by several numbered items. For each numbered item select the **one** lettered choice with which it is **most** closely associated. Each lettered choice may be used once, more than once, or not at all.

Questions 42–45

For each manifestation of hypercalcemia listed below, match the causative agent.

(A) Primary hyperparathyroidism
(B) Renal cell carcinoma
(C) Multiple myeloma
(D) Paget's disease of the bone
(E) Metastatic breast cancer

42. Osteoclast activation

43. Excessive bone resorption resulting from excessive production of parathyroid hormone

44. Bone destruction and calcium release

45. Hyperactivity of the bone resorption-formation sequence

Questions 46–50

For each tumor that is listed below, match the causative agent.

(A) External irradiation
(B) Herpesvirus
(C) Estrogen
(D) Epstein-Barr virus
(E) Ultraviolet light

46. Papillary carcinoma of the thyroid

47. Squamous cell carcinoma of the cervix

48. Burkitt's lymphoma

49. Clear cell carcinoma of the cervix and vagina

50. Malignant melanoma

Questions 51–55

Match the following tumor-associated antigens with the tumors in which they are most likely to be found.

(A) Carcinoma of the pancreas
(B) Hepatoma
(C) Oat cell carcinoma of the lung
(D) Fibrous mesothelioma
(E) Hydatidiform mole

B 51. Alpha-fetoprotein
E 52. Chorionic gonadotropin
A 53. Carcinoembryonic antigen
C 54. Antidiuretic hormone
D 55. Hypoglycemic principle

Questions 56–60

For each tumor that is listed below, match the purported causative agent.

(A) Dietary fat
(B) Vinyl chloride
(C) Asbestos
(D) Cigarette smoking
(E) Cyclamates

B 56. Angiosarcoma of the liver
E 57. Cancer of the urinary bladder
A 58. Carcinoma of the colon
C 59. Mesothelioma
D 60. Carcinoma of the lung

ANSWERS AND EXPLANATIONS

1. The answer is D. (*Chapter 3 III A, B*) Numerous studies have shown that most pleural effusions that are caused by malignant disease in patients without known cancer contain adenocarcinoma cells. Statistically, the usual primary sites for such tumors are the breast in women and the lung in men.

2. The answer is B. (*Chapter 1 I D 3*) During the vascular stasis stage of hyperemia, neutrophils and monocytes adhere to the vascular endothelium prior to migration into the extravascular space in a process known as margination. Leukocytes emigrate (diapedesis) through gaps between the endothelial cells. Chemotaxis is the process by which leukocytes undergo unidirectional migration toward a specific target. Various chemotactic substances or factors influence the rate of movement of the cells. Several chemotactic factors have an apparently specific action on selected cell types.

3. The answer is A. [*Chapter 4 II A 3 a (3)*] Significant irreversible myocardial ischemia causes myocardial infarction, which is death of myocardial muscle fibers. Angina pectoris refers to the severe chest pain that may accompany myocardial ischemia but is not always associated with permanent myocardial damage. Ischemic heart disease is an inclusive term for all types of cardiac disease due to insufficient blood supply and, again, is not exclusive for permanent myocardial damage. Paroxysmal nocturnal dyspnea is sudden difficulty in breathing, occurring during the night when the patient is usually asleep and lying flat. While a ventricular aneurysm may be the eventual outcome of myocardial infarction, it is not the best descriptor of permanent ischemic myocardial damage.

4. The answer is D. (*Chapter 5 III B 1*) When thrombi form in the veins of the lower extremities and embolize, the emboli travel to the right side of the heart and enter the pulmonary arterial tree. Pulmonary emboli can cause pulmonary infarction, leading to necrosis of the lung tissue that is served by the occluded pulmonary artery branch. These emboli could not cause infarction of the brain, kidney, heart, or intestines unless a right-to-left shunt is present to allow emboli access to the systemic circulation.

5. The answer is B. (*Chapter 5 V B*) Glomus tumors originate from a structure known as the neuro-myoarterial glomus, which is an arteriovenous structure rich in autonomic nerves of the related artery. The cutaneous glomus organ has a function in temperature regulation.

6. The answer is E. (*Chapter 5 V C*) Osler-Rendu-Weber disease is the hereditary form of multiple aneurysmal telangiectasias. This condition is inherited as an autosomal dominant trait. Patients typically have telangiectasias of the lips, tongue, and nasal mucosa. Bleeding from these lesions is a common clinical presentation.

7. The answer is B. (*Chapter 6 IV H*) Pneumoconiosis is a pathologic condition of the lungs produced by chronic inhalation of particulate or gaseous matter, which generally occurs in the course of certain occupations. Anthracosis (black lung) is observed in miners and occasionally in dwellers of congested urban environments. Silicosis is seen in miners, metal grinders, and others who are chronically exposed to silica particles. Asbestosis is a particularly widespread form of pneumoconiosis and can lead to the development of malignant mesotheliomas.

8. The answer is E. (*Chapter 6 VIII B 2 b*) Bronchioalveolar carcinoma is a special type of adenocarcinoma that is composed of tall columnar or cuboidal epithelial malignant cells. The cells line respiratory spaces without invading the stroma of the lung. This tumor usually arises from bronchiolar epithelium, including that comprised of the Clara cells, and then spreads to and intermixes with the alveolar epithelium. The tumor can present radiographically as a single peripheral nodule, multiple nodules, or as a diffuse, pneumonia-like infiltrate.

9. The answer is D. (*Chapter 6 V A*) Emphysema is the most common cause of chronic obstructive pulmonary disease in the United States. It is characterized by over-distended lung alveoli with variable amounts of alveolar septal wall destruction. Although the exact mechanism that produces emphysema is unclear, there is a strong association with cigarette smoking and living in an urban environment with its attendant air pollution.

10. The answer is E. (*Chapter 9 IV C 1 a*) This history is suggestive of pancreatic cancer with abdominal pain and weight loss, and the least invasive technique likely to yield the most diagnostic information is the computed axial tomography scan, which has been shown to detect small mass lesions (tumors) with great accuracy. The diagnosis of chronic cholecystitis is unlikely in view of the relatively recent onset of symptoms and the weight loss. Carcinoma of the ampulla of Vater and the head of the pancreas would most likely produce clinical evidence of jaundice, which was not present in this patient.

11. The answer is E. (*Chapter 10 VII A*) Hemangiomas are the most common tumors of the liver and are found in all age groups. Only rarely do these lesions reach sufficient size to cause problems due to rupture and hemoperitoneum. Usually, liver hemangiomas are incidental findings at surgery or autopsy.

12. The answer is B. (*Chapter 10 V C*) Hepatocellular adenoma is a very rare neoplasm of the liver, occurring in women with a peak incidence between the third and fourth decades of life. Liver cell adenoma is a recognized complication of oral contraceptive use. The neoplasm is prone to hemorrhage and necrosis, which lead to pain in the right upper quadrant of the abdomen. Sometimes it ruptures and results in intraperitoneal bleeding, requiring emergency surgery.

13. The answer is C. (*Chapter 11 IX B 3*) The term malacoplakia originally referred to a distinctive type of cystitis of the urinary bladder. However, the condition has been shown to occur in several locations along the urinary tract where *Escherichia coli (E. coli)* infects the lining epithelial layers. Grossly, these focal thickenings of the mucosa (and sometimes submucosa) may be mistaken for cancer. Microscopically, these lesions are seen to be produced by accumulation of granular histiocytes beneath the surface epithelial cell layer.

14. The answer is D. (*Chapter 11 III C 3*) Granular subendothelial immune deposits and proliferation of mesangial and endothelial cells is nearly diagnostic of systemic lupus erythematosus. In systemic lupus erythematosus the immune complexes are located between the endothelial cells and the glomerular basement membrane. Later in the course of this disease, the immune complexes may also be seen subepithelially.

15. The answer is B. (*Chapter 12 II E*) Of patients with testicular malignancies, those with seminomas have the best prognosis for survival. Survival of patients with seminomas is 90 to 98 percent at 5 years; with teratomas, 70 percent at 2 years; with embryonal cell carcinomas, 35 percent at 5 years; infantile embryonal cell or yolk sac tumors, 50 percent at 5 years; and choriocarcinoma, less than 5 percent at 2 years.

16. The answer is A. (*Chapter 12 II E 3*) Seminomas are the most common of the testicular tumors and account for approximately 70 percent of primary germ cell neoplasms of the testes. Teratomas are the next most common testicular tumor; however, they account for only 20 to 25 percent. Yolk sac tumors, choriocarcinomas, and embryonal cell tumors occur with much less frequency.

17. The answer is C. (*Chapter 12 IV C 1, 2, 3, 4*) Chronic prostatitis, resulting usually from extension of an inflammatory process in the urethra or bladder, is a troublesome condition because it is frequently recurrent and is probably the most common cause of relapsing urinary tract infections in males. Immune deficiency diseases are relatively rare in the population; however, when they are present in individuals, they may cause recurrent urinary tract infections. Malacoplakia is an unusual inflammatory reaction produced by *Escherichia coli (E. coli)* infections of the urinary bladder and prostate; it is characterized by large numbers of histiocytes and Michaelis-Gutmann bodies.

18. The answer is E. (*Chapter 14 VIII B 2*) Infiltrating ductal carcinoma is the most common form of breast carcinoma, encompassing nearly 70 percent of breast cancers. Intraductal carcinoma constitutes only 5 to 10 percent of cancers of the breast; medullary carcinoma also constitutes about 5 to 10 percent. Papillary and mucinous carcinomas each account for less than 3 percent of malignant breast tumors.

19. The answer is D. (*Chapter 15 VI F 2*) Because of the age of the patient, islet cell carcinoma can be virtually eliminated as a diagnosis. Calcification is diagnostic of neuroblastoma; Wilms' tumor, hepatoblastoma, and pancreatoblastoma do not show this finding.

20. The answer is B. (*Chapter 16 II H 1 e*) Severe head trauma, as would be expected to have occurred in this patient, leads to bruising of the brain against the bony skull. Cerebral edema ensues with consequent caudal displacement of the midbrain and pons; transtentorial herniation then takes place. The latter results in stretching and tearing of brainstem arteries and veins, producing parenchymal hemorrhages (Duret's). Although a ruptured aneurysm and malformation could result in findings similar to Duret's lesion, these diagnoses would not apply in this instance. Neither a severed medulla oblongata nor a cerebral infarct are reasonable expectations.

21. The answer is E. (*Chapter 17 IV C*) Hodgkin's disease almost never involves the gastrointestinal tract or the reproductive (pelvic) organs. However, the possibility of a smoldering periappendiceal abscess must be considered. Burkitt's lymphoma is a lymphoma that commonly involves the gastrointestinal tract, especially in children. Crohn's disease can produce inflammatory fibrous masses. Finally, ovarian cysts occur in young girls and must be considered in the diagnosis of this case.

22. The answer is E. (*Chapter 17 IV B*) Mongolism, Fanconi's anemia, Wiskott-Aldrich syndrome, and sideroblastic anemia all show high incidences of acute leukemia. Genetic (and chromosomal) abnormalities are found in patients with mongolism, Fanconi's anemia, and Wiskott-Aldrich syndrome and may predispose to neoplastic transformation. Sideroblastic anemia has a prolonged smoldering phase, which in many cases ultimately blossoms into acute leukemia. No higher incidence of leukemia is noted in sickle cell patients.

23. The answer is E. [*Chapter 17 II A 3 b (1)*] Megaloblastic anemia is characterized by intestinal malabsorption of vitamin B_{12}, and *Diphyllobothrium latum* infection, intestinal bypass surgery, gastric atrophy, and oral contraceptives all interfere with vitamin B_{12} or folate absorption or metabolism. The parasite *Diphyllobothrium latum* interferes with absorption of vitamin B_{12}. Patients who undergo intestinal bypass surgery have part of the ileum bypassed, which is the site of vitamin B_{12} and folate absorption. Severe gastric atrophy demonstrates an absence of intrinsic factor, a substance that is needed for vitamin B_{12} absorption. Ingestion of oral contraceptives may result in megaloblastic anemia via interference with folate metabolism. However, none of these abnormalities is found in chronic pancreatitis.

24. The answer is C. (*Chapter 18 II B 2*) Moniliasis, commonly called thrush, is an acute infection of the oral cavity caused by *Candida albicans*. This oral fungal infection typically occurs in infants but can occur in immunocompromised, debilitated, and diabetic adults. The acute infection produces white elevated patches distributed through the oral mucosa. The mucosa is eroded beneath these patches, producing a bleeding superficial erosion.

25. The answer is B. (*Chapter 19 I H 2 c*) Osteochondroma is also referred to as exostosis. It is a benign new bone growth that often protrudes from the outer contour of bones and is capped by growing cartilage. The multifocal and clearly hereditary form of this lesion is known as hereditary multiple cartilaginous exostosis. Whether multiple or isolated, nearly 80 percent of these lesions are noted prior to the age of 21 years.

26. The answer is E (all). (*Chapter 1 I A 1*) The inflammatory response is a direct reaction against injurious agents or organisms threatening the homeostasis of the host. It has multiple actions, including isolation of infected tissues, inactivation of noxious agents and organisms, neutralization of toxins, and cleanup of devitalized tissues in preparation for tissue repair.

27. The answer is E (all). (*Chapter 7 II B 2*) Long-standing hypertension leads to anatomic changes in the heart, involving, in part, concentric hypertrophy of the left ventricle, including hypertrophy of the papillary muscles. Until later decompensation causes ventricular dilatation, ventricular wall hypertrophy decreases the intraventricular volume. Endocardial fibrous thickening also is noted occasionally.

28. The answer is E (all). (*Chapter 6 II B 3 b*) Adult respiratory distress syndrome (ARDS) is a model of acute alveolar injury with pulmonary edema and respiratory failure. A number of preexisting conditions can lead to ARDS, particularly if high concentrations of oxygen are used as supportive respiratory therapy. Focal atelectasis and alveolar collapse occur with the development of pulmonary edema; hyaline membranes appear, type II pneumonocytes proliferate, and there is variable damage to the alveolar walls. The mechanisms of ARDS are not completely understood.

29. The answer is E (all). (*Chapter 10 IV A 1*) The fecal-oral route is a known mode of transmission of hepatitis A virus infection. Ingestion of raw shellfish from contaminated waters is also reported to cause outbreaks of hepatitis. Hepatitis B infection is more often acquired from viral contamination of blood or blood products (fibrinogen and antihemophilic factor). Drug abusers who share hypodermic needles are at risk of acquiring hepatitis from a contaminated needle.

30. The answer is D (4). (*Chapter 10 III B 2*) Severe prolonged right-sided heart failure produces chronic venous congestion of the liver, which can progress to cardiac cirrhosis. The result is a firm liver, which shows the characteristic nutmeg pattern when cut surfaces are examined. This pattern is produced by congested and hemorrhagic centrilobular areas alternating with paler midzones with a yellowish tinge produced by fatty changes.

31. The answer is A (1, 2, 3). (*Chapter 11 III B 4*) Amyloid is a pink, eosinophilic, acellular material produced as part of several disease processes. Plasmacytoma, medullary carcinoma of the thyroid, and chronic infection of the kidney may lead to amyloidosis or be associated with amyloid deposition in various tissues. However, the Kimmelstiel-Wilson lesions that are found in the glomeruli of diabetic patients are composed of an acellular hyaline material in the glomerulus.

32. The answer is D (4). (*Chapter 12 II D 1*) Acute orchitis commonly involves the testis and often also the epididymis when infectious organisms, particularly *Escherichia coli* (*E. coli*), staphylococci, and streptococci, enter the testis via the vas deferens or via lymphatics. Acute orchitis is actually a rare complication of mumps. The condition does not increase the likelihood of later testicular malignancy.

33. The answer is E (all). (*Chapter 13 V B 6 b*) Squamous cell carcinoma of the cervix usually originates at the squamo-columnar junction, which is the dividing line between the endo- and exocervix. Because the tumor arises in this site, it can be detected by cytologic recovery screening tests, such as Papanicolaou's (Pap) test. Early detection has decreased the incidence of invasive squamous cell carcinoma of the cervix over the past 25 years so that it now occurs with an incidence equal to that of endometrial cancer. The treatment for squamous cell cervical carcinoma includes hysterectomy for the microinvasive form and radiotherapy for frankly invasive forms.

34. The answer is A (1, 2, 3). (*Chapter 13 IV C 2; II C 3*) Gonorrhea produces an extensive purulent infection when a fallopian tube becomes involved. The infection destroys the tubal epithelium, causing the tubal plicae to adhere together, effectively blocking the fallopian tube. If the infection extends outside the tube, both paratubal and tubo-ovarian abscesses and adhesions can occur. These adhesions and tubal stenoses are a major cause of sterility. Cervical stenosis is not a complication of gonorrheal infection.

35. The answer is E (all). (*Chapter 13 V B 6*) Epidemiologic studies of large populations of patients with cervical carcinoma show a higher incidence in individuals who engaged in early, promiscuous intercourse. A higher incidence has been noted in groups of low socioeconomic status. Having a large number of children also seems to increase the likelihood of developing squamous cell carcinoma. These epidemiologic findings have led to an ongoing search for a transmissible causative agent, which as yet has not been clearly identified.

36. The answer is A (1, 2, 3). (*Chapter 14 III B; VIII A 2*) Amastia is the rare congenital absence of one or both breasts, and breast carcinoma is no more likely to occur in an individual with only one breast due to this congenital abnormality than in an individual with two breasts. Epidemiologic studies have shown an increased incidence of breast carcinoma in nulliparous women, in women with fibrocystic disease, and in women with a strong family history of breast cancer.

37. The answer is A (1, 2, 3). (*Chapter 18 IV B 7*) Laryngeal papillomatosis is a true neoplasm that is postulated to be of viral origin. Malignant change is very rare. The papilloma is composed of a central core of fibrous tissue covered by stratified squamous epithelium. Surgical therapy is sufficient for the laryngeal polyps that do not regress spontaneously.

38. The answer is B (1, 3). (*Chapter 19 I H 3 a*) Osteogenic sarcoma affects predominantly men, with a peak incidence at about 20 years of age. Osteogenic sarcoma in older patients is often associated with Paget's disease of the bone. The tumor has also been associated with large doses of therapeutic radiation. Only anecdotal information links bone trauma to later development of osteogenic sarcoma.

39. The answer is A (1, 2, 3). [*Chapter 19 I F 1 c (3)*] Pott's disease or tuberculous spondylitis is a destructive infection of the spinal vertebrae. The long bones of the extremities are also commonly affected by tuberculosis of the bone. Bone involvement occurs by hematogenous spread of organisms originating in the primary lung focus of infection. Occasionally bone infection can occur because of direct spread from infected lymph nodes in the mediastinum.

40. The answer is E (all). (*Chapter 19 I G 1*) This patient is likely to have Paget's disease (osteitis deformans). This disease produces an accumulation of woven bone, which is characterized by a mosaic pattern created by a cement-like substance between the original bone and the new bone formation. Osteoblasts and osteoclasts are abundant, and there is excessive fibrosis in the marrow spaces between the cancellous bone spicules.

41. The answer is B (1, 3). (*Chapter 20 III D 1 b*) Leprosy is caused by *Mycobacterium leprae,* and although the disease is first manifested in the skin, parenchymal organs may also harbor the bacteria. In the lepromatous form of the disease, the bacteria multiply rapidly, presumably because of inadequate host defenses. Microscopically, lepra cells are seen to be filled with acid-fast bacilli. In the tuberculoid form of this disease, bacilli are difficult to detect. However, there is a prominent, noncaseous granulomatous reaction, which involves nerves as well as other tissues.

42–45. The answers are: 42-C, 43-A, 44-E, 45-D. (*Chapter 15 IV C 4; IV C 4; IV C 3, D 2; IV B*) Osteoclast-activating factor is released locally by tumors of lymphoid-plasma cell lines and causes calcium release due to excessive bone resorption. Parathyroid hormone activates bone resorption and formation, but the resorption exceeds the formation. The activation of osteoclastic resorption leads to bone mineral (i.e., calcium) release. Mass lesions in bone (mostly metastatic cancers) release calcium to the bloodstream by destroying bone. Whether this is a direct mechanical destruction or (more likely) results from the release of local factors and prostaglandins and from tumor cells or reactive neighboring lymphocytes, remains unknown. In pagetic bone, marked activity of resorption and formation occur; often a net loss of bone mineral (i.e., calcium) results.

46–50. The answers are: 46-A, 47-B, 48-D, 49-C, 50-E. (*Chapter 15 III B 7 b; Chapter 13 V B 6; Chapter 17 IV C 2 b; Chapter 13 IX C 2 b; Chapter 20 III G 4*) External irradiation to the neck (usually low dose) has been implicated in papillary thyroid cancer, although doses of radiation high enough to destroy the thyroid do not have this neoplastic effect. Most series have reported the association of thyroid cancer and radiation to be strongest when the radiation exposure occurred in childhood.

There are strong indications for a viral etiology of neoplasia. Epidemiologic, serologic, and refined biochemical evidence closely link cervical cancer and herpesvirus. Another neoplastic-viral association is Burkitt's lymphoma and Epstein-Barr virus, and although the evidence of the association is less strong than that for cervical cancer and herpesvirus, it is nonetheless intriguing.

Clear cell carcinoma of the cervix and vagina is a very rare tumor, and until recently it was virtually unheard of in young women. When a series of these tumors was diagnosed, epidemiologic evidence was obtained, which showed that the patients were the products of pregnancies in which there had been exposure to diethylstilbestrol (DES), a synthetic estrogen.

Melanoma may be related to ultraviolet light since epidemiologic studies indicate that the tumor is more common in areas of strong sunlight; it is almost epidemic in Australia.

51-55. The answers are: 51-B, 52-E, 53-A, 54-C, 55-D. (*Chapter 10 VI A; Chapter 13 III B 6 a; Chapter 9 IV C 1; Chapter 6 VIII B 3 b; Chapter 4 II E 1, Chapter 6 IX C 2*) Alpha-fetoprotein is found in the serum of adult patients with hepatoma and germ cell tumors.

Chorionic gonadotropin is a normal product of trophoblast. In neoplastic disorders of trophoblast, such as hydatidiform mole, chorionic gonadotropin is elevated, usually beyond the levels found in normal pregnancy.

Carcinoembryonic antigen can be elevated in patients with a variety of neoplasms, although it is most often found in patients with adenocarcinomas, frequently found in primary sites in the gastrointestinal tract and the pancreas.

Antidiuretic hormone is one of the common polypeptide hormones elevated in lung cancers, which are usually small (oat) cell carcinomas.

A tumor product that has the capacity to lower blood sugar is occasionally elaborated by tumors of mesenchymal origin. Many of these tumors that cause hypoglycemia are of mesothelial origin, and although the substance that they produce has not been fully characterized, it is known not to be insulin.

56–60. The answers are: 56-B, 57-E, 58-A, 59-C, 60-D. (*Chapter 10 VII C; Chapter 11 IX C; Chapter 8; Chapter 4 II E 1, Chapter 6 IX C 2; Chapter 6 IV H 3*) An association between a very rare liver tumor, angiosarcoma, and occupational exposure to vinyl chloride has been established. The epidemiology was indicated by the unusual histology of the tumor.

Although furor raged over governmental studies showing the development of bladder cancer in animals fed large amounts of cyclamates, this association in man is far from clear.

Epidemiologic studies from many areas of the world have indicated an association between diet and colonic neoplasia. One dietary agent implicated is fat; the incidence of colon cancer is high in countries in which the diet is rich in fat.

Asbestos exposure has been implicated in a variety of cancers, especially cancer of the lung. Mesothelioma, however, has been developed by a disproportionate number of individuals who have been exposed to asbestos. The rarity of mesothelioma supports a theory of "causative" association with asbestos.

Of great emotional and economic importance is the association of lung cancer (usually squamous and small cell types) with cigarette smoking.

1
Inflammation and Thrombosis

I. FUNDAMENTALS OF INFLAMMATION

A. Inflammation is the directed tissue responses to noxious and injurious external and internal stimuli, whether caused by toxic and chemical agents, physical factors (heat, cold, electricity, irradiation, and trauma), or microorganisms and their metabolic by-products. Inflammation and infection may coexist.

1. Advantages of Inflammation.
   a. It serves to localize and isolate the injured (or infected) tissue area, which protects the surrounding healthy tissue.
   b. It tends to neutralize and inactivate the toxic substances that are produced by humoral factors and enzymes.
   c. Inflammation counteracts, destroys, or limits the growth of infecting microorganisms.
   d. It sets the stage for wound healing and repair by clean-up of devitalized tissue and cell debris.

2. Disadvantages of Inflammation.
   a. It causes pain (dolor), swelling (tumor), heat (calor), and redness (rubor), which lead to varying degrees of disability.
   b. It may lead to viscus rupture (e.g., perforated appendicitis) and serious hemorrhage (e.g., an enlarging pulmonary tuberculous granuloma).
   c. A consequence of inflammation is excessive scar tissue formation with contracture, cicatrix formation (which can result in adhesive bowel obstruction), and keloid formation.
   d. Fistula formation in the abdominal-perineal area can occur as can bronchopleural fistula formation and pleural empyema, with accompanying normal tissue breakdown by neutral proteases.
   e. Inflammation may propagate further inflammation by destruction of the surrounding healthy tissue (biologic vicious circle).
   f. Specific examples of inflammation-damaged tissue include the following.
      (1) Renal disease (e.g., glomerulonephritis)
      (2) Arthritis
      (3) Fatal allergic reaction
      (4) Myocarditis
      (5) Encephalitis

B. CELLULAR COMPONENTS INVOLVED IN INFLAMMATORY PROCESSES

1. Circulating Blood–Derived Cell Elements.
   a. The **polymorphonuclear leukocytes**, which are variably known as neutrophils, granulocytes, "poly," and pus cells, are the predominant cells in acute inflammation, in abscess formation, and in loculation and empyema. They are also the first cells to arrive at the injured area. These cells are most likely responsible for the peripheral blood leukocytosis that occurs in response to a crisis.
      (1) Intracellular granules contain the following active enzymes.
         (a) Acid hydrolases act on organic matter, including bacteria.
         (b) Proteases cause degradation of the proteins of basement membranes, of elastin, and of collagen.
         (c) Lysozyme (muramidase) acts on microorganisms through hydrolysis; it is found in monocytes-macrophages-histiocytes as well.

(d) Myeloperoxidase, the major active component product of granulocytes, is the main antibacterial enzyme, operating with hydrogen peroxide (H_2O_2) and a halide ion.

(e) Cationic proteins inhibit bacterial growth, cause monocyte chemotaxis, and increase vascular permeability.

(2) **The neutrophils** leave the vascular system by diapedesis and are directed to the tissue site by chemotaxis; their major activity consists of phagocytosis and the extracellular release of lysosomal enzymes.

b. Basophilic Granulocytes.

(1) Basophils are granulocytic leukocytes containing specific basophilic granules that stain blue with Wright's stain. The granules consist of packets of histamines and heparin.

(2) They are involved in type I immunoglobulin E (IgE)-mediated hypersensitivity reactions [see C 3 b (1)]. When a specific antigen to IgE (the cytotrophic antibody, reagin) enters the body, basophils stimulate the formation of IgE, which binds to the surface of the cells. A cellular response can occur, and the granules release histamine and other vasoactive amines to produce anaphylactic reactions in sensitized individuals.

c. Eosinophilic Granulocytes.

(1) These cells have cytoplasmic granules, which stain orange with Romanovsky's stain and orange-red with eosin, and a characteristic bilobed nucleus. Eosinophils are increased in the peripheral blood in the presence of allergy and parasitic infestations.

(2) The granules consist of packets of hydrolytic enzymes, histaminase, peroxidase, and a poorly understood major basic protein. Although they can be found in the peripheral blood, the majority of the body's eosinophils are found within the tissues.

(3) Eosinophils are readily chemotactic upon the release of eosinophil chemotactic factor, which is due to anaphylaxis as a result of IgE-sensitized mast cells and are also phagocytic, although phagocytosis is a minor function. They are found in hypersensitivity sites in tissues and are able to abort hypersensitivity reactions.

2. Blood- and Tissue-Derived Cell Elements.

a. The **monocyte-macrophage system** is synonymous with reticuloendothelial cells and histiocytes.

(1) Monocytes are larger than granulocytic leukocytes. They are derived from bone marrow stem cells, which differentiate into peripheral blood monocytes, some of which migrate into tissues and become histiocytes. These include those of the

(a) Lungs—pulmonary-alveolar macrophages

(b) Abdominal cavity—peritoneal macrophages

(c) Liver—Kupffer's cells

(d) Mesenchymal and connective tissue—histiocytes

(2) Macrophages involved in inflammation are derived from blood monocytes and are characterized by abundant cytoplasm, indented nuclei, and cytoplasmic lysosomes.

(a) They ingest micromolecules by a process of pinocytosis. Engulfment of the particles occurs by cytoplasmic membrane extension, which surrounds the particles.

(b) The macrophages phagocytose larger fragments, foreign material, blood and cell debris.

(c) They have surface receptors for Fc, one of the two segments for immunoglobulin G (IgG) molecule, and complement component (C3b).

(d) They contain or produce hydrolytic substances similar to those contained by neutrophils (i.e., acid hydrolase, protease, lysozyme, complement, colony stimulating factor, lymphocyte mitogenic protein, pyrogen, and prostaglandin).

(3) **Monocyte-Macrophage Functions.**

(a) Immunologically, macrophage mobilization and metabolic activation in response to inflammation are influenced by the lymphokines.

(i) The **macrophage migration inhibition factor** is a low molecular weight protein that arrests the intrinsic mobility of macrophages and is produced by stimulation of sensitized T lymphocytes, as may occur through mitogenic or specific antigenic activity.

(ii) The **macrophage activation factor** stimulates macrophage growth with consequent increase in cell size and with a concomitant increase in the number of mitochondria, hydrolytic enzymes, and lysosomes. This factor also stimulates the bactericidal and tumoricidal activities of macrophages.

(iii) Macrophages interact with sensitized immune T lymphocytes. Macrophages present the antigen to immune lymphocytes and with mediation by sensitized lymphocytes begin endocytosis (phagocytosis-pinocytosis) of microorganisms and their metabolic by-products, cell debris, foreign material, and other cells. Macrophages prolong the inflammatory process by release of vascular permeability factors and chemotactic factors. They also release pyrogens and prostaglandins, which induce acute phase signs such as fever and peripheral blood leukocytosis (a left shift of immature neutrophilic granulocytes).

   (b) The monocyte-macrophage system aids in healing after inflammation subsides by
      (i) Cellular débridement through phagocytosis
      (ii) Release of fibroblast proliferating factor
   (c) The antimicrobial effects of the system include
      (i) Direct phagocytosis and digestion
      (ii) Antibacterial lysozyme release
      (iii) Interferon release

 b. Lymphocytes and Plasma Cells.
  (1) Tissue lymphocytes and plasma cells are derived from circulating blood lymphocytes, bone marrow, the spleen, lymph nodes, and germinal center lymphoid aggregates throughout the body (e.g., tonsils, Peyer's patches of the gastrointestinal tract, and the appendix).
  (2) They are primarily of immunologic importance, but they are found in the tissue sites of all types of inflammation, especially after the acute ingress of neutrophils.
   (a) B lymphocytes, named for the bursa of Fabricius, are morphologically identical to T lymphocytes and are found in lymphoid follicles with germinal centers. Antigen receptors are found in the immunoglobulin molecules that are part of the lymphocyte membrane. B cells differentiate into morphologically distinct immunoglobulin-producing plasma cells. Each plasma cell produces only one type of immunglobulin: IgG, IgM, IgA, or IgD. Like macrophages, B cells also have cell receptors for the Fc portion of IgG and complement component C3b. Erythrocyte-antibody-complement (EAC) rosettes (IgM-coated sheep erythrocytes) identify B cells.
   (b) T lymphocytes are found between the follicles of lymph nodes (in the interfollicular T zone) and comprise 70 percent of peripheral blood circulating lymphocytes. They function in cell immunity (in transplant rejection and delayed hypersensitivity reactions) and in immune regulation responses (as helper and suppressor cells). Because T lymphocytes have cell surface receptors for sheep erythrocytes, they form visible microscopic rosettes when reacted with reagent sheep red cells in vitro. This T-cell rosetting with sheep red cells is the main laboratory test for separating T from B lymphocytes.
   (c) Killer (K) and natural killer (NK) cells are small lymphocytes that are not definable by T- and B-cell criteria.
     (i) K cells are null cells that have Fc receptors but no immunoglobulins in the cell membrane. They are able to lyse antibody-coated cells, a capability that is known as antibody-dependent cytotoxicity.
     (ii) NK cells are thought to be bone marrow dependent and capable of lysing leukemia-lymphoma cells experimentally. They are important in the rejection of bone marrow transplants.

C. VASCULAR CHANGES OF INFLAMMATION. The definition of inflammation as a tissue and physiologic response to injury includes the vascular system in a role in the response phenomenon. Inflammation is dependent on the integrity of the circulatory system and occurs almost synonymously with alterations in the blood vessels and capillary beds of the injured site.

  Microcirculatory response occurs immediately within the site of primary injury and variably within the peripheral tissue adjacent to the site.

 1. Arteriolar constriction occurs in variable fashions and lasts from seconds to minutes; it may be influenced neurogenically.

 2. Vasodilatation occurs after the initial constriction phase, leads to postcapillary venule dilatation, and allows increased blood flow to the site (flare phenomenon). It is reflected clinically by heat and erythema (hyperemia). If intracapillary hydrostatic pressure exceeds the capillary bed tissue pressure, edema may result by the movement of fluid, **transudate**, into the tissue, which results in a wheal.

 3. There is an **increase in vascular permeability** with passage of plasma (colloid and water) through the vessels into the tissue, resulting in further edema and vascular stasis. Fluid at this stage is an exudate of higher specific gravity than the early transudate due to plasma proteins and leukocytes.

    a. Vascular permeability is probably affected in part by widened junctions between the vascular endothelial lining cells.

    b. There are three types of increased vascular permeability.

       (1) **Immediate-transient response** is caused by heat and histamine and involves small- and medium-sized venules. It is caused by contraction of endothelial cells, resulting in widened intercellular gaps. This is type I hypersensitivity.

       (2) **Immediate-sustained response** is caused by severe vascular injury (as occurs in severe burns) with vascular permeability continuing beyond 1 day. It affects venules, arterioles, and capillaries alike.

       (3) **Delayed-prolonged response** begins after a delay of several hours. It is seen in type IV hypersensitivity, in overexposure to ultraviolet light, in irradiation, and in moderate thermal burns.

    c. Loss of plasma due to increased vascular permeability leads to vascular stasis and the sludging of red cells through the microcirculation.

D. ACTIONS OF LEUKOCYTES IN INFLAMMATION. During the vascular stasis stage of hyperemia, leukocytes begin to line the endothelial surfaces of the affected vessels.

  1. Margination and Pavementing. Neutrophils and monocytes adhere to vascular endothelium preparatory to migration into the extravascular space.

    a. Microcirculation stasis aids in the margination of leukocytes along the endothelial surface.

    b. Chemotactic factors probably influence the attraction to the vessel periphery. Cell membrane electronegativity and divalent calcium (Ca^{++}) probably play a role in adherence to endothelium.

  2. Diapedesis.

    a. Leukocytes develop pseudopods and emigrate, without accompanying loss of fluid, through gaps between the endothelial cells. The emigration is purposeful, directed, and ameboid; however, it is independent of endothelial cell contraction.

    b. Neutrophils are the first to emigrate. They are short-lived, with a life span of 24 to 48 hours, and contain a chemotactic factor for monocytes.

    c. Monocytes then follow the neutrophils into the site, apparently on cue from the elaborated neutrophilic factor.

    d. All leukocytes (neutrophils, basophils, eosinophils, lymphocytes, and monocytes) emigrate in the same manner.

  3. Chemotaxis is the process by which leukocytes are directed to a specific target.

    a. The **chemotactic factors for neutrophils** are

       (1) **Bacterial proteases**—soluble, low molecular weight factors, which are elaborated from both gram-positive and gram-negative organisms

       (2) **Components of the complement system**, which are activated by the complement cascade

    b. Inhibition of active leukocyte esterase (serine esterase) suppresses chemotaxis of leukocytes.

    c. Leukocytes appear to have cell surface binding receptors for peptides of chemotactic factors. Following exposure to a chemotactic agent, random motion of the leukocyte begins. The microtubular system and contractile proteins are involved in cell locomotion.

    d. **Monocyte-macrophage chemotactic factors** involve and are released in response to the following.

       (1) The third and fifth components of complement (C3a and C5a)

       (2) Bacteria-related substances

       (3) Sensitized lymphocytes

       (4) Antigen-antibody complexes

    e. The **Eosinophil Chemotactic Factor of Anaphylaxis.**

       (1) Eosinophils are attracted to sites of hypersensitivity, antigen-antibody anaphylaxis, and parasitic infestations.

       (2) The chemotactic factors are emitted by basophils, mast cells, and sensitized lymphocytes.

  4. Endocytosis mainly involves the actions of neutrophils and monocytes-macrophages, which discern the particles to be ingested and then engulf and degrade them.

    a. **Identification and recognition** of the particles to be phagocytosed involve cell surface receptors that attach to coated material prior to ingestion. These are receptors for

       (1) IgG opsonin

(2) C3 component of complement opsonin
   b. Phagolysosomes result when the cytoplasmic membranes of macrophages and neutrophils extend around the attached particles and form vacuoles that connect with the lysosomes.
   (1) Phagolysosome formation is accompanied by release of peroxides and hydrolytic enzymes into the extracellular space, which may cause tissue damage.
   (2) Acid hydrolases are then released into the phagolysosomes.
   (3) Both Ca^{++} and divalent magnesium (Mg^{++}) are required for phagocytosis.
   c. Degradation of the Phagocytosed Particles.
   (1) Oxidase-mediated bactericidal activity, which is initiated from cell membrane oxidase and is oxygen-dependent, converts O_2 to H_2O_2.
   (2) H_2O_2 then combines with neutrophilic myeloperoxidase and chloride ion for bactericidal effects in the phagolysosome; the combination constitutes the most important leukocytic bactericidal mechanism.
   (3) Superoxide radical formations are dependent upon and are stimulated during oxidative metabolism following phagocytosis. They are independent of myeloperoxidase and have bactericidal activity.
   d. Leukocyte bactericidal activity independent of oxygen involves lysozymes, cationic proteins, and hydrogen.
   (1) Lysozymes hydrolyze bacterial wall glycopeptides in a powerful bactericidal activity.
   (2) Cationic proteins also have a deleterious effect on bacterial cell walls.
   (3) Hydrogen ions are released into the phagolysosome, creating an acid pH to suppress bacterial growth.

E. BIOCHEMICAL-PHYSIOLOGICAL ACTIVATORS OF INFLAMMATION. Tissue responses to injury, circulatory alterations, activation and mobilization of leukocytes, and immunologic reactions occurring in inflammation are all under the control of physiologic substances that are stimulated, synthesized, and emitted during inflammation. Observable edema and erythema are examples of chemically mediated reactions to injury.

   1. Amines are responsible for hemodynamic and vascular changes. Histamine and serotonin, which are contained within the granules of mast cells, basophils, and platelets, are released immediately in response to injury (degranulation). If levels of intracellular adenosine 3':5'-cyclic monophosphate (cAMP) decrease during some inflammatory states, the release of vasoactive amines is enhanced. If cAMP is increased by prostaglandin or epinephrine, degranulation of mast cells and basophils is inhibited, with consequent reduction in histamine and serotonin release.
   a. There are direct vascular reactions after degranulation of mast cells and basophils. Some degree of vasoconstriction (which varies according to animal species) almost always occurs, followed by vasodilatation, which is the stage of observable hyperemia. There is also increased vascular permeability of the small veins and venules.
   b. Physical factors (heat, cold, and irradiation), drugs, immunoglobulins, C3a and C5a complement components, and cationic proteins all may cause histamine release from mast cells.

   2. Leukocyte substances, such as proteases, hydrolytic enzymes, and cationic proteins, are activators of inflammation and are discussed under the section on cells of inflammation (I B).

   3. Slow-reacting substance is a **low molecular weight lipid** found within mast cells. It accounts for many of the clinically dramatic (and potentially lethal) reactions during anaphylaxis by bronchial smooth muscle contraction and for edema due to increased vascular permeability.

   4. Kinins.
   a. Contact of plasma with collagen, endotoxin, and basement membrane proteins (vimentin and laminin) activates clotting factor XII (Hageman factor).
   b. This is followed sequentially by kallikrein formation, which then converts kininogen into bradykinin.
   c. Bradykinin
   (1) Increases vascular permeability
   (2) Is responsible for smooth muscle contraction
   (3) Causes vasodilatation
   (4) Causes pain
   (5) Is influenced by phospholipase A in the production of prostaglandin

   5. Prostaglandins are tissue hormones with multiple physiologic functions that are derived from arachidonic acid.
   a. Prostaglandin E (PGE) is found in exudates as a secondary response to the acute phase of inflammation.

(1) It increases vascular permeability through vasodilatation.
(2) It acts on the hypothalamic mechanism of fever production.
b. Most mammalian cells, including endothelial and inflammatory cells, have the potential to produce prostaglandin.

6. Components of complement function in antigen-antibody complexes, which are involved in immunologic reactions to inflammation.
    a. Circulating immune complexes activate the complement system and, by successive steps of cleavage and combination, generate complement components C3a and C5a.
        (1) Both C3a and C5a are chemotactic components for neutrophils.
        (2) They have an important role in the increased vascular permeability resulting from histamine release from mast cells.
    b. Nonimmunologic injury reactions will activate the alternate pathway of complement cascade.
    c. After complement cascade activation, C5, C6, and C7 in combination also become chemotactic.

7. Lymphokines are biologically active factors that are produced by T lymphocytes.
    a. They permit chemotaxis of macrophages and granulocytes.
    b. Macrophage migration inhibition factor serves to keep the monocyte-phagocyte elements in the area of inflammation.

II. TYPES OF INFLAMMATION

A. ACUTE INFLAMMATION is the hallmark of mammalian tissue response to injury. It is reflected by, in order of occurrence, vasodilatation (redness), edema (swelling), and ingress of neutrophils, followed by ingress of monocytes-phagocytes. Every organ and tissue type is susceptible to inflammation; the previous state of health, nutrition, immunity, and the nature and severity of the noxious stimuli govern the degree and type of inflammatory response.

    1. Exudate consists of the fluid and cells of acute inflammation and contains protein in excess of 3.0 g/dl and has a specific gravity over 1.015. There are four specific types of acute inflammatory exudate.
        a. Purulent (suppurative, pyogenic) exudate consists of large amounts of neutrophils, often accumulated in response to bacteria, which may lead to abscess formation (Fig. 1-1).

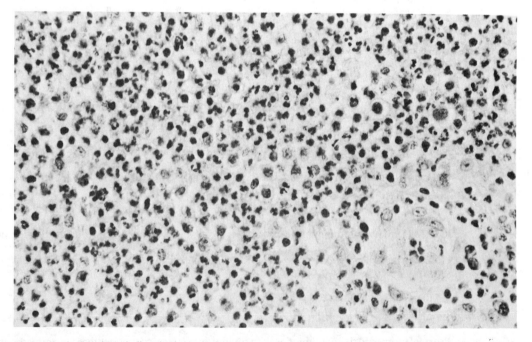

Figure 1-1. The histologic hallmark of acute inflammation is the presence of numerous acute inflammatory cells in the form of neutrophils with multilobated nuclei. Monocytes and phagocytes are also scattered throughout and are readily visible by their single oval and round nuclei. A reactive capillary is seen in the *lower right*.

   b. **Fibrinous** exudate is characterized by high protein (albumin, fibrinogen) from plasma with visible deposits of fibrin coagulum, and it is often bloody (sanguineous). Examples of fibrinous exudate include tuberculous pleuritis and rheumatic pericarditis. The coagulum exudate may become organized by neovascularity and fibroblast formation, with consequent scarring.

   c. **Serous** exudate occurs in mild degrees of inflammation and is characterized by fewer cells and less protein than the other types. It is generally in body (pleural, pericardial, and peritoneal) cavities or in the spinal fluid. Examples are the fluids in second-degree thermal burns and viral meningitis and joint and pleural effusions.

   d. **Inflammation of mucous membranes** (catarrhal) produces an exudate that is high in mucus. This type of exudate occurs in allergic rhinitis (coryza) and bronchitis.

   2. **Transudate** is noninflammatory fluid, characterized by few cells, protein less than 3.0 g/dl, and specific gravity less than 1.015.

B. **CHRONIC INFLAMMATION** occurs when incomplete healing, ongoing noxious stimuli, or responses to immunologic reactions are present. Tissue healing and scarring may be concurrent.

   1. Cells of chronic inflammation are monocytes-phagocytes, lymphocytes, and plasma cells. Monocytes that are derived from the peripheral blood become tissue macrophages.

   2. Granulation tissue forms from budding capillaries with fibroblast proliferation and variable degrees of collagen deposition. Granulation tissue response may be slight and inapparent.

   3. Chronic inflammation may coexist with acute inflammation, as in repeated episodes of acute cholecystitis (with gallstones), osteomyelitis, and pilonidal sinus.

C. **GRANULOMATOUS INFLAMMATION** is an important type of chronic inflammation, and its presence implies some degree of immune capability. It is characterized by granulomas that are discrete aggregates of epithelioid macrophages, lymphocytes, and multinucleated giant cells. The main cell of the granuloma is the epithelioid macrophage, which may have a secretory function. The giant cells are formed by fusion of multiple macrophages. Blood monocytes transform into epithelioid cells at the tissue site. The granuloma forms in response to a persistent antigen.

   1. **Infectious granulomas** form in response to the following conditions.
      a. **Mycobacterial infection** is caused by acid-fast bacilli. Examples of the infection include tuberculosis, leprosy, and intracellular infections caused by *Mycobacteria avium, kansasii,* and *marinum.* Tuberculous granulomas have central caseous necrosis.
      b. **Brucellosis** is a granulomatous condition as are glanders, caused by *Pseudomonas mallei,* and tularemia.
      c. Lymphogranuloma venereum is an infectious disease of **viral origin**.
      d. Cat-scratch fever is caused by a newly discovered bacteria that stains with silver.
      e. **Fungi**, such as *Coccidioides, Actinomyces, Cryptococcus,* and *Histoplasma capsulatum* can produce infectious granulomas.
      f. *Treponema,* a type of spirochete, causes syphilis, pinta, and yaws.
      g. **Parasitic infestation**, resulting in schistosomiasis, also produces granulomatous formation.

   2. **Foreign-body granulomas** form in the presence of the following.
      a. **Particulate matter**—glass, soil, gravel, and metal (Fig. 1-2)
      b. **Synthetic material**—surgical sutures
      c. **Vegetable matter**—cellulose, which may develop from fecal contamination of tissues as occurs in fistulae formation and in perforated bowel
      d. **Beryllium poisoning**

   3. **Lipoid granulomas** react to various insoluble lipids, waxes, and oils.

   4. **Unknown. Sarcoidosis** is characterized by epithelioid granulomas that may involve the lungs, liver, spleen, lymph nodes, and skin. The granulomas are non-necrotic, uniformly sized, and multiple.

III. CONSEQUENCES OF INFLAMMATION

A. **EVENTUAL HEALING** is the goal of all inflammatory processes.

   1. Factors that inhibit the desired tissue restoration after inflammation are listed below.
      a. **Old age**—the ability to mount an adequate inflammatory response decreases with advancing age.

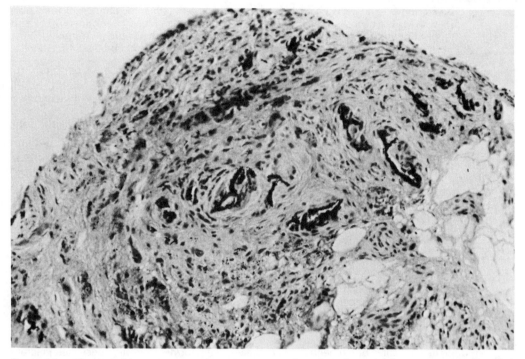

Figure 1-2. Chronic inflammation—granulomatous type. Multinucleated giant cells are seen engulfing dark-staining particulate foreign material. The granuloma is also rimmed by fibrous connective tissue and chronic inflammation.

    b. Nutrition—cell metabolism and activation for defense is affected adversely by malnutrition.

    c. Immune depression—cell-mediated immunity is decreased in familial and acquired states of reduced immunity [e.g., aquired immune deficiency syndrome (AIDS)], which may allow inflammation to become chronic-active or to disseminate (e.g., as in disseminated tuberculosis).

    d. Malignancy—malignant neoplasms, including leukemias and lymphomas, adversely affect mobilization and activation of leukocytes.

    e. Drugs—anti-inflammatory drugs and antineoplastic agents cause bone marrow suppression with leukopenia and reduced response to noxious stimuli.

    f. Superimposed infection—opportunistic secondary invasion of injured tissue by bacteria, yeasts *(Candida)*, and fungi can occur.

    g. Inflammation progressing to formation of fistulous tracts, perforations, and abscesses inhibits healing.

2. Mechanisms of Healing. The first stage of tissue restoration begins almost at the onset of inflammation itself. Healing is dependent on an antecedent inflammatory stage.

    a. Restoration occurs by regeneration of cells and tissue specific for the damaged site.

        (1) There is direct regrowth of hematopoietic and epithelial lining cells in gastrointestinal mucosa, the urinary bladder, the skin, and uterine endometrium. These tissue cells are referred to as **labile cells** because they possess a constant capacity to regenerate.

        (2) Limited regrowth capacity of organ parenchymal cells, which are able to undergo cell division in order to replace dead cells, describes the situation of **stable cells**. For normal structural restoration to occur, basement membrane zones and the supporting stroma of the organs must be intact. This type of restoration occurs in the liver, pancreas, kidney, and blood vessels.

    b. Healing by granulation tissue formation is effective where large tissue defects need repair. Necrotic debris and abscesses must be diminished before granulation tissue formation can occur.

        (1) Neocapillary growth (buds of endothelial proliferation) and fibroblastic proliferation begin during the macrophage activity stage (36 hours after injury).

        (2) By 100 hours after injury, inflammation is accompanied by well-developed granulation tissue formation, unless abscess formation causes delay (Fig. 1-3).

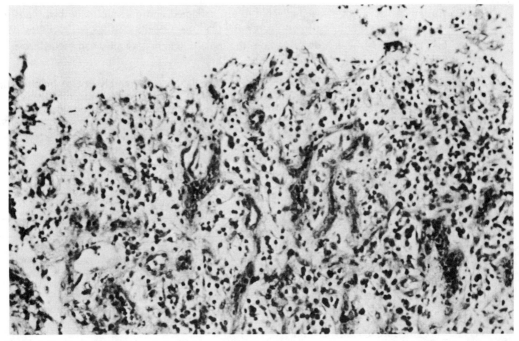

Figure 1-3. Granulation tissue is instantly recognized by numerous budding capillaries (neovascularization), stromal edema, fibroblasts, and red cells. Accompanying the granulation tissue are persistent chronic inflammatory cells. This reaction is the type that heals large tissue defects.

   (3) Fibroblasts synthesize collagen and glucosaminoglycan ground substance.
   (4) Eventual fibrosis (scar tissue) occupies the defect left by the inflammation.

B. UNTOWARD EFFECTS OF INFLAMMATION AND HEALING

   1. Perforation. Expanding masses of inflamed tissue in the acute inflammatory phase may lead to viscus wall weakening with rupture.
      a. A ruptured appendix with spillage of the contents into the abdominal cavity results in purulent peritonitis.
      b. Exudative perihepatitis can occur secondary to tubo-ovarian pyogenic infections (e.g., pelvic inflammatory disease) due to gonorrhea.
      c. Chemical peritonitis can occur as a sequela to a perforated posterior duodenal ulcer.

   2. Advancing planes of inflammatory tissue (fistulous tracts) are adverse effects of inflammation.
      a. A bronchopleural fistula can form from pulmonary staphylococcal abscess, with consequent purulent pleuritis (empyema).
      b. Acute mediastinitis can result from eroding inflammatory tracheal-esophageal fistulae.
      c. Perirectal and ischiorectal fossa fistulae can form from expanding perineal abscesses.

   3. There are problems related to **fibrosis and scar formation** after healing.
      a. Keloids, excessive collagen deposition in the dermis of susceptible individuals, can form.
      b. Bowel obstruction can occur due to adhesive fibrous bands forming from repair of abdominal trauma (e.g., surgery and knife wounds).
      c. Sterility can result from fibrous obliteration of the fallopian tubes after healing of salpingitis.

   4. Complications resulting from sequelae to an inflammatory process include the following.
      a. Ascending pylephlebitis of the portal vein system and cholangitis can be caused by a ruptured appendix.
      b. Any large abscess formation, occurring in the liver, brain, and body cavities, with a thickened fibrous capsule on the exterior preventing resolution and healing is a complication.
      c. There can be spread of infection through the draining lymphatics and regional lymphadenitis. It appears as reddish streaking, which is visible through the skin.

5. **Thrombosis** of larger vessels adjacent to any inflamed and necrotic tissue bed leads to a vicious circle of additive tissue ischemia and necrosis, causing possible further thromboses.

6. Infected thrombi, which dislodge from the initial inflammatory site, can **metastasize vascularly** to other parts of the body.

IV. THROMBOSIS AND COAGULATION.
Blood coagulation is intimately tied to inflammation and tissue necrosis because vessels within and contiguous to the damaged site frequently demonstrate thromboses. Sludging and stasis of blood in the microcirculation with increased viscosity play a role in inflammation as well. It is also known that fibrinogen and platelets increase in these areas. Fibrinolysis begins almost as soon as clots begin to form and is an important system in generating plasma, which has a multifunctional role in inflammation.

A. Coagulation factors are **interdependent**, and the activation of each generally requires activation of its antecedent factor. Enzymes and Ca^{++} are required for the activation of some stages.

Factor		Function
I	Fibrinogen	Fibrin precursor protein
II	Prothrombin	Thrombin precursor; requires dietary vitamin K
III	Tissue thromboplastin	Activates extrinsic clotting system
IV	Calcium	Required in several steps
V	Labile factor (proaccelerin)	Required in prothrombin activation stage
VI	Regarded as activated form of factor V	
VII	Proconvertin stable factor	Important in the extrinsic clotting system
VIII	Antihemophilic factor (von Willebrand factor–related)	Important in the intrinsic clotting system
IX	Christmas factor (plasma thromboplastin)	Involved only in intrinsic clotting system
X	Stuart-Prower factor (thrombokinase)	Pivotal step in extrinsic and intrinsic clotting systems
XI	Plasma thromboplastin antecedent	Involved in intrinsic system activation
XII	Hageman factor (contact factor)	Initial step in the cascade of the intrinsic factor system
XIII	Fibrin stabilizing factor	Stabilizes the fibrin clot

B. Coagulation proceeds after tissue injury via the extrinsic clotting system or with activation of the Hageman factor (intrinsic system).

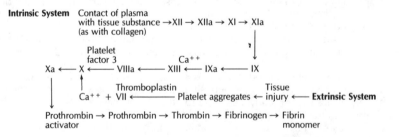

Thrombin further acts on factor XIIIa to stabilize the fibrin clot by polymer formation.

C. Fibrinolysis begins by the time thrombin is generated. Clot lysis is homeostatic if it is controlled and modulated, but it may become pathologic, which occurs in disseminated intravascular coagulation:

$$\text{proactivator} \rightarrow \text{tissue activators} \rightarrow \text{plasminogen} \rightarrow \text{plasmin.}$$
$$\text{(urokinase)}$$

Plasmin then degrades the fibrin clot through proteolysis into measurable fibrin split products, which are designated by D, E, X, and Y. If the plasmin system was not operative, fibrin clots would not be lysed after they have served their homeostatic purpose.

In general, fibrinolysis has vascular effects through the actions of plasmin.

1. **Bradykinin** (which causes vasodilatation and increased vascular permeability) is generated by the activated Hageman factor.

2. Plasmin also cleaves chemotactic complement component C3a from C3.

STUDY QUESTIONS

Directions: Each question below contains five suggested answers. Choose the **one best** response to each question.

1. Fluid that collects during acute inflammation and that has a protein content in excess of 3.0 g/dl and a specific gravity over 1.015 is termed

(A) exudate
(B) transudate
(C) coagulation
(D) lymphokine
(E) wheal

2. Which of the substances listed below exerts an apparent influence on metabolic activation and mobilization of macrophages?

(A) Lysozymes
(B) Lymphokines
(C) Proteases
(D) Thrombokinases
(E) Coagulation factor XIII

3. Of the cell types listed below, which differentiates into morphologically distinct cells capable of immunoglobulin production?

(A) Polymorphonuclear leukocytes
(B) Basophils
(C) B lymphocytes
(D) T lymphocytes
(E) Plasma cells

4. The term that describes the margination and adherence of neutrophils and monocytes to the vascular endothelium prior to movement into the extravascular space is

(A) sludging
(B) diapedesis
(C) pavementing
(D) emigration
(E) clotting

5. In blood coagulation, which of the following coagulation factors links fibrin monomers to stabilize the early fibrin clot?

(A) Ia
(B) III
(C) VIII
(D) Xa
(E) XIIIa

6. Which of the following coagulation factors is reduced or absent in classic hemophilia?

(A) I
(B) III
(C) VIII
(D) X
(E) XIII

7. In the process of fibrinolysis, which of the following substances acts on the fibrin molecule and splits it into products of varying molecular size?

(A) Proactivator
(B) Activator
(C) Plasminogen
(D) Plasmin
(E) Antiplasmin

Directions: Each question below contains four suggested answers of which **one or more** is correct. Choose the answer

    A if **1, 2, and 3** are correct
    B if **1 and 3** are correct
    C if **2 and 4** are correct
    D if **4** is correct
    E if **1, 2, 3, and 4** are correct

8. Cells that participate most actively in the body's defense through endocytosis and phagocytosis include

(1) neutrophils
(2) monocytes
(3) macrophages
(4) basophils

9. Of the following infectious agents, those that typically can produce a granulomatous reaction include

(1) *Treponema pallidum*
(2) *Mycobacteria tuberculosis*
(3) *Coccidioides immitis*
(4) *Actinomyces bovis*

ANSWERS AND EXPLANATIONS

1. The answer is A. (*II A 1*) Exudate is the fluid and cells that collect during acute inflammation in excess of 3.0 g/dl and with a specific gravity over 1.015. The term transudate is reserved for fluid expressions with few cellular elements, protein content less than 3.0 g/dl, and a specific gravity less than 1.015. A wheal is a focus of tissue swelling that is produced by a local transudate. Lymphokines are products of T lymphocytes.

2. The answer is B. [*I B 2 a (3)*] Macrophage mobilization and metabolic activation in response to inflammation are influenced by the group of substances known as lymphokines. Lymphokines are soluble substances produced by various lymphocytes to direct, regulate, and modify a variety of immune responses, including macrophage function.

3. The answer is C. (*I B 2 b*) B lymphocytes differentiate into plasma cells, which produce immuno-globulins. Each plasma cell apparently manufactures only one class of immunoglobulin. Plasma cells are the mature and already differentiated form of cells; they are so-called "end-cells" because they no longer divide. B lymphocytes are stimulated to differentiate into plasma cells under the influence of antigens, T lymphocyte interaction, and macrophage interaction.

4. The answer is C. (*I D 1, 2*) As the vascular changes of inflammation evolve, leukocytes and monocytes pavement or adhere to the vascular endothelium prior to migration into the extravascular space by the mechanism of diapedesis. Leukocytes develop pseudopods and emigrate, without accompanying loss of fluid, through gaps between the endothelial cells. Loss of plasma due to increased vascular perme-ability leads to vascular stasis and the sludging of red cells through the microcirculation.

5. The answer is E. (*IV A*) Factor XIII—fibrin stabilizing factor—is activated by the enzymatic action of thrombin and becomes factor XIIIa or transglutaminase, which binds to fibrin monomers and forms cross-links between the gamma and alpha chains of the polymerizing fibrin molecules. Patients with factor XIII deficiency have a mild bleeding tendency, particularly following trauma. Wound healing is delayed, and irregular scar formation is also common in these individuals.

6. The answer is C. (*IV A*) The coagulation factor VIII complex is under the control of the X chromosome and is reduced or absent in classic hemophilia, which is a sex-linked disorder. Factor VIII is also reduced in von Willebrand's disease.

7. The answer is D. (*IV C*) Plasmin, derived from plasminogen, acts on both the fibrinogen molecule and on fibrin. Once the fibrin is cross-linked, however, the breakdown process is slower because plasmin cannot gain access to the stable fibrin polymer as readily as it can to the unstable, non–crossed-linked fibrin mesh. The proteolysis caused by plasmin produces the various fibrin split products that can be detected.

8. The answer is A (1, 2, 3). (*I B 1 a, 2 a*) Neutrophils and the monocyte-macrophage cell line participate most actively in endocytosis and phagocytosis of particulate matter. Cell surface receptors on these cell lines are responsible for identification of opsonized material, which is to be ingested and destroyed enzymatically. Basophils are concerned with the release of vasoactive amines after complexing with immunoglobulin E (IgE) to promote type I IgE-mediated hypersensitivity reactions.

9. The answer is E (all). (*II C 1*) Several infectious agents evoke the distinctive inflammatory reaction pattern that is termed a granulomatous inflammation. The granulomas consist of 1-mm to 2-mm diameter nodules, which are composed of modified macrophages-histiocytes. The macrophages-histiocytes usu-ally are surrounded by a mononuclear cell infiltrate, which typically is composed mainly of lympho-cytes. While tuberculosis usually is cited as the classic example of an infectious granulomatous disease, *Treponema pallidum*, *Coccidioides immitis*, and *Actinomyces bovis* can produce granulomas as well.

2
Neoplasia

I. INTRODUCTION

A. Neoplasia is a general term for any proliferation of cells that lack the control of the normal mechanisms governing their growth. However, as used by most investigators and clinicians alike, neoplasia is equated with the term cancer as understood by the general public.

B. The importance of cancer can be assessed from several viewpoints.

    1. In the United States, cancer is the **second leading cause of death**, accounting for 20.4 percent of deaths in 1977, compared to 37.8 percent due to cardiac causes, 9.6 percent to cerebrovascular disease, and 5.4 percent to accidents of various types. For perspective, however, one should recognize that cancer is less significant worldwide; in so-called underdeveloped countries, malnutrition and parasitic infections (e.g., malaria) still account for more deaths than cancer does.

    2. The **cost** of cancer per year in the United States is counted in billions of dollars if one includes about $300 to $500 million for cancer research (government sources only; the amounts of private contributions are unknown) and millions for diagnostic tests, surgical, radiological, and drug therapies, physicians, laboratory fees, and the costs of rehabilitation and long-term care facilities.

    3. The **psychosocial costs** remain immeasurable. Public awareness of cancer is increasing, and people are unduly pessimistic about cancer mortality; 40 percent of people regard the therapy of cancer as "very painful," and the majority of people do not view any treatment as effective, perceiving only a 20 percent cure rate for all cancers. Whereas heart attacks and stroke are viewed as natural hazards of old age or as the result of overeating or high living, cancer is regarded as **unpredictable**, striking indiscriminately at rich and poor, fat and thin, young and old.

C. EPIDEMIOLOGY. Four important factors believed to be associated with the increasing incidence of cancer are age, diet, environment, and heredity.

    1. Age. With the population increasing in age, carcinogens are thought to have more time to exert their effects; additionally, the immunologic capacity of the elderly may be less effective than that of young people. However, it is crucial to realize that cancer can occur at any age. There are congenital neoplasms, and cancer accounts for 11 percent of deaths in the 1- to 14-year-old age group, second only to accidents as a cause of death.

    2. Diet. Geographical differences in cancer rates can be explained partially by dietary differences.

        a. The smoking of foods is associated with the production of known chemical carcinogens. Icelandic people, who have an exceedingly high rate of esophageal cancer, eat large amounts of smoked fish.

        b. A diet very rich in fiber and low in animal fat and refined carbohydrates seems to discourage colorectal cancer. The African Bantus, on such a diet, have almost no incidence of colorectal cancer.

        c. Japanese people who live in Japan have a very high rate of cancer of the stomach, twice the rate of Japanese who have migrated to Hawaii and have adopted a Western diet. However, diet alone cannot be the total answer, since Japanese in Hawaii still have a higher rate of gastric cancer than do nonJapanese in the same environment.

        d. Alcoholic beverages affect carcinogenesis when consumed frequently and excessively over long periods. This carcinogenic impact is especially pronounced on hepatic cells as well as on the mucosae of the esophagus, pharynx, and oral cavity. When combined with tobacco use, alcohol yields an excess cancer risk of 14 for the mouth and pharynx and over 40 for the esophagus. Coexisting cancers, sometimes termed multiple primary cancers, occur with twice the frequency among cirrhotic as among noncirrhotic persons. Although alcohol per se appears not to be carcinogenic, it may potentiate the effects of substances in alcoholic beverages or allow for the increased absorption of carcinogens.

3. Environment. The environmental agents associated with high cancer incidences include radiation and chemical pollution. Industrialization or development, along with the conquest of infection and malnutrition, is associated with increases in cancer incidence.
  a. An urban setting, with higher air and water pollution indices than a rural environment, leads to higher cancer rates, especially of lung cancer.
  b. Smokers get lung cancer much more frequently than do nonsmokers. Smoking has been linked to oral, pharyngeal, laryngeal, and bladder carcinoma.
  c. Industrial workers, exposed to certain specific agents such as asbestos and vinyl chloride, develop cancer more often than do control groups.
  d. Sexual activity may be related to cancer.
    (1) Viruses or other carcinogens may be venereally transmitted.
    (2) The uterine cervix has the highest association with malignant disease and its precursors in the female reproductive tract. The cervix has an increased vulnerability to neoplasia after it is exposed to infection, particularly infection in which herpesvirus 2 can be demonstrated. Since squamous cervical neoplasia begins in the squamocolumnar junction, the enlargement of this area as a result of the irritation of infection may be causative. Only viruses such as herpesvirus 2 or papilloma virus appear to be able to reprogram the nuclei of growing cells and perhaps lead to cervical cancer.

4. Heredity. Patients with genetic abnormalities show higher incidences of cancer than those without genetic abnormalities.
  a. Familial multiple colonic polyposis is often associated with colorectal cancer.
  b. Patients who have Down's syndrome (mongolism) have an incidence of acute leukemia that is 4 to 30 times higher than in the normal population.
  c. Children with immunologic deficiencies have an extremely high rate of lymphoid malignancies.

D. CHARACTERISTICS OF NEOPLASIA. Certain characteristics are shared by neoplasms, both in vitro and in vivo. The main ones include **clonality, autonomy,** and, in malignant neoplasms, the capacity to invade local normal tissue and disseminate (**metastasize**) to other tissues and organs. Groups of abnormally proliferating cells arise in any part of the body. Those that cannot invade the surrounding tissues are called **benign**.

1. In theory, a neoplasm represents the progeny of one cell, a **clone**, and in many neoplasms all cells show the same abnormal karyotype. Even when several chromosome patterns are present, marker chromosomes in each cell suggest that different subpopulations derive from a common stemline. Cell products (immunoglobulins) from a myeloma (plasma cell neoplasm) display a homogeneity that is characteristic of a single clone. Glucose-6-phosphate dehydrogenase studies in heterozygous women with neoplasms indicate that the same number of the X-chromosome pair is functional in all cells of a given lesion, suggesting descent from a common precursor.
  a. A neoplastic cell acquires a growth advantage over adjacent normal cells, and proliferation proceeds either immediately or after a latent period.
  b. Because of genetic instability (apparently greater in the neoplastic state), mutant cells are produced. Some of these are destroyed either by metabolic disadvantage or immune mechanisms, but an occasional cell will express a selective advantage over the original neoplastic cells and will give rise to the predominant subpopulation. In time, this selection process leads to increasingly abnormal cells with the acquired properties of the fully developed cancer.

2. These abnormal cells exhibit autonomy or uncontrolled proliferation, free of the control of normal mechanisms. The properties of the autonomous clone include changes in morphology and alterations of membrane composition and, hence, receptor sites. Thus, normal inhibitory influences may not be effective. A response to inhibitory influences is a property that classically is associated with benign growth, accounting for the stoppage of cell movement when two cells growing in tissue culture collide. Malignant cells, in contrast, tend to grow over one another, although not all cancer cells behave so predictably.

E. THE ETIOLOGY OF CANCER is unknown and little understood.

1. The initial transformation of a normal to a neoplastic cell involves changes within the genetic apparatus of the cell (mutation). Heredity, chemicals, physical agents, radiation, and viruses may be involved in this change.

2. Most investigators feel that neoplasia involves a multifactorial, staged process of progressive mutation in the genetic makeup of cells. Cancer is not one disease but many with different manifestations and prognoses.

3. A constant feature of all agents that are known carcinogens is their demonstrated interaction with DNA; this interaction patently is obvious for the three major classes of carcinogens: chemicals, viruses, and ionizing radiation. Each of the classes can intercalate with, modify, or damage nuclear DNA. Cancer cells divide rapidly and therein lies their invasive potential. Rapidly dividing cells that retain their malignant persuasion demonstrate that this persuasion is heritable.

   a. **Genetic instability** is unique to cancer cells. It is only in cancer cells that broken sets, stray components, and ectopic gene products are found.

   b. **Clonal Instability.** The cancerous phenotype itself is very unstable. As a function of time, with continued cell division and progression of the neoplastic process, a variety of clones appear as progeny of a single cancer. This clonal heterogeneity may be manifested in a morphologic or biochemical sense. Each of the clones can show differences in morphology, special product elaboration, and antigenicity. This genetic instability bespeaks a change in the regulation of gene expression from that encountered in differentiated eukaryotic cells. In differentiated cells there is a lock on gene expression. For reasons that are not well understood and that are of fundamental importance, this lock has been damaged if not opened in the process of oncogenesis (carcinogenesis).

   c. Cancer cells display a type of **clonal evolution** that allows for the insidious selection of the most aggressive, rapidly growing, and invasive clones. It is this feature that gives rise to clones that are fiercely resistant to all known modes of therapy and eventually prove lethal.

II. DEFINITIONS

A. HYPERTROPHY is an enlargement in individual cell size. The proliferation is controlled.

B. HYPERPLASIA is any abnormal or unusual increase in the number of cells in a tissue or part of a tissue, which results in an increase in tissue mass. There are two types: physiologic and neoplastic.

   1. **Physiologic** hyperplasia is due to an external stimulus and subsides when the stimulus is removed.

   2. **Neoplastic** hyperplasia is due, at least in part, to a heritable abnormality within the involved cells.

   3. Both physiologic and neoplastic hyperplasia are often present in a tissue simultaneously.

C. METAPLASIA is the replacement of one adult tissue type by another; usually the replacement (metaplastic tissue) is simpler in form.

D. DYSPLASIA is any abnormal growth. This term can be used for congenital defects such as dysplastic (malformed) kidneys, but more commonly it connotes cytologic abnormalities in cells that are believed to be precursors of neoplastic cells. The term dysplasia has been overused and abused so that its clinical meaning has been somewhat obscured; however, it is a term so ingrained in the literature that it will continue to be used.

E. ANAPLASIA is the property of abnormal cells whereby their morphology resembles more primitive cells of similar tissue; the more primitive (embryonic) that cells appear, the more anaplastic they are said to be. In practice, anaplasia is equated with malignant neoplasia (i.e., cancer).

F. NEOPLASIA is the proliferation of cells without response to normal control mechanisms (i.e., autonomous proliferation). Neoplasms are commonly divided into two categories.

   1. **Benign** neoplasms cannot invade local tissues and are generally associated with a good prognosis.

   2. **Malignant** neoplasms, commonly called cancers, can invade tissues and generally are associated with a poor prognosis.

      a. **Carcinomas** are malignancies of tissues that are derived from the ectoderm and endoderm.

      b. **Sarcomas** are malignancies of tissues of mesodermal origin.

      c. Carcinomas and sarcomas are further designated by descriptive terms to indicate the histopathology [i.e., leiomyosarcoma (smooth muscle), squamous cell carcinoma, or adenocarcinoma (glandular)].

    d. Tumors of the hematopoietic series are termed **leukemias,** and those of the immune system are called **lymphomas.** Many exceptions have been established by long use. The peculiarities of terminology become familiar with use. (A tumor is, technically, any swelling, but the term is often used interchangeably with cancer, especially by the laity).

III. ORIGIN OF NEOPLASMS

    A. Most lesions that are classified as neoplasms actually are associated with a heritable alteration in the involved cells. The change from normality to malignancy is associated with increasing inflexibility of enzyme patterns, the reasons for which are unknown but may be related to the fact that malignant cells often have many more free ribosomes than normal cells.

    B. It is possible that all tumors pass through stages when they are still dependent upon physiologic factors, but this has only been documented in cases of the endocrine-dependent tissues, such as the female breast. With time, due to tumor progression, a tumor loses its endocrine dependency, and hormonal manipulation ceases to influence its growth.

    C. The prime feature of neoplastic progression is the stepwise loss of characteristics of the tissue of origin; malignancies tend to show abnormal mitoses and large nuclei. Karyotypic analysis shows that most malignant tumors are aneuploid.

    D. A variable number of steps occur during the change from the normal to the fully malignant cell.

        1. The first step apparently occurs in a single cell (i.e., cancer is a clonal disease). The change (mutation) in the first neoplastic cell is a random process. Any given etiologic factor simply increases the probability that any particular cell will be transformed, but how this is done is still not known.

        2. Many of these factors (often chemicals by nature) must be metabolically activated by cellular enzymes. In the absence of the appropriate enzymes, transformation cannot occur.

        3. This **mutation hypothesis** is favored by several arguments.
            a. All oncogenes (including chemicals, radiations, and viruses) are mutagenic.
            b. Defective DNA repair mechanisms, as occur in xeroderma pigmentosa, are associated with an increased risk of neoplasia.
            c. Neoplasia is a clonal disease.

        4. Neoplastic transformation can be caused by viruses, either of the DNA or RNA varieties, and in some systems, the viral genes seem necessary to maintain the transformed state. The neoplastic change depends upon new genetic information from the virus—a virus whose DNA (or the cellular DNA programmed by viral RNA in the case of RNA viruses) is integrated into the host's cellular genome.

        5. Whether an etiologic factor influences anything more than the first step of transformation is not known. Perhaps the etiologic agent starts the process and then the inevitable consequence of neoplastic independence occurs without further exogenous stimulus.

        6. This complex area remains poorly understood. However, neoplasia is at least a two-stage process (at least in experimental settings): **initiation** (primary insult) and **promotion** [other agents are required for full expression of the neoplasm (e.g., proper hormonal milieu for breast cancer)]. To be effective as a carcinogen, a compound almost certainly acts both as an initiator and as a promotor. An initiator causes alterations in DNA structure and is mutagenic. Alone, initiators or promoters are not carcinogens, but acting together in proper sequence, they can produce cancer in nearly 100 percent of cases.

IV. PROPERTIES OF CANCER CELLS

    A. Solid neoplastic growth requires **neovascularization** (i.e., the development of a blood supply to the neoplasm). In the absence of such a blood supply, solid neoplasms cannot grow beyond 2 mm to 3 mm in diameter. Various experiments have shown that neovascularization does not require direct cell-to-cell contact either between neoplastic cells or between the latter and endothelial cells in blood vessels near the lesion. A protein called **tumor angiogenesis factor** that stimulates endothelial cell mitosis and new vessel growth has been discovered.

B. The major characteristic of cancer and the only sine qua non for diagnosis is **metastasis**.

   1. As the neoplastic clone undergoes mutation, the more aggressive subpopulations selected tend to be those with metastasizing potential. Such groups must attain the capacity to blind the body's defense mechanisms as well as have the ability to penetrate lymphatic and vascular channels.

   2. Not only do such groups travel through the bloodstream away from the initial focus of cancer, but these cells also are able to transfer to organs other than those of their origin (i.e., liver, lung, and lymph nodes). Reasons for this ability remain unknown.

   3. Metastasis is not exclusively found in malignancy or even in neoplasia. Endometriosis, for example, involves the metastasis of apparently quite normal endometrium tissue to distant sites.

   4. The probability of metastasis is expressed by terming a lesion as either benign or malignant and can be estimated by the knowledge of the histopathology of a specimen combined with a knowledge of the behavior of similar lesions.

   a. The **gross anatomy** of a lesion may be suggestive of the degree of malignancy.

   (1) Benign lesions usually tend to grow by expansion, compress surrounding structures, and often produce a well-defined capsule.

   (2) Malignant lesions, in contrast, tend to infiltrate the surrounding tissues so that the borders of the lesions are not discrete, and no capsule is formed.

   b. Differences in mode of growth can often be seen **histologically**.

   (1) The edges of malignant lesions are usually poorly demarcated, and individual neoplastic cells infiltrate the surrounding normal tissue.

   (2) There is invasion into lymphatic channels and blood vessels.

   (3) Cells of malignant lesions tend to be large. The nuclear/cytoplasmic ratio is higher than normal, and chromatin clumping is seen. Multiple and prominent nucleoli may be present.

   (4) Mitotic figures, some abnormal, are usually prominent in a histologic section of a malignancy.

   (5) The percentage of differentiating cells is a very important criterion of the growth potential of a neoplasm and is a good indicator of the degree of malignancy. Many studies have shown that in a variety of types of tumors, a good prognosis correlates with a low grade (i.e., better differentiation toward normal).

   (6) While many criteria correlate well with the propensity of a lesion to metastasize, it should be emphasized that no one criterion is absolute. However, a lesion that has already metastasized will have a poorer prognosis than one that has not yet spread.

   c. The **biochemical** basis of invasion and metastasis has several factors.

   (1) Cells of a malignant neoplasm are less tightly adherent than are normal cells; calcium content in the malignant cell walls is lower than that in normal cells.

   (2) The negative surface charge of malignant cells tends to be high, and the cells tend to repel one another.

   (3) Some neoplasms have been shown to produce hyaluronidase, which may facilitate invasion through tissue ground substance.

   d. Each neoplasm tends to have **certain sites of predilection** for spread or metastasis. Some of these patterns are determined by purely anatomic considerations; for example, the lung capillary bed is the first vascular sieve that catches intravenous tumor cells. However, some patterns of tumor metastasis are explained only on the basis of more favorable sites for that particular neoplasm.

   e. The morphologic alterations of cancer allow the trained eye to recognize not only the invasive malignant process (diagnosis) but also the **preinvasive** lesions. Developments in histopathology and cytopathology have allowed for the screening of preinvasive (usually asymptomatic) cancer; once such a lesion is recognized, it can be effectively treated.

C. The process of neoplasia is accompanied in some instances by an expression or elaboration of proteins or other substances, which may be normal or abnormal counterparts of known body components or the re-expression of a fetal or embryonic substance. These substances are called **tumor markers** and are measurable in the serum or plasma of patients with certain neoplasms. Such markers serve predominately a diagnostic or post-therapeutic use. Three examples follow.

   1. In 40 percent to 90 percent of primary liver cancers, there is an associated elaboration of α-**fetoprotein**, a substance regularly made by developing embryonic liver cells but not by normal adult tissue.

   2. The hormone **calcitonin**, normally produced by thyroid parafollicular cells, is elevated in neoplasms of such cells (medullary thyroid cancer).

   3. Calcitonin or other peptide hormones such as **adrenocorticotropic** (ACTH) and **antidiuretic**

hormone (ADH) may be increased in some forms of lung cancer. The production of these hormones may be accompanied by symptoms of hormone excess. These so-called paraendocrine syndromes suggest that the regulation of differentiation tends to be deranged in a variety of bizarre and unexpected ways. These changes are not completely random, however, since particular types of tumors show particular patterns of aberrant differentiation.

V. HOST RESPONSE

A. Host reactions to neoplasms include lymphoid cell infiltrates into tumors and fibrous stromal responses.

1. Autoimmune reactions to cancer cells are common. However, the cancer cells' ability to stimulate the immune mechanism is usually quite small and probably inconsequential as a defense mechanism. The antigens on the surface of the cancer cell are, at least in part, of the same specificities as those in normal cells (e.g., organ-specific antigens and histocompatibility antigens). Most cancer cells also appear to possess antigenic specificities that are nonexistent in normal cells. Some of these may result from derepression of parts of the genome that are normally functional only in the embryonic life, producing so-called **carcinoembryonic antigens** (CEAs). When any of these antigens are capable of stimulating a tumor-destructive immune reaction, they are called **tumor-specific transplantation antigens** (TSTAs). Although immunologic surveillance may be weak to the point of nonexistent, immunotherapy of cancer may be possible, especially in certain tumors such as osteosarcoma. Since most and perhaps all tumors have TSTAs, it may be possible to activate the impotent surveillance mechanism to greater effectiveness.

2. Fibrosis (stromal response to infiltrating tumor cells) may reflect an attempt of the host to confine the tumor, but such tissue reaction may interfere with normal structures and function (e.g., cancers in the retroperitoneum may obstruct the ureters and produce uremia).

B. Host factors that predispose to cancer, both genetic and acquired, have been identified. Clinical observations indicate that cancer can have a mendelian basis of inheritance. Examples include xeroderma pigmentosum, familial polyposis of the colon, and multiple endocrine neoplasia syndromes. In affected families, neoplasms are common, multiple, and often found at an early age.

VI. PRECANCER. In many if not all systems (cervix, lung, colon), clinicopathologic studies have demonstrated that initial neoplastic change can be recognized in a **preinvasive** stage (precancer). Such changes can progress over a prolonged time span. Whether all malignant neoplasms arise as benign lesions, which then undergo progression, or whether some are highly malignant from the start is debatable. However, it seems probable that all neoplasms go through a benign preinvasive phase, even if this phase often is not recognized clinically.

VII. CLINICAL ASPECTS

A. Benign neoplasms can

1. Be **asymptomatic** and be noticed incidentally at physical examination, unrelated surgery, or at autopsy

2. **Obstruct** a hollow viscus, such as a leiomyoma of the small bowel occupying the lumen and producing obstruction

3. **Bleed**

4. Produce a **lump**

5. Produce abnormal **function**. The best example of this is found in endocrine organs, where a neoplasm can produce an excess of a specific hormone since the neoplasm is not bound by normal feedback control mechanisms. Symptoms resemble those associated with hormonal excess. Examples include parathyroid adenoma with hypercalcemia and adrenal adenoma with Cushing's syndrome.

B. Malignant tumors (i.e., cancers) are associated with the following problems.

1. **Masses.** A lump can occur anywhere, usually on an exposed or easily palpable structure such as the breast.

2. **Obstruction.** Malignant tumors, just like benign ones, can occupy the lumen of and obstruct a hollow viscus, as in malignant lymphoma of the small intestine.

3. **Bleeding.** Whereas benign neoplasms usually produce bleeding by expansive growth and

erosion of the overlying surface, cancers often invade and ulcerate the surface tissues over them, as in adenocarcinoma of the stomach. They also can infiltrate vessels and rupture them.

4. **Anemia.** As a consequence of chronic low-grade blood loss, usually associated with gastrointestinal or genitourinary neoplasms, anemia of an iron-deficiency type may be responsible for the initial symptoms (weakness and fatigue) of a cancer. Anemia also may result from poor nutrition, especially in oral and esophageal cancers, and from replacement of red cell–producing bone marrow by metastatic tumor.

5. **Nutritional deprivation** is most often noted in patients who have head and neck and upper gastrointestinal tract cancers. However, many other cancer patients also exhibit poor nutrition. Sometimes malnutrition is associated with the gastric distress, nausea, and vomiting resulting from radiotherapy and chemotherapy. Carcinomas also may produce substances (not characterized) that interfere with intestinal absorption or produce anorexia.

6. **Loss of function** can result from the mass effect of cancer or the replacement of normal tissue at various sites.

7. **Ectopic hormone production.** Various paraneoplastic syndromes can be produced by malignant tumors. Because the hormones produced are not controlled by normal mechanisms (tumors being autonomous), the symptoms of excess hormones (e.g., ACTH or ADH) may become the major clinical and life-threatening problem.

8. **Infection.** A neoplasm may be obstructive (e.g., of a bronchus) and lead to postobstructive infection (e.g., pneumonia). Infections are common in general in patients who have cancer and may occur for several other reasons.
   a. **Altered host resistance,** due to serologic or cellular factors, may permit relatively avirulent organisms such as normal bacterial bowel flora, common fungi, parasites, or viruses to cause infection and death.
      (1) **Serologic Factors.** In lymphomas and leukemias, normal immunoglobulins are decreased, resulting in an increased susceptibility to and increased severity of infection.
      (2) **Cellular Factors.** Decreased total mature granulocyte counts often are associated with intensive chemotherapy and are found in patients with acute leukemia or with various types of neoplasia involving bone marrow. The function of the neutrophils, not only their total count, is critical since immature granulocytes phagocytize and kill bacteria less efficiently than mature leukocytes. Quantitative and qualitative abnormalities of neutrophil function include defects in chemotaxis, phagocytosis, and bactericidal capacity.
      (3) Patients with lymphoid malignancies (especially Hodgkin's disease) have alterations of cell-mediated immunity. Cytotoxic chemotherapy has significant adverse effects on both B- and T-cell functions, resulting in diminished opsonization, inadequate lysis of bacteria, and defective neutralization of bacterial toxins.
   b. **Integumentary and mucosal barriers** can be disrupted by a tumor or by its treatment (surgery and radiation), providing a nidus for microbial colonization and a portal for invasion. Breakdown of mucous membranes may lead to sepsis with normal bowel flora.
   c. **Malnutrition** promotes infection by contributing to the loss of integrity of the skin and mucosal barriers, imparing phagocytosis, and depressing lymphocyte function.
   d. **Microbial Flora.** Eighty percent of infections that occur in cancer patients arise from endogenous flora. Numerous factors contribute to this, including the use of special equipment and surgical procedures. Endogenous flora can be altered by antibiotic and chemotherapeutic agents, and when these microbial changes occur in conjunction with other host defects, life-threatening infection can result.

VIII. THE DIAGNOSIS OF CANCER. The pathologist must be able to

   A. Define the nature of the process. Is it a neoplasm or some other process.

   B. Determine if the process is a neoplasm. Is it benign or malignant.

   C. Define the type if malignant: Is it carcinoma, sarcoma, or lymphoma.

   D. Define the grade (equivalent to degree of differentiation). In many organs, a good correlation exists between the grade of a tumor, its stage, and the ultimate prognosis.

   E. Define the stage (extent of tumor). Pathologically this involves determination of metastasis and the extent of invasion into surrounding tissues. The extent of tumor is the most important factor in prognosis.

F. Describe associated lesions that may be of clinical or epidemiologic importance. For example, in medullary carcinoma of the thyroid, the finding of multiple nodules of tumor or hyperplastic parafollicular cells strongly suggests the presence of multiple endocrine neoplasia syndrome, and family members of an affected patient also may be affected and so should be evaluated.

IX. **SUMMARY.** Neoplasia remains a complex constellation of problems; it requires understanding of its causes, explanations of associated epidemiologic data, and elucidation of host-reactive mechanisms and immunity. Only then can reasonable hope be offered for control of cancer by prevention, early diagnosis, and finally, therapy.

STUDY QUESTIONS

Directions: The question below contains five suggested answers. Choose the **one best** response.

1. The most important prognostic factor for human cancer is the

(A) grade
(B) stage
(C) lymphocytic infiltration
(D) vascular invasion
(E) mitotic index

Directions: The question below contains four suggested answers of which **one or more** is correct. Choose the answer

A   if **1, 2, and 3** are correct
B   if **1 and 3** are correct
C   if **2 and 4** are correct
D   if **4** is correct
E   if **1, 2, 3, and 4** are correct

2. Histologically, benign neoplasms most often prove fatal because they

(1) transform into carcinomas
(2) do not invoke a host immune response
(3) are multifocal
(4) may interfere with the functioning of a vital structure

ANSWERS AND EXPLANATIONS

1. The answer is B. (*VIII E*) In most human cancers, stage (i.e., the extent of the disease) is the most important prognostic factor. Tumor grade (or differentiation), mitotic count, and invasion may correlate with stage in that the higher-grade tumor (i.e., the less differentiated) tends to be a higher-stage lesion.

2. The answer is D (4). (*VII A 2*) Although rare examples of transformations into carcinomas do occur, fatality results when benign neoplasms interfere with the functioning of a vital structure. Any neoplasm may invoke an immune response, and occasionally multifocal benign neoplasms are found.

3
Special Diagnostic Techniques

I. ELECTRON MICROSCOPY. Studying tissues at the ultrastructural level by means of both transmission and scanning electron microscopy (EM) allows a better understanding of normal disease, disease processes, functional derangements, and neoplasia. EM can be used to study acute cellular injury, infectious agents, and neoplasms.

A. ACUTE CELLULAR INJURY. The initial events involve cessation of respiration and depletion of substrates. The oxygen content of tissues and cells rapidly goes to zero, and mitochondrial function ceases. With this cessation, calcium apparently is redistributed in the mitochondria and probably leaks into the cell sap. Fatty acids no longer can be oxidized by the mitochondria, and perhaps because of the calcium release from the mitochondria, activation of phospholipase in the cell membrane and mitochondria occurs, resulting in the further accumulation of fatty acids. Contraction of muscle filaments and of filaments in other cells probably soon ceases.

1. Morphologic Changes.
   a. There is nuclear chromatin clumping, probably associated with decreased RNA synthesis, as the condensed chromatin fibrils become more inactive.
   b. Cytoplasmic glycogen decreases.
   c. Mitochondrial granules disappear.
   d. There is formation of blebs and invaginations in cell membranes, giving the appearance of apical vacuoles, and distortion of villose contours.
   e. There is dilatation of both rough and smooth endoplasmic reticulum (ER) and often of Golgi cisternae and vesicles, the latter frequently taking on concentric lamellar profiles. This dilatation is correlated with inward movement of water and ions into the cisternae.
   f. Prominent condensation in inner mitochondrial compartments occurs, with the mitochondrial matrices appearing dense and the interstitial space enlarging; tiny flocculent densities may occur within the swollen mitochondria, which indicates irreversible cell damage.
   g. Breaks in the plasmalemma may be observed at this stage; necrosis with karyolysis and cellular disruption follows.

2. Biochemical Alterations.
   a. Changes in activity of membrane enzymes
   b. Accumulation of toxic products in the cytoplasm
   c. Release of lysosomal enzymes with further cellular disruption

B. INFECTIOUS AGENTS. Screening for detection of microorganisms always should be done by light microscopy, not by EM. Proper uses for EM include

1. Confirmation of the initial light microscopy impression, especially when cultures are not available (some organisms such as *Pneumocystis carinii* cannot be cultured)

2. Searching for tumor-specific viral particles thought to be factors in the induction of benign and malignant tumors

3. Correlation of the changes found in tissues infected with a variety of microorganisms, including fungi

C. NEOPLASMS. At the ultrastructural level, neoplastic cells may be difficult to distinguish from regenerative cells. Ultrastructural analysis is helpful in identifying the nature of neoplasia and the cell of its origin, but it must be combined with gross microscopy and light microscopy, and the biological characteristics of the cells must be considered to establish the presence of a neoplastic disease.

1. **Usual Changes in the Cell Membrane and Its Components.**
   a. Distribution of the intercalated particles is seen by freeze-etching, which may be associated with the transformed state of the cell membrane.
   b. There are changes in the configuration of surface villi.
   c. There are changes in the mitochondria of tumor cells as compared with that of the cell of origin.
   d. The ER in tumor cells develops poorly. (The exact disposition of ER can be of great importance for diagnosis.)
   e. Secretory granules of a characteristic type are present. The dense core of granulated vesicles that are typical of endocrine cells often can permit recognition of carcinoids when the light microscopic morphology is deceptive. Diagnosis of melanomas can be a problem when they are undifferentiated (inconspicuous pigment). Melanosomes and premelanosomes, however, often can be recognized by their characteristic appearances in electron micrographs and can be of great help in the diagnosis.
   f. Changes in the nucleus of the malignant cell include the following.
      (1) The nuclear envelope is very irregular, showing deep invaginations with numerous pseudoinclusions, which often degenerate and result in true inclusions of lipid and other debris.
      (2) The pattern of chromatin clumping is different from that in the normal cell.
      (3) The nucleoli are typically large, often multiple, and attached to the inner surface of the nuclear envelope.

2. **Diagnosis by EM**. EM is becoming a useful adjunct in the diagnosis of tumors, but it is no substitute for the light microscope. Ultrastructural features of the cell membrane may be helpful in establishing the diagnoses of squamous cell carcinoma, adenocarcinoma, mesothelioma, thymoma, lymphoma, sarcoma, meningioma, and neurogenic tumors.
   a. The ultrastructural diagnosis of **squamous cell carcinoma** is based on the presence of desmosomal attachments and cytoplasmic tonofibrils, the morphologic ultrastructural counterparts of keratinization. Desmosomes abound in well-differentiated tumors but not in poorly differentiated neoplasms. However, desmosomes persist even in the poorly differentiated squamous cell carcinomas, as exemplified in the lymphoepithelial carcinoma of the nasopharynx, a neoplasm often difficult to differentiate from lymphoreticular lesions.
   b. **Adenocarcinomas** present, in addition to desmosomes, tight junctions between neighboring cells with the formation of true acini. Microvilli are usually present, recapitulating the glandular formations of the parent tissue.
   c. In diffuse pleural **mesotheliomas**, mesothelial cells are joined by desmosomes with abundant tonofilaments, studded with long microvilli, and adjacent cells delineate systems of communicating channels.
   d. The presence of desmosomes almost always excludes the possibility of sarcoma or lymphoma, although focal thickening of opposed cell membranes is not uncommon in sarcoma.
   e. EM studies may be of value when the surgical pathologist is confronted with any of the following situations.
      (1) The differential diagnosis of carcinoma, sarcoma, and lymphoma
      (2) Confirmation of the diagnosis of thymoma
      (3) The unequivocal diagnoses of histiocytosis X, melanoma, rhabdomyosarcoma, leiomyosarcoma, angiosarcoma, and neurogenic sarcomas
      (4) Differentiation between fibrous histiocytoma and liposarcoma
      (5) Identification of cell type in islet cell tumors, carcinoid, and other related tumors and their discrimination from poorly differentiated ductal carcinomas
      (6) The differential diagnosis of undifferentiated small round cell tumors

3. **Disadvantages of EM for Tumor Diagnosis.**
   a. Instrumentation, technical assistance, and special processing is expensive.
   b. Special preparation of tissues is needed.
      (1) For optimal results, the freshly removed sample should be placed in appropriate fixative immediately.
      (2) If EM examination is considered, after routine tissue processing for conventional microscopy, the artifacts of inadequate tissue preservation make the examination suboptimal at best.
   c. Although some rapid methods for EM techniques are available, many laboratories require several days for processing and diagnostic interpretation.

D. SPECIFIC ORGAN SYSTEMS

1. **Liver**. Many hepatic diseases are impossible to diagnose precisely by light microscopy, and new pathologic entities are being revealed through the use of EM. Hepatic parenchymal cell damage also can be estimated with the EM, and in the future, as morphometric techniques are applied, it should be possible to provide more accurate correlations with liver function tests.

2. **Kidney**. Renal pathology has been redefined by ultrastructural analysis. Often correlated with immunologic results, the classification of renal diseases has important clinical and prognostic relevance. Indeed, modern nephrology could not exist without EM diagnosis of the primary lesion, analysis of therapeutic effects, and analysis of types of rejection in transplant patients. Certain renal disorders (lipoid nephrosis and minimal lupus nephritis) show no light microscopic lesions, yet they exhibit ultrastructural abnormalities.

3. **Hematopoietic System**. Ultrastructural studies of hematopoietic tissues, particularly blood buffy coat and marrow samples, have helped pathologists reach more precise diagnoses in a variety of serious hematological conditions, including the acute leukemias, hairy-cell leukemia, Sézary syndrome, granulocytic sarcoma, and "nonsecretory" myeloma. Two main objectives can be met through the ultrastructural studies of hematopoietic tissues.
   a. The solution of diagnostic problems that cannot be resolved by routine light microscopic studies
   b. A better understanding of both cytogenesis and pathogenesis

4. **Nervous System**. EM has replaced the special stains of the past because of the ease of use and the reproducibility of the results. EM permits not only the characterization of poorly definable light microscopic abnormalities, such as inclusion bodies and storage substances, but also, even in autopsy material, the identification of virions, of other infectious agents, and of cytopathic effects that are currently attributed to "slow" viruses.

5. **Urinary System**. EM of the urothelium can alert the urologist to a high risk of cancer.

6. **Female Reproductive System**. Through EM, histologically undifferentiated cancers may be classified into epithelial tumors (carcinomas) and mesenchymal tumors (sarcomas), and they can be subclassified according to their histogenetic differentiation (i.e., adenocarcinoma, squamous cell carcinoma, leiomyosarcoma, and endometrial stromal cell sarcoma). EM also helps to differentiate early endometrial adenocarcinoma from hyperplastic lesions that may be mistaken for neoplasms and noninvasive borderline lesions of the ovary from their frankly malignant counterparts.

7. **Skin**. Ultrastructural investigations have shed new light on the pathogenesis of skin disease. EM of skin biopsy specimens may be classified by the type of structure identified.
   a. Intracellular virus particles: particles of variola virus, vaccinia, molluscum contagiosum virus, and herpesvirus can be identified readily in infected cells through EM, although not all viruses can be distinguished structurally from others of the same group.
   b. Cell types in cutaneous neoplasms: insufficiently differentiated tumors frequently may be identified by EM demonstration of specific organelles or other ultrastructural features. Malignant melanoma may be identified by the presence of melanosomes or unpigmented premelanosomes, even when too little melanin is formed to be seen through light microscopy. This is especially valuable in the differential diagnoses of metastatic tumors when no primary tumor has been identified because a metastatic melanoma is more frequently unpigmented than a primary malignant melanoma. Metastases may become manifest clinically years after the removal of a presumed mole or in the absence of any known primary lesion in patients with metastatic melanoma.

8. **Endocrine System**. An endocrine cell exhibited through light microscopy often is distinguished by the number of endosecretory granules in the cytoplasm. However, EM is necessary for adequate evaluation of the granules, especially when they are sparse. EM has identified previously unrecognized tumors as probably derived from endocrine cells. Direct EM, along with silver stains and immune techniques examined at the ultrastructural level, may permit early identification of endocrine cells in utero and help to determine the origin of such cells. EM is helpful in the identification of all tumors that occur in families with multiple endocrine adenomatosis, but it has not demonstrated any difference between tumors that are associated with the syndrome and those that occur separately. Correlation with immunohistochemical results allows even better definition of the cell type and product.

9. **Soft Tissue Tumors**. The major benefit of EM of soft tissue tumors is derived from the light microscope. Through correlation between the features of light microscopy and EM, EM can extend diagnostic acumen in identifying a given tumor.

II. IMMUNOHISTOCHEMISTRY

A. IMMUNOFLUORESCENCE. Antisera can be combined chemically with small quantities of certain dyes without loss of their specific antibody properties. Fluorescent dyes [usually fluorescein isothiocyanate (FITC)] can be detected in a fluorescence microscope since the visible light generated in the tissue does not have to contrast with any visible incident light. It is thus possible to use fluorescein-conjugated antisera for histological localization of the corresponding antigens.

1. The immunofluorescence technique has wide applications for the **detection of autoantibodies** in human sera. In clinical practice the specificity of these reactions is deduced from the histological localization of the patient's antibody on the substrate tissue. In the indirect technique that is used generally, the tissue is treated first with the patient's serum, and after removal of uncombined serum proteins by washing, the attached human antibody is demonstrated by a fluorescent antihuman immunoglobulin serum.

2. The immunofluorescence technique can be used to **localize tissue antigens** (serum proteins and certain hormones) and to **identify microorganisms** in tissues. Since few properly characterized sera are available commercially, immunofluorescence techniques largely are used as research tools and have little application to clinical practice.

3. **Disadvantages** of this technique include the following.
   a. Special equipment (fluorescence microscope) is needed.
   b. Samples fade, requiring photography to document results.
   c. There is difficulty in reading slides because of autofluorescence.
   d. Fresh frozen tissue is required for reliable results.

B. IMMUNOPEROXIDASE TECHNIQUES

1. The enzyme bridge method involves the use of three antisera. The marker enzyme is rendered visible or electron opaque by an appropriate histochemical technique. If autoantibodies are present in the first antiserum (e.g., human antinuclear factor), the appropriate antigen is stained selectively in the substrate tissue (e.g., nuclei). Fortunately, nonorgan-specific autoantibodies are not species specific, and therefore rodent substrate tissue can be used for detecting human autoantibodies in this test. The three antisera are flooded onto a test substrate tissue in the order listed below.
   a. An antiserum to the antigen to be demonstrated
   b. An antiserum (from a different species) to the immunoglobulin component of the original antigen (**a**)
   c. An antiserum from the original species (**a**) to a marker enzyme, in this case, horseradish peroxidase

2. The enzyme bridge method has four advantages over fluorescent techniques.
   a. It gives a permanent preparation.
   b. Only a conventional light microscope is necessary for examining the stained sections.
   c. Conjugation procedures are not required, thus the risks of denaturing sera and reducing their antigenicity are avoided.
   d. A range of antihuman sera to different immunoglobulins may be used with just one antibody—antiperoxidase.

3. The technique has two disadvantages.
   a. It requires more time to complete than do immunofluorescence techniques.
   b. The pale background staining makes weakly positive antibodies more difficult to detect.

C. IMMUNOCYTOCHEMISTRY, especially the unlabeled-antibody method of immunoperoxidase techniques, has made it possible to demonstrate the presence of antigens in a tissue section, thus allowing pathologists to investigate the functional aspects and histogenesis of many diseases. Immunocytochemical techniques have contributed to the identification of neoplastic and hyperplastic lesions of endocrine organs. Identification of tumor-specific markers also has helped pathologists in cases of difficult differential diagnoses. Immunocytochemical methods provide a bridge between the morphological and functional aspects of a lesion since they permit examination in situ.

1. The **major applications** of the methods are
   a. Identification of the cell of origin of an antigen (e.g., endocrine neoplasms)
   b. Detection of abnormal distribution or number of cells producing an antigen in a lesion (e.g., hyperplasia or hypoplasia of endocrine cells)
   c. Detection of loss of a normal antigen in a neoplasm (e.g., blood group antigens in bladder and breast neoplasms)

    d. Identification of oncofetal antigens in neoplasms [e.g., α-fetoprotein (AFP) and carcinoembryonic antigen (CEA)]

    e. Identification of tissue-specific markers in soft-tissue neoplasms

    f. Detection of microorganisms

    g. Detection of autoantibodies

  2. Specific Uses.

    a. Lymphomas. The immunoperoxidase method can be used in the following ways.

      (1) To distinguish a B-cell lymphoma from a reactive proliferation by the detection of a single class of an immunoglobulin light chain in the lymphoma, thus establishing its monoclonal nature

      (2) To distinguish a large B-cell lymphoma from an undifferentiated carcinoma by detecting intracytoplasmic immunoglobulins

      (3) For retrospective studies of lymphomas, plasma cell myelomas, and macroglobulinemias

    b. Hormones. Detection of hormones in neoplasms gives information about the neoplastic histogenesis. The immunocytochemical procedure is so sensitive that an extremely small amount of hormone can be detected in cases of clinically nonfunctioning neoplasms. There is now evidence that many neoplasms of endocrine organs contain multiple hormones.

    c. Enzymes. Many enzymes have been localized in tissue sections by immunocytochemistry. Some enzymes can be detected by standard enzyme histochemical methods, but these methods necessitate fresh or specially handled tissue. Enzymes, such as prostatic acid phosphatase or lysozyme, are used as tissue-specific markers to ascertain the histogenesis of neoplasms.

    d. Oncofetal antigens, such as AFP and CEA, are fetal substances that are synthesized during gestation and appear in adults in association with certain types of tumors. A variety of neoplasms can be associated with elevated levels of these antigens.

    e. Tissue-specific markers are antigens that are present in only a few tissues; thus, they are extremely useful in diagnostic pathology since they may be used to determine the histogenesis of a neoplasm. Some enzymes and immunoglobulins are also tissue specific because they are produced by particular organs or cells and are present in neoplasms derived from these organs. Detection of myoglobin, factor VIII, or lysozyme in soft tissue neoplasms by immunocytochemical methods serves to indicate the differentiation of the neoplasms toward skeletal muscles, blood vessels, or histiocytes, respectively.

    f. Microorganisms. If antibodies against microorganisms are available, a specific method to identify these microorganisms can be developed.

    g. Viral Antigens. Many studies have been done describing localization of hepatitis B surface (HB$_s$Ag) and core (HB$_c$Ag) antigens both at the light microscopic and EM levels. HB$_s$Ag represents excessive capsular material of the hepatitis B virus (HBV). This antigen is present in the cytoplasms of hepatocytes but not in the nuclei. Although immunocytochemical methods of HB$_s$Ag staining correlate well with histochemical methods (orcein staining), positive cells are demonstrated more intensely by immunocytochemical staining.

III. CYTOLOGY. Cytological techniques of scrapings and brushings from minimally invasive lesions allow for the early diagnoses of cancers of the bronchus, esophagus, stomach, colon, breast, and many other sites. The value of diagnostic cytology in modern cancer detection cannot be overemphasized.

  A. NEOPLASTIC CELLS CAN BE IDENTIFIED in several ways, including morphologically. The interpretation of cytologic smears depends on the differences between benign and malignant cells.

    1. Nuclear changes enable distinction between benign and malignant elements.

    2. The **appearance of cytoplasm** distinguishes the type of malignancy and also reflects genetic abnormalities.

    3. Malignancy is associated with **changes in chromosomal** and **biochemical composition.** Visually, these changes are reflected in the nucleus and nucleolus of the cells and in cellular and nuclear shapes, sizes, and configurations.

  B. CELL MEMBRANE BIOCHEMISTRY. Recent research has attempted to elucidate such phenomena as cell-to-cell communication, contact inhibition, and the development of metastases. In vitro, normal cells cease dividing when they become crowded together (contact inhibition). Malignant cells do not stop dividing, despite cell-to-cell contact; instead, they pile up. The uncontrolled, often rapid growth of neoplastic tissue presents a problem to the neoplasm—how to obtain and maintain adequate nutrients. Necrosis is observed commonly in malignant tumors. Neoplastic cells, because of loss of contact inhibition, tend to be less sticky and are exfoliated and scraped off more easily than their normal counterparts.

C. **THE EXAMINATION OF ISOLATED CELLS IN SMEARS**, which forms a basis of modern diagnostic cytology, must be appreciated from several standpoints.

 1. Cells may be collected from areas where they normally exfoliate, such as the vagina and cervix uteri.

 2. Cells from sites where they normally desquamate but remain for periods of time may be examined (e.g., cells from sputum and urine specimens).

 3. Cells may be coaxed to exfoliate, for example, through various washing methods (such as bronchial or bladder washings).

 4. Cells may be brushed or scraped directly from lesions visualized through endoscopes. This method has gained favor for pulmonary, gastrointestinal, and oral lesions.

 5. Aspirations of various sites, such as breast masses, thyroid nodules, salivary gland tumors, and enlarged lymph nodes, may be performed.

D. **FINE-NEEDLE ASPIRATION BIOPSY**

 1. Fine-needle aspiration biopsy is a sampling of a palpable or roentgenographic mass by means of a fine needle with negative pressure supplied by an attached syringe.

 2. This technique can be used in the following ways.
    a. Aspiration of superficial lumps and bumps from the breast has proved particularly advantageous.
    b. During a laparotomy, the pancreas may be examined safely and suspicious hepatic nodules may be aspirated. The diagnosis should be rapid to determine the extent of surgery.
    c. The lung may be aspirated during fluoroscopy.
    d. Deep organs can be penetrated by cutaneous biopsy with the aid of ultrasonography and computed tomography.

 3. A few **complications** have been reported.
    a. Pulmonary hemorrhage is very rare, although pneumothorax (spontaneously resolving) occurs in 10 percent to 30 percent of the cases.
    b. The thousands of biopsies reported from Scandinavia have shown that seeding through the needle tract is of no significance.

 4. The **advantages** of the technique are myriad.
    a. The equipment and technique are simple.
    b. The procedure can be done in the office on any superficial lesion the first time a patient is seen.
    c. The biopsy takes 1 minute and can be processed and interpreted within 15 minutes.
    d. The procedure is safe.
    e. The procedure has an accuracy of 80 percent to greater than 95 percent.
    f. For some patients aspiration biopsy may eliminate hospitalization or surgery, and for others it may shorten their hospital stay.

STUDY QUESTIONS

Directions: Each question below contains five suggested answers. Choose the **one best** response to each question.

1. A 54-year-old woman has a positive sputum cytology but no apparent lesion on x-ray. The best procedure to clarify her condition would be to

(A) perform a repeat sputum cytology
(B) perform a bronchoscopy
(C) perform a mediastinoscopy
(D) perform a lobectomy
(E) plan for surgical exploration

2. Cytologic examination of pleural effusions in a woman without a known primary cancer is most likely to reveal which of the following malignant cells?

(A) Lymphoma
(B) Mesothelioma
(C) Carcinoma of the breast
(D) Carcinoma of the lung
(E) Leiomyosarcoma

3. Urinary cytology can detect all of the following disorders with great accuracy EXCEPT

(A) prostatic carcinoma
(B) lead poisoning
(C) papillary transitional carcinoma of the bladder
(D) cytomegalovirus
(E) in situ carcinoma of the bladder

4. A 70-year-old asymptomatic man is found to have bilateral inguinal hernias. At operation for hernia repair, an enlarged lymph node is removed. Pathologic evaluation disclosed a metastatic adenocarcinoma. The primary site of such a tumor can best be determined by

(A) barium enema
(B) exploratory laparotomy
(C) immunoperoxidase localization of specific tumor markers
(D) computed axial tomography (CAT) scan of the pelvis
(E) electron microscopic (EM) examination of the node

5. Cytologic abnormalities, which are recognized morphologically in many malignant cells, can be explained best by

(A) chromosomal anomalies
(B) excessive mucin content
(C) cell surface alterations
(D) a decrease in cellular glycogen content
(E) abnormal mitotic figures

ANSWERS AND EXPLANATIONS

1. The answer is B. (*III C*) Cytologic screening programs for detection of early, radiologically occult lung cancer occasionally produce a dilemma in that abnormal cells may be shed into a sputum sample but a lesion cannot be detected by chest x-ray. Bronchoscopy, especially that employing flexible fiberoptic scopes, can be used to detect early lung cancer either by direct visualization of mucosal abnormalities or by biopsy. If no abnormal area is seen, systematic brushings of the bronchial mucosa, separating samples from each lobe, can localize [i.e., by lobectomy (surgical excision of the involved area)] the tumor cells to a specific area of the lung that can be treated. Merely repeating the sputum cytology will not localize the lesion. Mediastinoscopy can be used to stage (evaluate the extent of) the lesion and assess operability. Lesions so small as to be picked up by screening only are unlikely to spread (metastasize) to the mediastinum, and hence mediastinoscopy would not be needed in this patient at this time in her evaluation.

2. The answer is C. (*III C 5*) Numerous studies have shown that pleural effusion caused by malignant disease in patients without known cancer contain adenocarcinoma cells. Statistically, the usual primary sites for such tumors are the breast in women and the lung in men. Lymphoma, mesothelioma, and leiomysarcoma are rarely diagnosed by cytological studies.

3. The answer is A. (*III A; III C 2*) Normally, very few prostatic cells, whether benign or malignant, are exfoliated into the urine. Bladder lesions, in situ cancer, invasive papillary or nonpapillary cancer, and lead poisoning can be detected readily by appropriate examination of urine specimens prepared and screened adequately. Cytomegalovirus inclusions in bladder epithelium also have a characteristic cytologic appearance, which can be readily diagnosed.

4. The answer is C. (*II B 1*) The most likely primary site for the metastatic lesion in an elderly man as described is the prostate. Immunochemical localization of prostatic acid phosphatase (an enzyme acting as a tumor marker) or prostatic-specific antigen will provide the least invasive, least expensive solution. The other choices, barium enema, laparotomy, computed axial tomography (CAT), and electron microscopic (EM) examination, are less specific and more expensive and uncomfortable for the patient.

5. The answer is A. (*III A 1, 2, 3*) Although cell surface alterations can explain cytologic abnormalities, cytologically the alterations are not reflected uniformly. Cytologic abnormalities can also be explained by abnormal mitotic figures, although mitotic figures are not specific for cancer since such changes are seen also in granulation, tissue repair, and so forth. The presence or absence of glycogen or mucin may aid the pathologist in defining tumor type, but not in determining malignancy.

4
The Heart

I. THE CIRCULATORY SYSTEM. The circulatory system is composed of the heart, arteries, veins, and lymphatics, all of which function as an entity. (The vascular system is outlined in Chapter 5.) The heart functions as a muscular pump for the circulatory system. A brief review of the normal heart is described below.

A. Knowledge of the **embryology** of the normal heart is essential to understanding the multiple congenital anomalies that present clinical problems.

1. Paired primitive heart tubes fuse to form the **bulboventricular tube**. The cephalic portion dilates to form the aortic sac, which develops into the first through the sixth aortic arches. The caudal portion forms the embryonic ventricle.

2. Sigmoid folding of the bulboventricular tube forms the **bulboventricular loop**; the atrium and sinus venosus become more cephalic than the ventricle and bulbus cordis.

3. A transverse septum divides the atrium and the ventricle, forming two chambers, between the fifth and eighth weeks of gestation.

4. An interventricular septum develops as the two ventricles enlarge by centrifugal growth of the myocardium; fusion of the medial walls of the ventricles forms the muscular ventricular septum. Conal cushions fuse to form the basilar septum.

5. The **bulbus cordis** forms the primitive truncus arteriosus, which the aorticopulmonary septum splits to form the aorta and the pulmonary artery. The fourth aortic arches align with the aortic channel, and the sixth aortic arches align with the pulmonary artery.

6. Atrioventricular valves are formed mainly from "skirts" of ventricular muscle, which develop at the atrioventricular junctions and are attached to the ventricle walls by trabeculae. These trabeculae will become the papillary muscles. The primitive valves change from thick muscular structures to thin fibrous cusps, with the chordae tendineae connecting the valve cusps and papillary muscles.

B. Knowledge of the **normal anatomy** of the heart is essential to clinical understanding and diagnostic evaluation of diseases affecting the heart.

1. The heart lies enclosed within the pericardial sac in the middle mediastinal compartment. The pericardial sac is lined by a serosal membrane and contains up to 30 ml of clear serous fluid, which acts as a lubricant. Inflammation of the pericardium often leads to accumulation of and changes in this fluid and may result in fibrous adhesions between the parietal pericardium and the epicardium of the heart.

2. The normal heart weighs about 250 g to 300 g in females and 300 g to 350 g in males, but this varies with age, body size, nutritional status, and the amount of epicardial fat deposits that are present.

3. Normal cardiac valves are described as follows.
   a. The **mitral valve** is approximately 10 cm in circumference and has two major leaflets to direct blood flow from the left atrium into the left ventricle.
      (1) The **anteromedial leaflet** extends from the posteromedial aspect of the muscular ventricular septum to the anterolateral wall of the left ventricle.
      (2) The quadrangular **posterolateral leaflet** controls about two-thirds of the mitral valve orifice from the anterolateral to the posteromedial portion of the **annulus fibrosus**. This is the larger, less mobile of the two mitral valve leaflets.
   b. The **tricuspid valve** has a circumference of about 12 cm, and it directs right atrial blood

flow anteroinferiorly and to the left into the right ventricle. There are normally three tricuspid leaflets, which are of unequal size.
  (1) The **anterior leaflet** is usually the largest and extends from the infundibulum to the inferolateral ventricular wall.
  (2) The **septal** (or **medial**) **leaflet** attaches to the membranous and muscular portions of the interventricular septum.
  (3) The **posterior leaflet** is usually the smallest and is attached to the posterior inferior part of the tricuspid valve ring.
  c. The **aortic valve** is about 7.5 cm in circumference and is a semilunar valve composed of three fibrous cusps. Because the coronary arteries originate in the sinuses of Valsalva of two of the aortic cusps, the aortic cusps are named the right coronary cusp, the left coronary cusp, and the noncoronary or posterior cusp.
  d. The **pulmonic valve** is about 8.5 cm in circumference and also contains three cusps: anterior, right, and left. Like those in the aortic valve, each cusp has a concave free edge with a central fibrous **nodulus Arantii**. During ventricular diastole, the cusps passively fall together to support the column of blood and the noduli Arantii meet in the center to help support the leaflets in closure.

4. Blood supply to the heart is provided chiefly by the three major coronary arteries.
  a. The left main coronary artery originates from the aorta in the sinus of Valsalva behind the left aortic valve cusp. This divides into two main branches.
    (1) The first branch of the left main coronary artery is the **left anterior descending coronary artery**, which commonly supplies the left ventricular apex, the medial half of the anterior surface of the left ventricle, a portion of the medial anterior wall of the right ventricle, and the anterior portion of the interventricular septum.
    (2) The **left circumflex coronary artery** is the other large branch of the left main coronary artery in most individuals. It supplies blood to the anterolateral walls of the left ventricle and to a portion of the posterior wall.
  b. The **right coronary artery** originates from the aorta behind the right aortic valve cusp. It supplies a large part of the right ventricle as it passes to the right and then posteriorly along the posterior-inferior heart surface. The right coronary artery commonly provides the circulation to the posterior portion of the interventricular septum, to adjacent parts of the posterior left ventricle, and sometimes to the apex of the left ventricle.
  c. Because the coronary artery "watersheds" are highly variable, each patient may have a slightly different blood flow distribution, which becomes important in considering coronary artery atherosclerotic disease.

II. MAJOR CLASSIFICATIONS OF CARDIAC DISEASE. The four major classifications of cardiac disease described here are based upon data from the United States and western Europe and are not necessarily reflective of the incidence of cardiac disease in other parts of the world.

A. **CORONARY ARTERY ISCHEMIC HEART DISEASE** is the collective term applied to several conditions that produce cardiac dysfunction because of reduction or absence of the blood supply required by the myocardium.
  The **epidemiology** of ischemic heart disease shows that the atherosclerotic type predominates, affecting the population to such a degree that it is the leading cause of cardiac-related death in the United States. Coronary artery ischemic heart disease accounts for 80 percent to 90 percent of all heart disease mortality.

  1. In 1980, ischemic heart disease produced a death rate of 343 per 100,000.

  2. Deaths from ischemic heart disease occur in a range from 35 to 65 years of age. More men than women die from this disease, although this differential decreases as age increases.

  3. The age-adjusted death rate for ischemic heart disease, at least for white men in the susceptible age group, declined somewhat since the late 1960s. It is possible that this is a reflection of better medical care now afforded to victims, especially in view of the massive effort toward rapid diagnosis and intensive care, which is available in modern coronary care units. Changes in smoking habits, diet, and exercise also are postulated as modifiers of the death rate from atherosclerotic ischemic heart disease.

    a. **Atherosclerotic disease** (see Chapter 5, "The Vascular System") is the most common lesion affecting the coronary arteries with resultant ischemic heart disease. It may be limited to the blood vessels without associated cardiac disease until the metabolic demands of the heart muscle exceed the blood flow available through the affected coronary arteries. Three types of ischemic heart disease may result.

(1) Ischemic atrophy and **fibrosis** of the myocardial muscle fibers occur, often silently, when blood supply is insufficient to maintain the required metabolic demands of the myocardium.

   (a) Diffuse myocardial fibrosis is present throughout the ventricle, and there may be associated degenerative fibrocalcific changes in the heart valves of the left ventricle. The heart is commonly smaller than normal because of progressive muscle loss. Grossly evident disease appears as diffuse, gray-white streaking of the normally red-brown myocardium. This diffuse scarring is apparent microscopically as perivascular fibrosis with increased fibrous tissue along the supportive connective tissue framework of the myocardium, sometimes to the point of separation of myocardial fibers.

   (b) Clinical Data. Compensated ischemic disease may present no symptoms until the cardiac function is challenged by an additional disease or stress, which can then precipitate left ventricular failure (i.e., absence of left ventricular output that is sufficient to meet the blood supply needs of the body).

(2) Angina pectoris is the clinical syndrome of paroxysmal substernal or precordial chest pain, which is commonly provoked by a temporary increase in cardiac demand for blood flow. This form of cardiac ischemia is reversible when it is precipitated by exercise or emotional stress. Angina pectoris can also be produced by a coronary artery spasm, with or without atherosclerotic coronary artery disease.

   (a) No anatomic changes are specific for angina pectoris. It is a clinical syndrome of pain representing cardiac ischemia, which is no longer silent ischemic atrophy but is not so severe or irreversible so as to produce myocardial infarction.

   (b) Angina pectoris is usually relieved by decreasing the cardiac metabolic level (i.e., cessation of exercise or relief of emotional stress) or by the therapeutic administration of drugs such as nitroglycerin.

(3) Myocardial infarction (Fig. 4-1) is permanent myocardial damage due to irreversible myocardial ischemia, which is produced most often by atherosclerotic coronary artery disease. The result is ischemic coagulative necrosis of myocardial fibers with loss of the normal conductive and contractile responses of the affected myocardium.

   (a) Clinical Data. Myocardial infarcts are described in several ways.

   (i) Location within the heart (e.g., anterolateral left ventricle infarct)

   (ii) Degree of depth of ventricular wall involvement (e.g., transmural infarction, which implies necrosis of more than one-half of the thickness of the ventricular wall)

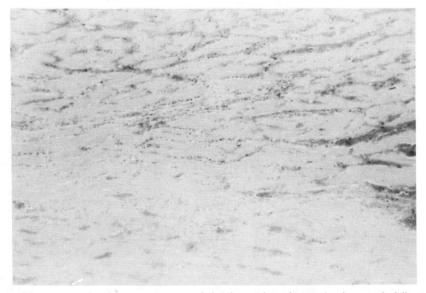

Figure 4-1. Photomicrograph of an acute myocardial infarct taken during the first week following onset. Coagulative necrosis of myocardial fibers is apparent. Edema and focal hemorrhage have caused separation of individual myofibrils. The dark nuclei of leukocytes, which have entered the zone of infarction, are seen between individual myocardial fibers.

      (iii) Association with complicating factors such as arrhythmias or life-threatening hypotension

      (iv) Association with obstruction of a particular coronary artery (e.g., a left anterior descending coronary infarct)

  (b) The **morphologic features** of myocardial infarcts are similar regardless of their location, but they are highly time-dependent.

      (i) First Week. Five to six hours after infarction, coagulative necrosis of myocardial fibers becomes apparent, with signs of hyaline change, loss of myocardial fiber striations, deep eosinophilic staining, karyolysis of myocyte nuclei, and pyknosis and karyorrhexis. Between 12 and 24 hours, neutrophils begin to enter the infarct from its periphery. This infiltrate increases from the second through the fourth days. Removal of dead myocardial fibers is mediated through the release of catalytic enzymes by the leukocytes and phagocytosis by histiocytes that enter the infarct. Edema and focal hemorrhage are often present. By the end of the first week after onset, new capillaries and fibroblasts enter the infarct from the periphery to begin reconstruction.

      (ii) Second Week. There is continued removal of necrotic myocardial fibers with progressive replacement by highly vascularized fibrous collagen "scar" tissue. The necrotic area is filled with pigmented macrophages containing yellow-brown lipofuscin granules from the phagocytosis of necrotic myocardial fibers and erythrocytes from the hemorrhage. The cellular infiltrate now includes eosinophils, lymphocytes, and plasma cells.

      (iii) Third Week. There is progression of phagocytosis, centripedal ingrowth of vascularized connective tissue, decreasing numbers of eosinophils, and prominent collagen synthesis, particularly at the periphery of the infarcted zone.

      (iv) Weeks Four through Six. There is a gradual accumulation of newly synthesized collagen, forming the connective tissue scar present in the site of infarction. This is followed by a gradual decrease in the proliferation of new capillaries, and fewer macrophages and lymphocytes are now present. This zone of myocardial fibrosis or scar slowly contracts as it matures. Any viable myocardial fibers that remain are microscopically apparent within this fibrous tissue.

  (c) Complications of the myocardial infarct that produce anatomic signs may also cause clinical symptoms (e.g., the auscultated pericardial friction rub is a sign of pericarditis, which can accompany the myocardial infarct). Other complications may be extremely dangerous clinically (e.g., severe arrhythmias) but often do not leave any histologic sign. Some of the anatomically apparent complications are listed below.

      (i) Fibrinous or **fibrinous** and **hemorrhagic pericarditis** can develop in the region overlying the myocardial infarct or it may become generalized. The pericarditis may resolve completely or can produce fibrous adhesions between the heart and the pericardium.

      (ii) **Mural thrombi** can form on the disrupted endocardial surface over areas of myocardial infarction. Because these thrombi are quite friable prior to fibrous organization, portions of a thrombus may break off and enter the peripheral circulation as emboli.

      (iii) **Peripheral artery embolism**, which can result from the presence of a mural thrombus, may obstruct blood flow to an extremity, a part of the brain, the kidneys, spleen, or a part of the intestine and thus produce clinical signs that are consistent with infarction of the involved part of the body.

      (iv) **Rupture** of the myocardium at the site of infarction can occur at any time within 3 weeks or so after infarct onset, but it tends to occur more frequently at the end of the first week or at the beginning of the second week, when the infarcted zone has minimal structural strength.

      (v) Myocardial rupture often produces intrapericardial hemorrhage, which causes **cardiac tamponade** if the rupture is through any portion of the ventricular wall other than the septum. Rupture of the septum will produce left-to-right intracardiac shunts.

      (vi) A **ventricular aneurysm** develops when the fibrous scar that is formed after infarction has insufficient structural strength to withstand the intraventricular chamber pressures. The result is extreme thinning of the ventricular wall with progressive convex deformity of the external cardiac surface. The aneurysm cannot contract naturally in phase with the remaining normal ventricle and thus is a potential site of blood stasis. Mural thrombi may form in a ventricular aneurysm.

b. Ischemic cardiac disease may also result from the **spasm** of otherwise apparently normal coronary arteries, from **thrombosis** of a coronary artery—most often in an area that is affected by atherosclerotic coronary artery disease, from **stenosis** of the ostia of the coronary artery, from inflammatory **arteritis**, and from a host of uncommon conditions with the common result of compromising coronary artery blood flow to the point of myocardial ischemia.

B. HYPERTENSIVE HEART DISEASE is the result of sustained systemic **hypertension**, which is usually above 90 mm Hg diastolic or 140 mm Hg systolic. The result is **left ventricular hypertrophy**.

1. **Systemic hypertension** is classified into two broad groups.
   a. Primary (idiopathic or essential) **hypertension** is a disease for which the underlying cause is unknown. Unfortunately, nearly 90 percent of patients with systemic hypertension fit into this category.
   b. Secondary hypertension is disease with a known etiology, generally from one of the following categories.
   (1) Renal—due to vascular, parenchymal, or obstructive lesions
   (2) Cerebral—usually secondary to increased intracranial pressure from various causes such as neoplasms and hemorrhage
   (3) Endocrine—due to causes such as functioning tumors of the adrenals or the pituitary gland
   (4) Eclamptic—occurs with pregnancy
   (5) Cardiovascular—due to malformations such as aortic coarctation or arteriovenous fistulae

2. The **morphologic criteria** for hypertensive heart disease include hypertrophy of the heart, which afflicts primarily the left ventricle. This hypertrophy can produce hearts that weigh two to four times the norm.
   a. Concentric hypertrophy of the left ventricle causes thickening to 25 mm or more (the norm is 13 mm to 15 mm), with hypertrophied papillary muscles and trabeculae carneae. This hypertrophy decreases the volume of the ventricular cavity. Endocardial fibrous thickening occasionally may be present.
   b. There are no microscopic findings that are characteristic of hypertensive heart disease, but enlargement of individual myocardial fibers may be seen.
   c. Before concentric hypertrophy of the left ventricle can be ascribed to hypertension alone, other abnormalities that might cause an increased cardiac workload must be excluded (e.g., valvular lesions or aortic malformation). The diagnosis of hypertensive cardio-myopathy is therefore one of exclusion for the pathologist.
   d. When the heart can no longer adequately compensate by hypertrophy alone, cardiac dilatation may occur.

3. **Clinical symptoms** may not be apparent during the period of compensated cardiac hyper-trophy. Eventually, the various signs and symptoms of the underlying hypertension will become manifest.
   a. Symptoms of cardiac decompensation initially are indicative of left ventricular failure; dyspnea, paroxysmal nocturnal dyspnea, orthopnea, cough, and hemoptysis—all reflecting increasing pulmonary congestion and edema. Signs of right ventricular failure may follow.
   b. Cardiac hypertrophy can be diagnosed by echocardiography, x-rays, electrocardiogram findings, and clinical examination; however, often diagnosis is not made until cardiac decompensation has alerted the physician.

4. **Epidemiologic studies** suggest that hypertension increases in incidence with increasing age. Depending upon the criteria that are chosen to define hypertension, about 20 percent of men under 30 years of age, 40 percent of men in the fifth decade of life, and nearly 60 percent in the seventh decade of life are affected.
   a. Heredity seems to play a role since nearly one-half of the children of hypertensive parents develop elevated blood pressure.
   b. Race is also apparently a factor since blacks in the United States are slightly more likely to have hypertension than whites. How much of this is the effect of cultural and envi-ronmental differences is unclear.

5. The **prognosis** for patients with hypertensive heart disease is highly variable, but there does seem to be a positive correlation between the severity of the hypertension and the onset of symptoms and eventual disability.

    a. These patients most often die of the cardiac complications of their disease, chiefly congestive heart failure.

    b. Hypertensive heart disease often is accompanied by atherosclerotic heart disease, with its associated problems.

C. INFLAMMATORY DISEASES OF THE HEART (Fig. 4-2) [**endocarditis, myocarditis, pericarditis,** and **pancarditis**] may affect any or all of the anatomic layers of the heart and may produce severe deformation of one or more of the valves, so that the valvular deformities become the most important clinical problem.

  1. Rheumatic heart disease follows rheumatic fever, which is a systemic, nonsuppurative, inflammatory complication that is linked to immunologic reactions following group A streptococcal infections of the pharynx.

    a. Five major manifestations may appear, but the cutaneous and subcutaneous signs are almost never seen alone. In each manifestation, inflammatory lesions are found in the connective tissues of the affected part of the body. The classic manifestations include

        (1) Erythema marginatum
        (2) Subcutaneous nodules
        (3) Chorea
        (4) Arthritis
        (5) Carditis

    b. In the United States, there has been a continuous decrease in the mortality from rheumatic fever since the beginning of this century. This has been attributed to the prevention and prompt antibiotic treatment of streptococcal pharyngeal infections.

    c. The precise **etiology** is unclear, so there is no single laboratory test or sign that is pathognomonic of rheumatic fever. The **diagnosis** is often based on the modified **Jones criteria**, which require the finding of at least one, and preferably two, of the five major manifestations listed above.

    d. Research has suggested that the myocardial lesions of rheumatic fever are the result of autoimmunity reactions induced by streptococcal antigens, which can share similarities with specific antigens in the body's connective tissues. These classic lesions are termed **Aschoff bodies** or nodules.

      (1) Aschoff bodies are found in the interstitial connective tissues of the heart, especially in the endocardium and myocardium, and are often in the vicinity of small blood vessels.

      (2) Three stages have been described in the development of an Aschoff body.

        (a) The early phase is thought to occur up to the fourth week of rheumatic carditis and is typified by fibrinoid degeneration—a nonspecific finding of altered collagen fibers and accumulated ground substance, including increased muco-

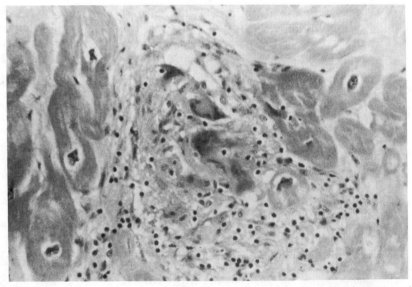

Figure 4-2. This photomicrograph shows a typical sarcoid granuloma within the myocardium. Sarcoidosis, which affects the heart directly, is recognized as a cause of heart failure that is distinct from cor pulmonale, which can accompany extensive sarcoid involvement of the lungs.

polysaccharides, which has an eosinophilic appearance resembling fibrin. This elliptical or globular zone is surrounded by a neutrophil infiltrate with a few lymphocytes, plasma cells, and histiocytes.

  (b) In the intermediate (proliferative or granulomatous) phase, the central focus of fibrinoid change is surrounded by mononuclear leukocytes, fibroblasts, large modified mesenchymal or histiocytic cells known as **Anitschkow's myocytes**, and a few multinucleated **Aschoff giant cells**. This phase is usually seen in heart tissues that have been obtained between the fourth and thirteenth week of the disease.

  (c) The late (senescent, fibrous, or healed) phase occurs at 3 or 4 months when there is regression and fibrosis of the Aschoff body with only a small number of lymphocytes and a rare plasma cell remaining.

  e. Rheumatic fever produces **pancarditis**—involvement of all three cardiac tissue layers (Fig. 4-3).

    (1) The endocarditis may be valvular or mural. The valvular disease is responsible for most of the deaths related to rheumatic fever.

      (a) The **mitral valve** is affected in almost 50 percent of cases. **Mitral plus aortic valve** involvement is the second most common pattern. Aortic valve disease alone ranks third, followed by trivalvular involvement of mitral, aortic, and tricuspid valves. The pulmonic valve rarely is diseased, either alone or in combination. _M A T_

      (b) Valvular lesions begin with thickening of the valve leaflets or cusps, followed by formation of characteristic wartlike nodules (verrucae), which are 1 mm to 3 mm in diameter, along the closure lines of the valves. The mechanism of verrucal development is unclear but may be the result of deposition of fibrin at erosion sites of inflamed endocardium followed by platelet deposition. Organization and fibrosis, which can cause adherence of the valve leaflets or cusps, then occur. Additional fibrosis causes thickening, shortening, and fusion of the valve's chordae tendineae. Eventual calcification of the valve may take place.

      (c) The result of this valvular damage is commonly mitral stenosis followed by aortic stenosis. The rigid, retracted valve leaflets can also be incompetent in closure so that mitral insufficiency is often combined with mitral stenosis.

      (d) The mural endocarditis produces lesions of thickened, plaque-like endocardium. These are common in the posterior wall of the left atrium above the posterior leaflet of the mitral valve, where they are called a McCallum's patch.

    (2) Rheumatic myocarditis is diagnosed histologically by the presence of Aschoff bodies in the myocardium, nonspecific inflammation of interstitial tissue between myocytes, and muscle cell damage, which varies from degenerative change to frank necrosis

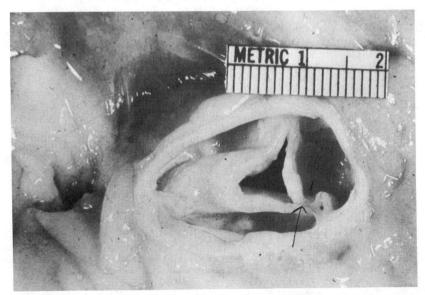

Figure 4-3. Photograph of an aortic valve from above showing partial fibrotic fusion of commissure following rheumatic fever.

of myocardial fibers. The Aschoff bodies and some nonspecific fibrosis remain even at resolution.

(3) The **pericarditis of rheumatic fever** is typified by an exuberant deposition of fibrin, which has led to the descriptions of "shaggy heart" and "bread and butter" pericarditis. The result is often formation of adhesions between the visceral pericardium and the parietal pericardium, leading to chronic adhesive pericarditis and sometimes to complete obliteration of the pericardial space.

f. The chief causes of morbidity and mortality following rheumatic carditis are cardiac failure, bacterial endocarditis, and peripheral embolism.

(1) Replacement with artificial valves has helped somewhat when diseased valves present the major clinical problem. Diseased valves may undergo slowly progressive stenosis over the course of their lives.

(2) The clinical course of rheumatic heart disease is variable for several reasons.

(a) The variability and severity of the rheumatic inflammation

(b) The degree of valve damage and scarring of the myocardium

(c) The location and severity of the hemodynamic problems due to valvular stenosis and insufficiency

(d) The frequency of recurrent attacks of rheumatic carditis

(e) The progression of the valvular fibrosis and calcification, which can continue in a damaged valve without any recurrent or persistent active rheumatic inflammation

2. **Syphilitic heart disease** is no longer very common because of the measures taken to control syphilis. However, it represents a type of cardiac inflammatory disease that is not autoimmune in origin but is related to infection.

a. Syphilitic cardiac problems are part of tertiary syphilis and may not become apparent until 15 to 20 years after the acute infection.

b. Syphilitic carditis occurs as a consequence of the spread of spirochetes from the mediastinal lymph nodes into the adventitia of the aorta. When the tunica media of the aorta is inflamed, disruption of the elastica and scarring lead to dilatation of the aortic valve ring and consequent narrowing of the coronary artery ostia.

c. The characteristic **obliterative endarteritis** of the aorta's vasa vasorum predisposes in some manner to the accelerated development of atherosclerotic lesions as well, especially in the root of the aorta. This contributes to the deformation of the aortic valve ring so that the leaflets become stretched and narrowed. The leaflets also undergo fibrosis. All of this leads to aortic insufficiency and strain on the left ventricle.

d. Left ventricular hypertrophy secondary to the aortic valve insufficiency may be so marked as to produce the "cor bovinum" of 1 kg or more.

e. Syphilitic carditis may remain clinically asymptomatic for many years, but eventually the aortic valve insufficiency, coronary ostia occlusion, and proximal aortic aneurysm lead to cardiac decompensation and death.

3. **Myocarditis** is a nonspecific term that is used to describe inflammation of the myocardium that is produced by infectious agents, physical or chemical agents, metabolic derangements, so-called collagen vascular diseases, and various idiopathic etiologies.

a. Myocarditis that is caused by infectious agents may result from actual invasion of the myocardium by the organisms or by the action of various toxins produced by the agents.

(1) **Histologic examination** may show either focal or diffuse inflammation with some muscle fiber degeneration and necrosis, especially in bacterial infections. Other agents produce only a nonsuppurative inflammation of the connective tissue elements with marked interstitial edema; this is typical of rickettsial infections. Small abscesses develop in pyogenic infections produced by staphylococcus and streptococcus and occasionally in infections by fungi such as actinomycosis and blastomycosis.

(2) The **gross appearance** is not usually distinctive for the causative organism. The myocardium becomes typically pale and flabby with dilatation of the ventricles and atria. Small granulomas may be present in myocarditis caused by tuberculosis, tularemia, or brucellosis.

b. **Acute viral myocarditis** may occur in a number of common viral infections and can lead to a debilitating loss of cardiac function. This is now the most common cause of myocarditis in the United States and western Europe. Because the link to viral infection is often difficult to prove, this disease often is termed idiopathic.

(1) Because the body needs time to create antibodies against the viral antigens, which then may cross-react with normal tissue antigens, a latency period exists between the systemic viral infection and the onset of clinically apparent myocarditis. There-

fore, an autoimmune mechanism has been suggested for the pathophysiology of this disease.

    (2) The clinical prognosis of postviral dilated cardiomyopathy and heart failure is unpredictable but generally poor.

  c. Other forms of infectious myocarditis are found commonly in areas endemic for specific organisms.

    (1) Chagas' disease is the most common form of heart disease in some parts of South America where *Trypanosoma cruzi* is endemic. More than 7 million individuals are affected—usually men in the third and fourth decades of life.

    (2) Echinococcal myocarditis is found in sheep-raising areas such as Uruguay, Australia, New Zealand, and some Mediterranean countries.

    (3) Trichinosis is the most common helminthic infection in the world, and myocarditis is its most serious and frequent complication.

4. Endocarditis is often a component of some of the diseases that have already been discussed, but there are several distinct endocardial lesions, especially those that primarily affect the cardiac valves, that deserve attention.

  a. Nonbacterial verrucous endocarditis **(Libman-Sacks disease)** is mitral and tricuspid valvulitis that is sometimes found in patients with disseminated lupus erythematosus.

    (1) The valvular connective tissues are affected by fibrinoid necrosis and subsequent fibrosis.

    (2) A frequent complication is the formation on the valve leaflet of flat, spreading vegetations. These may become infected secondarily to produce a bacterial endocarditis.

  b. Nonbacterial thrombotic endocarditis (marantic endocarditis) is characterized by fibrin and platelet vegetations on the mitral, aortic, and sometimes tricuspid valves. These lesions occur only on the valve surfaces that are exposed to the impact of the bloodstream.

    (1) Microscopically, these vegetations are small mounds of necrotic collagen fibers, serum proteins, fibrin, and platelets, with small ingrowths of capillary blood vessels but without appreciable inflammatory cells.

    (2) The pathogenesis is obscure, but these lesions may be clinically significant since they can be the source of peripheral emboli, leading to infarcts of such organs as the brain and kidneys. When marantic endocarditis is recognized, antibiotic therapy may be helpful to prevent the lesions from serving as sites for secondary bacterial infection.

  c. Bacterial endocarditis occurs when vegetations that are present on the heart valves are infected by bacteria. These vegetations may grow to a size sufficient to interfere with valve closure. In addition, the affected patient may have signs of septic emboli, which originated from the valve vegetation.

    (1) Acute and subacute forms of bacterial endocarditis are distinguished by the destructive ability of the causative organism. Some bacteria like staphylococci can produce extensive necrosis of the valves as well as abscesses in the myocardium and at sites of embolization. Less virulent organisms are less destructive but may not be detected as rapidly since symptoms and signs are delayed; this leads to the subacute designation.

    (2) Antibiotic therapy has been important in decreasing the incidence of this disease. If rapid diagnosis leads to prompt therapy, the degree of valvular damage can be minimized.

D. CONGENITAL HEART DISEASE results from the abnormal embryonic development of the heart and great vessels. This continues to be the most common form of cardiac disease encountered in young children.

  1. Acyanotic shunts (left-to-right) are the most common.

    a. Patent ductus arteriosus accounts for 15 percent to 20 percent of congenital heart anomalies. It may be encountered alone but often is associated with other congenital cardiac problems. The ductus connects the main or left pulmonary artery with the aorta in the fetus so that fetal blood bypasses the developing lungs while oxygenation occurs in the placenta. After birth, the lungs expand and decreasing amounts of blood pass through the ductus. Normally, functional closure and then anatomic closure occur in the ductus. If closure does not occur, a pressure gradient is established with blood flowing from the aorta into the pulmonary circulation, depriving the systemic circulation. Current therapy with drugs can facilitate closure in many instances so as to obviate the need for surgery.

    b. Atrial septal defects result from incomplete closure of either the ostium primum or ostium secundum to complete the separation of the two atria. The clinical consequences are largely determined by the volume of blood flow through the defects, which may lead to volume overload of the right side of the heart. This can result in right chamber enlargement, pulmonary hypertension, and dilatation of the pulmonary arteries. When pulmonary hypertension exceeds left-sided pressures, reversal of flow occurs with nonoxygenated blood now passing into the systemic circulation, causing eventual cyanosis. Surgical correction is required before irreversible pulmonary hypertension occurs.

   c. **Ventricular septal defects** are among the most common congenital heart anomalies and also occur in conjunction with other congenital anomalies. Again, the volume of the left-to-right shunt often determines prognosis. Large left-to-right shunts may cause death in infancy if they are not immediately corrected. Lesser shunts ultimately lead to right-sided heart failure with pulmonary hypertension and pulmonary artery system sclerosis. Vegetative endocarditis on the margins of the defect or at the site of bloodstream impact on the right ventricle can lead to septic emboli. Surgical closure is now common in childhood so that the prognosis is often excellent.

2. **Cyanotic shunts** (right-to-left) are less common statistically, but include some of the more complicated anomalies.

   a. **Tetralogy of Fallot.** If stenosis of the pulmonary artery infundibulum or valve area is severe or if pulmonary atresia is present, the child may survive only so long as the ductus remains patent. This permits blood flow from the aorta into the pulmonary circulation beyond the point of stenosis and thus allows the lungs to oxygenate the blood. The prognosis for these children is poor unless surgical correction is possible. The tetralogy of Fallot has four components.

      (1) A ventricular septal defect

      (2) Dextroposition of the aorta so as to override the septal defect, causing the aorta to receive blood from both ventricular chambers

      (3) Stenosis of the pulmonary artery infundibulum

      (4) Hypertrophy of the right ventricle

   b. **Eisenmenger's complex** is a congenital cardiac anomaly in which a ventricular septal defect is present in combination with pulmonary hypertension. This is a less common congenital cardiac anomaly than the tetralogy of Fallot and may have a slightly better prognosis since pulmonary artery flow may be adequate. However, cyanosis is seen because the left ventricle outflow tract receives unoxygenated blood from the right ventricle through the ventricular septal defect. Surgical correction is required to avoid eventual right-sided heart failure and bacterial endocarditis as may be found in tetralogy of Fallot.

   c. **Transposition of the great vessels** is present when the aorta develops in the anterior position that normally is occupied by the main pulmonary artery.

      (1) In the so-called corrected transposition, the aorta receives blood from a right-sided arterial ventricle while the pulmonary artery gets blood from the now left-sided venous ventricle. In effect, the ventricles have exchanged positions and each has a mirror-image proper valve. This is compatible with life unless other complications of ventricular septal defects or a patent ductus cause functional cardiac flow problems.

      (2) In **uncorrected transpositions**, the reversed aorta and main pulmonary artery receive blood from normally placed venous (right) and systemic (left) ventricles. This arrangement precludes survival unless septal defects, a patent ductus, or additional shunts provide sufficient cross-over circulation.

3. Other congenital anomalies are without circulation shunts but produce blood flow problems significant enough to require attention.

   a. **Coarctation of the aorta** is a discrete narrowing of the distal segment of the aortic arch.

      (1) **Infantile coarctation** may occur to the point of obliteration of the lumen. Since this occurs proximal to the insertion of the ductus arteriosus, a patent ductus may allow sufficient blood flow into the arterial side of the circulation until surgical correction can be achieved.

      (2) The **adult form of coarctation** is narrowing of the aorta distal to the ductus arteriosus. This narrowing is not so severe and usually involves a shorter segment of the aorta. The ductus arteriosus typically is closed; the point of maximal aortic constriction may appear as a ring or even as an incomplete membrane. When this constriction is sufficient to cause symptoms, they are symptoms of relative hypertension proximal to the obstruction (usually in the carotids and subclavian artery) with relative hypotension of the lower extremities.

   b. **Aortic stenosis** can present in three forms, all of which cause functional obstruction of left ventricular outflow.

      (1) **Aortic valvular stenosis** is the most common form. There is usually only one com-

missure in the aortic valve. This may cause left ventricular hypertrophy with left ventricular decompensation in infancy, or it may be silent until adult life, when dystrophic calcification following fibrosis leads to rigidity of the valve.

   (2) Subaortic valve stenosis and supravalvular aortic stenosis are the two other forms that cause functional obstruction. Poststenotic dilation of the aorta and coarctation are the common associated conditions.

E. MISCELLANEOUS CARDIAC DISEASES include a large number of conditions that are typically described according to the anatomic portion of the heart that is affected. The lesions reviewed here are the neoplastic diseases of the heart.

  1. Primary cardiac tumors arise from the cells that make up the various tissues of which the heart is composed.

   a. Primary pericardial tumors may arise from all of the tissues of the pericardium; and there are reports of fibromas, lipomas, angiomas, leiomyomas, mesotheliomas, and sarcomas of the pericardium.

   b. Primary intracardiac tumors are clinically more significant and can occur in both benign and malignant forms. The malignant cardiac tumors are usually sarcomas of the spindle cell type: fibrosarcomas, myxosarcomas, and leiomyosarcomas.

      (1) Myxoma is the most common primary cardiac tumor; it usually arises from the mural endocardium of the atria. Nearly 75 percent are found in the left atrium and may cause functional disturbances of blood flow and interfere with mitral valve function.

      (2) Rhabdomyomas grow within the myocardium but may reach a size sufficient to bulge into a chamber lumen. They usually occur in infants, often in association with tuberous sclerosis of the central nervous system.

  2. A variety of **metastatic tumors** occur in the pericardium and heart and are chiefly problems when the metastases interfere with the cardiac conduction system or when metastases cause pericardial effusions that compromise function.

STUDY QUESTIONS

Directions: Each question below contains five suggested answers. Choose the **one best** response to each question.

1. Which of the following coronary arteries supplies blood to the posterior portion of the interventricular septum?

(A) Left main coronary artery
(B) Left anterior descending coronary artery
(C) Circumflex coronary artery
(D) Proximal marginal coronary artery
(E) Right coronary artery

2. The classic lesion of rheumatic heart disease is

(A) Mallory's body
(B) Aschoff body
(C) psammoma body
(D) Negri body
(E) Anitschkow's myocyte

3. Of the following types of cardiac inflammation, which best describes that ongoing in rheumatic heart disease?

(A) Endocarditis
(B) Myocarditis
(C) Pericarditis
(D) Pancarditis
(E) Vasculitis

4. "Cor bovinum" is a Latin term that describes the appearance of a heart affected by which of the following heart diseases?

(A) Rheumatic
(B) Hypertensive
(C) Syphilitic
(D) Ischemic
(E) Atherosclerotic

5. The most common cause of myocarditis in the United States is

(A) Chagas' disease
(B) echinococcal infection
(C) trichinosis
(D) viral infection
(E) streptococcal infection

6. A patient who suffers from dizziness, occasional dyspnea, and intermittent claudication of the legs when running most likely has which of the following congenital abnormalities?

(A) Tetralogy of Fallot
(B) Coarctation of the aorta
(C) Eisenmenger's complex
(D) Ventricular septal defect
(E) Atrial septal defect

Directions: Each question below contains four suggested answers of which **one or more** is correct. Choose the answer

A   if **1, 2, and 3** are correct
B   if **1 and 3** are correct
C   if **2 and 4** are correct
D   if **4** is correct
E   if **1, 2, 3, and 4** are correct

7. Histologic signs that are produced by ischemic heart disease alone include

(1) diffuse myocardial fibrosis
(2) fibrocalcific change in valves
(3) perivascular fibrosis
(4) fibroelastosis

8. Complications of myocardial infarction include

(1) fibrinous pericarditis
(2) aortic aneurysms
(3) mural thrombi
(4) coronary atherosclerosis

9. Ventricular aneurysm formation following myocardial infarction may lead to

(1) enlarged cardiac silhouette on chest x-ray
(2) blood in the urine
(3) mural thrombi formation
(4) hemorrhagic pneumonia

10. Secondary hypertension may be related to conditions in which of the following organ systems?

(1) Central nervous
(2) Reproductive
(3) Urinary tract
(4) Intestinal tract

11. Anatomic anomalies that are associated with the tetralogy of Fallot include

(1) dextroposition of the aorta
(2) ventricular septal defect
(3) right ventricular hypertrophy
(4) pulmonary artery stenosis

ANSWERS AND EXPLANATIONS

1. The answer is E. (*I B 4*) In most individuals, the right coronary artery arises from the right aortic sinus and passes along the coronary sulcus onto the diaphragmatic surface of the heart ventricles. From the base of the ventricles to the cardiac apex, the right coronary artery is known as the posterior interventricular branch. Penetrating intraseptal branches usually supply the posterior part of the intraventricular septum. The anterior part of the intraventricular septum receives its blood supply from penetrating branches of the left anterior descending coronary artery.

2. The answer is B. (*II C 1 d*) Rheumatic pancarditis is classically identified histologically by the presence of myocardial Aschoff bodies. These lesions are a type of granuloma that shows fibrinoid degeneration of myocardial elements with a mononuclear cell infiltrate—Aschoff giant cells and Anitschkow's myocytes. These are large cells with one or more nuclei clumped together containing chromatin, giving an "owl's eye" appearance. There is still controversy as to whether Anitschkow's cells are really transformed muscle cells or are cells originating from a nonmyocyte progenitor.

3. The answer is D. (*II C 1*) Rheumatic heart disease can involve all layers of the heart—the endocardium, myocardium, and pericardium—thus it is pancarditic. It is a rather unusual inflammation with classic cardiac lesions and little effect on other organs.

4. The answer is C. (*II C 2*) Syphilitic carditis occurs as a consequence of the spread of the causative spirochetes from mediastinal lymph nodes into the adventitia of the aorta. Dilatation and scarring of the aortic valve ring leads to aortic insufficiency; in an attempt to compensate for this, the left ventricle hypertrophies to sometimes massive proportions. The very large heart that results is often nearly the size of a cow's heart, which has led to the descriptive terminology of "cor bovinum."

5. The answer is D. (*II C 3*) Myocarditis is a nonspecific term that refers to inflammation of the myocardium regardless of etiology. The frequency of infection by each specific etiologic agent varies with the population studied, but in the United States, viral infection is responsible for the majority of cases of myocarditis.

6. The answer is B. (*II D 3*) Coarctation of the aorta is a discrete narrowing of the distal segment of the aortic arch, usually occurring because of a deformity of the aortic tunica media. The characteristic clinical feature of coarctation is the significant difference in systolic blood pressure between that of the upper and lower extremities. A large proportion of coarctation patients have mild to severe hypertension with its array of symptoms. Claudication occurs when there is insufficient lower extremity blood flow to meet the metabolic needs of the leg muscles.

7. The answer is A (1, 2, 3). [*II A 3 a (1) (a)*] When the blood supply to the heart muscle is not sufficient to meet cardiac metabolic needs, ischemic atrophy and diffuse myocardial fibrosis occur—often without causing any symptoms. The valves of the left side of the heart frequently and concurrently can undergo degenerative fibrocalcific change. This diffuse ischemic scarring of the myocardium is recognizable microscopically by perivascular fibrosis and increased fibrous connective tissue between myocardial fibers.

8. The answer is B (1, 3) [*II A 3 a (3) (c)*] Fibrinous pericarditis and mural thrombi may occur as complications of myocardial infarction. Coronary atherosclerosis is a proposed etiology of myocardial infarction; it is not a complication. Aortic aneurysms are not caused by myocardial infarction but are usually the result of various infectious diseases, connective tissue abnormalities, congenital defects, or atherosclerosis.

9. The answer is A (1, 2, 3). [*II A 3 a (3) (c) (vi)*] If the aneurysm-distorted ventricular segment forms one of the heart margins seen on x-ray, the silhouette may appear enlarged. Mural thrombi may form within an infarcted ventricle in areas of akinesis and dyskinesis produced by the infarct. Portions of these thrombi may break away to embolize the kidneys, causing small renal infarcts, which can cause back pain and hematuria.

10. The answer is A (1, 2, 3). (*II B 1 b*) Secondary hypertension results from a primary disease of an organ or tissue, which in turn affects the systemic blood pressure. Increased intracranial pressure from a variety of causes, pregnancy complicated by eclampsia, and diseases of the kidneys all can cause secondary hypertension.

11. The answer is E (all). (*II D 2 a*) The tetralogy of Fallot is characterized by four congenital cardiac defects, which include an aortic root overriding a large ventricular septal defect, right ventricular hypertrophy, and anatomic obstruction of pulmonary flow.

5

The Vascular System

I. INTRODUCTION

A. The vascular system is composed of arteries, veins, and lymphatic vessels.

B. The conditions affecting these structures include arteriosclerosis, arteritis, aneurysms, thrombophlebitis, varicosity, various causes of primary and secondary lymphedema, and neoplasia.

II. THE ARTERIES

A. NORMAL STRUCTURE. Anatomic and histologic division of the arteries is important because each class of artery tends to have its own array of lesions.

1. Large elastic arteries include the aorta and its major branches. Histologic composition is defined by the three tunica.
   a. The **tunica intima** is made up of endothelial cells, myoepithelial cells, collagen, and longitudinally arranged elastic fibers forming a felt-like support layer.
   b. The **tunica media** is the muscular layer containing elastic fibers interspersed with fibrous connective tissues. The external limit is defined by the condensed layer of elastin fibers that form the external elastic membrane.
   c. The outermost **tunica adventitia** is a poorly defined connective tissue layer containing nerve fibers and the small, thin-walled vasa vasorum, which supply blood to the artery.

2. Muscular arteries are medium-sized vessels that distribute blood to specific organ systems. Like the large elastic arteries, they contain three histologic layers.
   a. The inner layer, the **tunica intima,** is more clearly defined than in large elastic arteries by a compact internal elastic membrane. Increased amounts of elastic tissue often reflect the abnormal stress of hypertension.
   b. The **tunica media** contains prominent smooth muscle cells arranged in concentric layers.
   c. The **tunica adventitia** contains more neural innervation than in the large arteries, reflecting the role of the muscular arteries in autonomic regulation of blood flow.

3. Small arteries, usually less than 2 mm in diameter, are defined histologically by the progressive loss of first the external elastic membrane and then the internal elastic membrane. These small arteries and the still smaller arterioles are located predominantly within organs and tissues.

4. Arterioles are richly supplied by the autonomic nervous system and thus constitute the major focus for autonomic control of blood flow.

B. ARTERIOSCLEROSIS is the generic term for three different patterns of arterial disease that produce narrowing of the lumina, thickening of arterial walls, and loss of elasticity.

1. Atherosclerosis is characterized by the formation of elevated plaques called atheromas in the intima. Atheromas narrow arterial channels, damage the underlying tunica media, and may progress to calcification, ulceration with thrombosis, and intraplaque hemorrhage.
   a. Epidemiology. Atherosclerosis is common in North America, Europe, and Russia and may be related to diet and other aspects of the cultures. The incidence is higher in men than in women and increases with advancing age and in the presence of hypercholesterolemia, hypertension, cigarette smoking, and diabetes mellitus.
   b. The **pathogenesis** of atherosclerosis still is not completely known.

(1) Two classic theories existed—the lipid infiltration or insudation explanation and the encrustation or thrombogenic hypothesis.

    (a) The lipid infiltration theory postulated that lipid accumulation in the intima was the result of either increased influx or decreased catabolism of serum lipoproteins.

    (b) The thrombogenic explanation saw atherosclerosis as the end product of multiple repeated episodes of intramural thrombosis with subsequent organization of the thrombi producing atheromas.

(2) The current **injury and repair** hypothesis invokes three essential steps in the formation of atheromas.

    (a) Proliferation of smooth muscle cells in the intima

    (b) Formation of excessive amounts of connective tissue matrix (collagen, elastic fiber proteins, and proteoglycans) by smooth muscle cells

    (c) Deposition of intracellular and extracellular lipid that results in the formation of a pool of lipid and cell debris within the plaque

c. The **clinical presentation** of atherosclerosis is most often reflected in ischemic injury of the organs that are supplied by the diseased arteries, in embolic injuries resulting from the "downstream" flow of components of an atheroma, or by local compromise of the circumferential strength of an artery, resulting in aneurysm formation.

d. Gross Pathology and Histology. Fatty streaks and atheromas are the two classic lesions. Controversy still exists regarding which is the primary lesion.

(1) Fatty streaks are slightly elevated, poorly demarcated, yellow intimal lesions, which are usually localized to the thoracic aorta and coronary arteries. Microscopically, fatty streaks are composed of lipid-containing cells, some extracellular lipid pools, and variable amounts of collagen, elastic fibers, and proteoglycans.

(2) Atheromas are elevated, fibrous, fibromuscular, or fibrofatty intimal plaques in varying shades of white-yellow coloration that are found in the abdominal aorta, coronary arteries, lower thoracic aorta, carotid arteries, and circle of Willis. Atheromas have a tendency to occur at points of arterial branching and around ostia of primary branches of the aorta. Microscopically, atheromas are composed of smooth muscle cells, connective tissue fibers and matrix, and lipid deposits; the three components are present in varying proportions depending upon the age of the atheroma.

(3) Complicated plaques are produced when atheromas undergo calcification, ulceration, superficial thrombosis, or intraplaque hemorrhage. These processes may cause either total occlusion in the smaller coronary and cerebral arteries or aneurysms, particularly in the aorta, when there is sufficient damage to the tunica media.

2. Mönckeberg's medial sclerosis, the second, much less common, histologic pattern of arteriosclerosis, is characterized by band-like calcifications within the tunica media of medium and small muscular arteries. Medial sclerosis and atherosclerosis may occur together in the same individual and even in the same artery, but these two disease processes are thought to be distinct entities.

a. Epidemiology. Medial sclerosis shows no sex predilection and is rare before the fifth decade of life.

b. The lesion of medial sclerosis is **circumferential calcification** of the tunica media with no associated inflammatory response. The endothelium remains intact, and the lesions of the tunica media do not encroach on the lumen of affected arteries to cause obstruction of blood flow. The lesions of medial calcific necrosis occasionally undergo ossification so that bone and bone marrow may be found within the arterial wall.

3. Arteriolosclerosis, the third form of arteriosclerosis, is characterized by proliferative fibromuscular and endothelial thickening of the walls of small arteries and arterioles. Two descriptive subtypes are encountered: hyaline arteriolosclerosis and hyperplastic arteriolosclerosis.

a. The **epidemiology** of both forms of arteriolosclerosis shows a relationship with hypertension.

(1) Hyaline arteriolosclerosis commonly affects older patients who have long-standing, mild-to-moderate hypertension. These patients have manifestations of prolonged hypertension, such as heart disease. Hyaline arteriolosclerosis also is found in diabetic patients who are normotensive.

(2) Hyperplastic arteriolosclerosis occurs in patients who have malignant hypertension, which may appear de novo or be superimposed upon preexisting mild or moderate hypertension. The clinical presentation of these patients usually is referable to cardiac decompensation or central nervous system disturbances. Rarely, patients with malignant hypertension will present in oliguric acute renal failure.

b. Hyaline arteriolosclerosis appears as a homogeneous, pink (when stained with hematoxylin and eosin), acellular thickening of the walls of arterioles with an apparent loss of structural detail and narrowing of the lumen. The result is decreased blood flow to the downstream tissues. This process is best seen in the kidneys; hyaline arteriolosclerosis is a major morphologic characteristic of nephrosclerosis, which produces symmetrically contracted fibrotic kidneys as the result of renal ischemia.

  c. **Hyperplastic arteriolosclerosis** appears as an onion-like concentric laminated thickening of arteriolar walls with resultant narrowing of the lumen. Frequently, these hyperplastic changes are accompanied by fibrinoid deposits and necrosis of the wall of the arterioles; this is termed **necrotizing arteriolitis.**

C. **ARTERITIS** refers to a variety of inflammatory or immunologic diseases that are primary lesions of the arteries. Focal inflammation of an artery due to spread of a contiguous inflammation, such as occurs in an abscess, is not considered an arteritis. Arteritis includes a number of entities, each with incompletely understood pathogenic mechanisms. The more common forms are briefly described below.

  1. The **polyarteritis nodosa** group of systemic necrotizing vasculitides has a widespread distribution of arterial lesions with involvement of multiple organ systems and signs of widespread ischemic tissue injury. These lesions often result in the formation of microaneurysms in affected vessels. The common thread among the polyarteritis nodosa group is the presence of necrotizing lesions of medium-sized and small muscular arteries.

  2. **Giant cell arteritides** include temporal arteritis and Takayasu's arteritis. The inflammatory lesion in both diseases usually contains multinucleated giant cells. However, the presence of giant cells is not required for either histologic diagnosis.
     a. **Temporal arteritis** usually involves branches of the carotid artery, particularly the temporal, hence its name, but the disease can be systemic and may affect any medium or large artery.
        (1) Temporal arteritis occurs most frequently in elderly women. The **symptoms** are variable and depend upon the site of arterial involvement; sometimes the only complaints are weakness, malaise, low-grade fever, and weight loss. More specific symptoms include headache with pain radiating to the neck, jaws, or tongue; and intermittent claudication of the jaw is quite characteristic. The scalp may be exquisitely sensitive to pressure, and, if the ophthalmic artery is involved, visual disturbances occur.
        (2) **Microscopically**, one sees partial destruction of the artery wall by an infiltrate of inflammatory cells including multinucleated giant cells of both the Langhans' type (peripheral nuclear necklace) and foreign body type (random distribution of nuclei). Phagocytic cells may contain fragments of the disrupted internal elastic lamina. These lesions are often segmental so that "skip areas" are present and can lead to false-negative temporal artery biopsies.
     b. **Takayasu's arteritis** is sometimes called pulseless disease because of the weakness of the pulse in the upper extremities of affected patients.
        (1) This process produces a pronounced irregular thickening of the wall of the aortic arch, the proximal segments of the great vessels, or both. In nearly half the cases, the main pulmonary artery also is involved. No particular age or sex predominance is known.
        (2) **Microscopic examination** shows an early mononuclear cell infiltrate surrounding the vasa vasorum in the tunica adventitia. This is followed by a diffuse polymorphonuclear leukocyte infiltration of and subsequent mononuclear cell influx into the tunica media. As in temporal arteritis, giant cells of both types have been seen. Temporal arteritis appears to begin in the tunica media, however, while Takayasu's arteritis seems to appear first at the junction of the adventitia and media.

  3. **Thromboangiitis obliterans (Buerger's disease)** is a recurrent inflammatory disorder of arteries that is characterized by thrombosis of medium-sized vessels, especially the radial and tibial arteries. Although the arteries are the primary sites of inflammation, adjacent veins and nerves can become involved.
     a. Thromboangiitis obliterans occurs almost exclusively in cigarette smokers and is prevalent in men between the ages of 25 and 50 years. It is extremely rare in nonsmoking men or in women, although as more women smoke cigarettes, this pattern may change. The etiology and pathogenesis are unknown.
     b. Affected patients may initially present with recurrent episodes of patchy thrombophlebitis of superficial veins. Once the actual arterial lesion develops, these patients usually complain of pain in the affected extremity brought on at first by exercise and eventually present even at rest. Ischemia may cause tissue ulcerations and gangrene. Because individual thrombi can recanalize, the symptoms can abate until a new thrombus forms and ischemia returns.
     c. **Histologically,** the involved arterial segment is occluded by a thrombus with varying degrees of organization, recanalization, or both. The thrombus contains microabscesses. A

nonspecific inflammatory infiltrate is found at first in the adjacent arterial wall, but, as the disease process advances, both inflammation and subsequent fibrosis extend through the tunica adventitia to envelop adjacent veins and nerves. This fibrous encasement of artery, vein, and nerve is the histologic hallmark of thromboangiitis obliterans.

4. There are a number of other specific disorders that have a necrotizing vasculitis as a component. These include Wegener's granulomatosis, systemic lupus erythematosus, rheumatoid arthritis, hypersensitivity vasculitis, and allergic granulomatosis of Churg and Strauss. These will be discussed elsewhere because arterial lesions are not the primary findings in these diseases, and thus these disorders are not classified as arteritides.

D. ANEURYSMS are abnormal dilatations of either arteries or veins but will be discussed in this chapter only under arterial diseases because arterial aneurysms are much more common and clinically significant than venous aneurysms. Arterial aneurysms are classified both in terms of etiology and anatomic form.

1. **Functional** or **etiologic** groupings of aneurysms include several types.
   a. **Atherosclerotic aneurysms** are the most common type and usually are located in the abdominal aorta below the origin of the renal arteries. The common iliac arteries often are involved as well. The complex atheromas that form in these areas lead to destruction of the tunica media, allowing aneurysm formation. Mural thrombi are common. Atherosclerotic aneurysms may dissect or thrombose to occlude renal artery blood flow, blood flow to the lower extremities, or both.
   b. **Syphilitic aneurysms** are not as common as in the past because of the decreased incidence of tertiary syphilis in today's population.
      (1) The **clinical** presentation of patients with syphilitic aneurysms is varied but can include respiratory difficulty because of compression of lungs, major bronchi, or both, dysphagia secondary to compression of the esophagus, persistent cough if there is pressure on the recurrent laryngeal nerve, possible bone pain caused by pressure erosion of ribs, vertebral bodies, or both, and aortic valvular disease secondary to dilatation of the aortic valve ring.
      (2) Syphilitic aortitis nearly always is confined to ascending and transverse portions of the thoracic aorta. Secondary atherosclerotic change often is superimposed.
      (3) Advanced syphilis occludes the vasa vasorum of the aorta through a proliferative endarteritis, including perivascular cuffing by plasma cells and gumma formation. The resulting ischemic injury of the aortic wall permits aneurysmic dilatation, which may extend to involve the aortic valve ring and the ostia of the coronary arteries.
   c. **Dissecting aneurysms** from **idiopathic cystic medial necrosis** are caused by multifocal destruction of elastic and muscular components of the tunica media of the aorta. Hemorrhage within the medial layer can cause longitudinal dissection until external rupture occurs.
      (1) **Epidemiologic studies** suggest that hypertension may be a cause of dissecting aneurysms. Possible enzymatic defects in connective tissue metabolism also have been postulated as a cause. Medial necrosis is more common in patients with Marfan's syndrome than in the general population and has been experimentally produced in the condition known as lathyrism.
      (2) **Clinical Data.** Affected patients usually present only after aortic dissection has started with complaints of episodic chest pain similar to that experienced in myocardial infarctions. Sensory and motor functions of the lower body become abnormal when vertebral arteries are compromised; hematuria and renal failure occur when the renal arteries are obstructed; and myocardial infarction can follow obstruction of the coronary arteries.
      (3) Dissection usually begins in the ascending aorta and extends both toward the heart and distally along the aorta. Typically, the plane of hemorrhagic dissection separates the outer one-third of the tunica media from the inner two-thirds. If both proximal and distal intimal tears occur, a double-barreled aorta is formed; but usually rupture is to the outside of the aorta, with subsequent hemorrhage.
      (4) **Histologic** examination of an affected aorta shows irregular clefts devoid of normal elastic tissue within the tunica media. There is no associated inflammatory process. These clefts contain metachromatic acid mucopolysaccharides, which can be identified using special staining techniques.
   d. **Cirsoid aneurysms** are aneurysmic arteriovenous fistulas in the form of a tangled mass of intercommunicating vessels. These aneurysms predispose to possible rupture with hemorrhage and can cause heart strain because of arterial-to-venous shunting of blood.

2. Aneurysms are classified according to anatomic form.
   a. **Saccular aneurysms** are balloon-like arterial dilatations in which the orifice may be small

compared to the diameter of the aneurysm. Because the blood is usually stagnant in these aneurysms, the lumen can contain a thrombus.

   b. Fusiform aneurysms are spindle-shaped dilatations of an artery; they need not be symmetric around the long axis of the affected artery. Fusiform aneurysms increase in size gradually to their maximum diameter and then taper back to the diameter of the normal portion of the artery. Thrombosis is variable.

   c. Cylindroid aneurysms are abrupt, cylindrical dilatations of an artery (Fig. 5-1). Again, symmetry and mural thrombosis are variable.

   d. Berry aneurysms are small saccular aneurysms, 0.5 cm to 2 cm in diameter, which resemble berries. They often are congenital and commonly are present in the smaller cerebral arteries, particularly in the circle of Willis.

III. THE VEINS

   A. NORMAL STRUCTURE. Veins are not as precisely characterized by size as are arteries.

   1. Histologic examination of veins shows relatively thin-walled vessels without the well-defined layers that are found in arteries. The tunica intima in veins is mainly an endothelial lining covering a scant layer of connective tissue. Only the largest veins have an internal elastic membrane or much supporting muscle and elastic tissue in the tunica media.

   2. Unlike the arteries, large veins, particularly those in the extremities, have **valves** formed by endothelial folds. These valves help to buttress the column of blood within the large veins, thereby reducing the hemodynamic load.

   3. Because there is so little normal supporting structure, veins are vulnerable to dilatation, compression, and easy penetration by neoplastic and inflammatory processes.

   B. THROMBOPHLEBITIS and **phlebothrombosis** both refer to thrombus formation within veins, which is the most significant clinical problem associated with the venous system.

   1. The most serious complication of venous thrombosis is **embolism** to the lungs. Occlusion of veins by thrombi also can cause tissue edema distal to the blockage, skin ulcerations, and additional venous thrombosis.

   2. Venous thrombi apparently can form in veins without endothelial damage initiating the event. Possible predisposing conditions include sluggish or static blood flow, so-called hypercoagulable states, and other poorly understood phenomena, such as the use of oral contraceptives.

   3. A majority of venous thrombi form in the deep veins of the legs, often in approximation to valves. The proposed formation sequence includes blood stasis, blood coagulation, and then

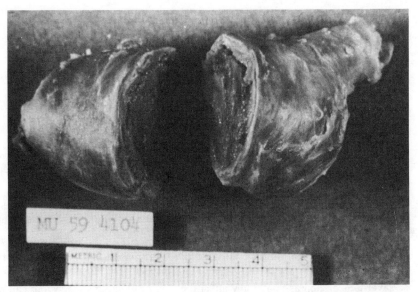

Figure 5-1. Cylindroid aneurysm of the femoral artery. Note the mural thrombosis.

thrombus formation. The outcome can be enzymatic dissolution, organization with recanalization, or detachment as thromboemboli.

C. **VARICOSE VEINS** are persistently dilated, tortuous veins, which are thought to result from chronically increased intraluminal pressure complicated by the loss of adequate structural support of the veins.

1. Superficial veins of the lower extremities are the most frequently involved, probably because of a high venous pressure resulting from upright posture and the relatively little support these veins receive from surrounding tissues. Elderly women with a positive family history are predisposed to varicose veins.

2. Special clinical problems occur with varicosities of the hemorrhoidal vein plexus at the anorectal junction and with esophageal varices, which can result from portal hypertension induced by cirrhosis of the liver. The typical pattern of increasing intraluminal venous pressure with resultant poor return blood flow leads to edema and congestion of distal tissues. Dystrophic tissue changes, stasis dermatitis, skin ulceration, and cellulitis may result.

3. Varicose veins have nodular or fusiform distentions and outpouchings with variable wall thickness. Valvular deformities and intraluminal thrombi are common. Adjacent zones along the vein may have a compensatory wall hypertrophy with increased smooth muscle content and subintimal fibrosis. In larger veins, degeneration of the elastic tissue and focal calcifications **(phlebosclerosis)** are commonly found.

IV. THE LYMPHATICS

A. **NORMAL STRUCTURE.** The lymphatics are essentially endothelial-lined spaces or canals through which lymph flows. Only the major lymphatic ducts have a small amount of smooth muscle and valves formed by endothelial folding.

B. **PRIMARY DISORDERS** of lymphatics are extremely uncommon; all result in dilated lymphatics with increased intraluminal pressure and resultant increased interstitial fluid pressure. The increased pressure in turn leads to interstitial fibrosis, particularly of the subcutaneous tissues, and can predispose to ulceration and cellulitis. Three primary forms have been described.

1. **Simple congenital lymphedema** occurs as an isolated limb abnormality, presumably because normal lymphatics have failed to develop.

2. **Milroy's disease** or **heredofamilial lymphedema** is a similar defect, but its occurrence follows a familial inheritance pattern.

3. **Lymphedema praecox** does not manifest until the second or third decade of life, usually occurs in females, and can result in progressive massive edema of one or both lower extremities with eventual involvement of the trunk.

C. **SECONDARY DISORDERS** of lymphatics causing lymphedema are much more common than any of the primary forms. Again, cellulitis, interstitial fibrosis, skin changes, and incapacitation of affected limbs can occur. Various causes include the following.

1. Postinflammatory fibrosis of lymphatics following soft-tissue infections

2. Obstruction of lymphatics or lymph nodes by spread of metastatic tumors

3. Surgical disruption of lymphatics, particularly with excision of lymph node groups (e.g., radical mastectomy with axillary lymph node dissection)

4. Postirradiation fibrosis with lymphatic obstruction

5. Filariasis in which parasites enter through the skin, find their way to regional lymph nodes, and cause obstructive fibrosis of lymphatics and nodes, resulting in edema of the extremity—elephantiasis

V. TUMORS OF THE ARTERIES, VEINS, AND LYMPHATICS will be considered together because both the morphology and outcome of these tumors are often the same regardless of their exact origin.

A. **ANGIOMAS** are benign tumors composed of either cavernous spaces or serpentine, capillary-like channels containing blood or lymph.

1. **Cavernous angiomas** commonly affect the skin or mucosal surfaces but can occur in deep tissues. These lesions are generally red-blue, sponge-like tumors, which may be several cen-

timeters in diameter and which have sharply defined margins. Histologic examination shows cavernous spaces, lined by normal endothelium, that contain liquid blood, a thrombus, or both. **Lindau-von Hippel disease** is the syndrome of multiple cavernous hemangiomas involving the cerebellum, brain stem, eyes, pancreas, and liver.

2. **Cavernous lymphangiomas** (cystic hygromas) are masses of lymphatic channels containing clear lymph fluid. They are located usually in the neck or axilla and rarely in the retroperitoneum. Although benign, these tumors grow by budding and expand into surrounding tissues, making total surgical excision difficult.

3. **Capillary hemangiomas** are unencapsulated skeins of capillaries separated by scant amounts of connective tissue. These tumors can occur in any tissue or organ but are common in the skin and mucous membranes. Because these vascular mazes contain liquid or clotted blood, they can vary from bright red to dusky blue in color. Clinical problems occur only if traumatic ulceration of these lesions causes bleeding.

4. **Capillary lymphangiomas** are the very uncommon lymphatic counterparts of capillary hemangiomas. The two tumors are differentiated by the absence of blood cells in the capillary lymphangioma. Presumably, only lymph is present in the fluid-containing spaces of lymphangiomas.

B. **GLOMANGIOMAS** (glomus tumors) are benign tumors composed of vascular channels in a connective tissue stroma that is surrounded by nests of glomus cells. These tumors originate from a neuromyoarterial glomus, which is an arteriovenous shunt that is richly supplied with nerve fibers. The glomus body has a function in temperature regulation. The typical location for glomangiomas is in the subungual part of a digit, but others occur in soft tissues and in the stomach wall. Subungual glomus tumors are quite painful because of their rich nerve supply and frequent contact trauma, which causes exquisite pain.

C. **TELANGIECTASIAS** are abnormal dilatations of preexisting small vessels and should not be considered true neoplasms. Often the lesions consist of a small central dilated vessel surrounded by radiating fine capillaries, thus the term spider telangiectasia. These lesions are common during pregnancy and in patients with chronic liver disease. Telangiectasias may be caused by altered estrogen levels. The hereditary form of multiple aneurysmal telangiectases is called **Osler-Rendu-Weber disease.**

D. **ANGIOSARCOMAS.** Malignant neoplasms of vascular tissues are termed angiosarcomas when they arise from the endothelial cells of vessels. These tumors grow as freely anastomosing, communicating channels lined by atypical endothelial cells. (See the section on soft tissue tumors in Chapter 21 for a complete discussion of these tumors and those that arise from the smooth muscle or connective tissues of vessels.)

STUDY QUESTIONS

Directions: Each question below contains five suggested answers. Choose the **one best** response to each question.

1. Which of the following processes typically gives rise to syphilitic arterial aneurysms?

(A) Cystic medial necrosis
(B) Fatty streaks
(C) Circumferential calcification
(D) Endarteritis of the vasa vasorum
(E) Congenital absence of the tunica media

2. In Lindau-von Hippel disease, the multiple vascular lesions involving several organs are known as

(A) necrotizing arteriolitis
(B) giant cell arteritis
(C) thromboangiitis obliterans
(D) cavernous hemangiomas
(E) telangiectasias

3. What is the common histologic finding in the various clinical presentations of polyarteritis nodosa?

(A) Aneurysms of large elastic arteries
(B) Circumferential calcification of arteries
(C) Necrotizing lesions of muscular arteries
(D) Hyaline arteriolosclerosis
(E) Fibrofatty intimal arterial plaques

4. Thromboangiitis obliterans occurs predominantly in individuals with

(A) congenital cardiac atrial defects
(B) atherosclerotic heart disease
(C) diets high in saturated fats
(D) heavy cigarette habits
(E) low exercise tolerance

Directions: The question below contains four suggested answers of which **one or more** is correct. Choose the answer

A   if **1, 2, and 3** are correct
B   if **1 and 3** are correct
C   if **2 and 4** are correct
D   if **4** is correct
E   if **1, 2, 3, and 4** are correct

5. Signs and symptoms of temporal arteritis include

(1) headache
(2) intermittent claudication of the jaw muscles
(3) low-grade fever
(4) bitter taste sensation

Directions: The group of questions below consists of lettered choices followed by several numbered items. For each numbered item select the **one** lettered choice with which it is **most** closely associated. Each lettered choice may be used once, more than once, or not at all.

Questions 6–10

For each vascular layer described below, select the correct histologic name.

(A) Tunica intima
(B) Tunica media
(C) Tunica adventitia
(D) Internal elastic membrane
(E) External elastic membrane

6. The layer in large elastic arteries that contains the bulk of the smooth muscle fibers

7. The arterial layer that contains the vasa vasorum

8. The arterial layer classically damaged in Mönckeberg's sclerosis

9. The arterial layer that shows the earliest signs of atherosclerosis

10. The venous layer that forms the valves in peripheral veins

ANSWERS AND EXPLANATIONS

1. The answer is D. (*II D 1 b*) Advanced syphilis may cause aortitis with aneurysm formation in the ascending and transverse parts of the thoracic aorta. Syphilitic aneurysms form because of loss of structural integrity of a part of the aorta due to ischemic injury. The ischemic injury is caused by the occlusion of the vasa vasorum supplying the aorta as the result of the proliferative endarteritis produced by the syphilitic infection.

2. The answer is D. (*V A 1*) Cavernous angiomas or hemangiomas are benign blood vessel tumors made up of cavernous vascular spaces and serpentine channels. If these lesions contain blood, they can appear as red-blue sponge-like tumors in various organs. In Lindau-von Hippel disease, patients have a large number of these lesions in multiple organs, especially the cerebellum, brain stem, eyes, pancreas, and liver.

3. The answer is C. (*II C 1*) Arteritis is a nonspecific term referring to any primary inflammatory lesion of the arteries. Polyarteritis nodosa is a subgroup of the arteritides, characterized by necrotizing lesions and microaneurysm formation in multiple small- and medium-sized muscular arteries. These lesions can involve arteries in multiple organs, leading to a complicated clinical presentation.

4. The answer is D. (*II C 3*) Although the exact pathogenesis of thromboangiitis obliterans (Buerger's disease) is unclear, the association with heavy cigarette smoking is inescapable. The disease occurs much more frequently in men than in women, and the onset of symptoms is typically before the age of 35 years. At least one study has shown that these patients may be hypersensitive to tobacco components.

5. The answer is A (1, 2, 3). (*II C 2*) As a specific clinical entity, temporal arteritis derives its name from its typical involvement of carotid artery branches, in particular, the temporal artery. The symptoms and signs depend upon which vessels are affected, but headache and intermittent claudication of the jaw muscles are often reported. Low-grade fever is not necessarily a manifestation of involvement of a particular artery, but perhaps is a reflection of the inflammatory disease process.

6–10. The answers are 6-B, 7-C, 8-B, 9-A, 10-A. (*II A 1, 2; II A 1 c; II B 2; II B 1; III A 1*) The tunica media in both large elastic arteries and medium-sized muscular arteries contains most of the smooth muscle fibers found in the arterial wall. These smooth muscle fibers are arranged in concentric layers. The tunica media is not exclusively smooth muscle, however; it also has elastic fibers and fibrous connective tissue elements.

The tunica adventitia is the outermost connective tissue layer of the large arteries and contains not only the vasa vasorum but also nerve fibers. The vasa vasorum are the small nutrient blood vessels that perfuse the thick walls of the larger arteries.

Mönckeberg's medial sclerosis is a type of arteriosclerosis that classically produces lesions in the tunica media of the muscular arteries. The lesions of Mönckeberg's sclerosis are band-like calcifications that involve the entire circumference of the artery. These lesions are often complicated by atherosclerotic lesions since the two diseases can occur together.

Although there are several lesions seen in atherosclerosis, the primary damage seems to be inflicted upon the tunica intima. Fatty streaks, atheromas, and the complicated plaques all primarily involve the tunica intima.

Although veins are without the precisely defined layers that are seen in the larger arteries, they do have internal structure. The largest veins can have an internal elastic membrane and some smooth muscle and elastic tissue in a tunica media. Infoldings of the tunica intima form valves within the lumens of the larger veins to aid in supporting unidirectional blood flow in these vessels.

6
The Lung

I. GENERAL CONSIDERATIONS

A. PULMONARY ANATOMY

1. The basic (terminal) respiratory unit is called an **acinus**. The terminal bronchi extend into respiratory bronchioles, which blend into alveolar ducts. Pulmonary lobules consist of several terminal bronchioles; each is connected to an acinus.

2. **Connective tissue** separates multiple lobules into compartments.

3. The **alveolar septa** are well structured, which allows gas exchange, and are composed of a thin lining of type I alveolar cells, a central basement membrane, and inner endothelial cell cytoplasm.

B. FUNCTION OF PULMONARY ACINAR CELLS

1. **Type I pneumonocytes** are the basic alveolar lining cells. They are flat in configuration, the nucleus is longitudinal, and the cytoplasm is thin and extends around the entire surface of the alveolus and adjoins adjacent type I cells. This thinness is optimal for gas diffusion and exchange.

2. **Type II pneumonocytes** are rounder in configuration than type I with large central, somewhat circular nuclei; ultrastructurally they have cytoplasmic extensions (microvilli) and contain osmiophilic lamellated bodies, which produce a granular appearance by light microscopy. These cells have an important synthetic function in that they make pulmonary surfactant and further serve as repair cells after alveolar membrane damage. **Pores of Kohn** are minute openings in the alveolar septae of adult lungs through which alveolar macrophages pass from one alveolar space to adjacent spaces.

3. **Alveolar macrophages** belong to the monocyte-phagocyte system and are derived from peripheral blood monocytes. They are recognized instantly by carbon particles and foreign material, which have been phagocytosed, in their cytoplasm. Alveolar macrophages have an antibody and immunity role in addition to their phagocytic properties (see Chapter 1, "Inflammation and Thrombosis"). Diffuse alveolar injury is reflected by proliferation of alveolar macrophages and type II pneumonocytes.

4. **Endothelial cells** of the alveolar septal capillary are involved in the metabolism of bradykinin, serotonin, acetylcholine, norepinephrine, and angiotensin I.

5. Bronchi and bronchioles are lined by **ciliated columnar epithelium** with intervening goblet cells, which moisten the inspired air and have a mechanical ciliary function in moving particles toward the larger airways. All types of injury to the ciliated columnar epithelium result in reversible squamous metaplasia. The ciliary function of respiratory epithelium may be compromised by viral infections and by inhalation of tobacco and toxins.

6. **Clara cells** are lining cells of bronchioles and have no cilia but have numerous electron-dense core granules. They are thought to be involved in the synthesis of lipoproteins.

II. PULMONARY BLOOD SUPPLY

A. SOURCE AND FUNCTION. Blood supply to the lungs has a dual source. One arises from the pulmonary artery, which emanates from the pulmonary outflow tract of the right ventricle; the second is from the bronchial arteries emanating from the aorta. This dual blood supply has a limited protective effect in the event of occlusion of one source. The bronchial arterial circulation delivers oxygenated blood while the pulmonary arterial system is returning hypo-oxygenated venous blood to the lungs.

B. VASCULAR DISORDERS OF THE LUNG

1. **Pulmonary hypertension** is morphologically represented by intimal proliferation, medial hypertrophy, and arterial sclerosis of the pulmonary vascular bed. Macroscopically, yellow linear intimal streaks are seen in the endothelial surfaces. If long-standing, this condition leads to right ventricular heart failure (cor pulmonale) and venous thromboses. The disorder is divided into primary and secondary forms.

   a. The **primary or idiopathic form** is found in young women and is rapidly fatal.

   b. The **secondary form** arises as a sequela to disorders that alter the intraluminal pulmonary pressure, volume, or flow, such as congenital heart disease (pulmonary stenosis, interventricular septal defects, and atrial septal defects), pulmonary arterial thromboemboli, left ventricular heart failure, aortic valve disease, chronic pulmonary diseases, such as chronic bronchitis and primary emphysema, pneumoconiosis, idiopathic interstitial fibrosis, sarcoidosis, tuberculosis, and vascular disorders, such as systemic polyarteritis nodosa and Wegener's granulomatosis. All of these conditions produce a vascular sclerosis of the pulmonary bed, with increased pulmonary artery pressures (as measured by wedge pressure) and eventual development of cor pulmonale.

   c. Recurrent and multiple **small pulmonary emboli** also lead to pulmonary hypertension because atheromas may develop over areas of clot organization.

2. **Pulmonary Infarction and Thromboembolism.**

   a. **Occlusion of pulmonary arteries** by in situ thrombosis or more commonly by embolism from sites such as pelvic and lower extremity veins may produce pulmonary parenchymal infarction. This is most often seen where clinical conditions exist that compromise the venous system, such as congestive heart failure, states of vascular insufficiency (shock), septicemia, inanition related to malignancy, and nonambulation and bed confinement.

   b. **Pulmonary thromboembolism** is a major cause of sudden death in hospitalized patients, especially if it involves the large pulmonary artery near its origin from the right ventricle (this is known as a saddle embolus). Important causes of this condition include fractures of long bones, age (elderly) of the patient, morbid obesity, and states leading to deep vein thrombosis of the lower extremities.

3. **Pulmonary Congestion and Edema.**

   a. Major causes of congestion and edema of proteinaceous fluid in the alveolar sacs include congestive heart failure with failure of the left ventricle, which results in increased pulmonary capillary pressure. There is consequent accumulation of fluid from regurgitation into the pulmonary capillary interstitial bed. Other conditions leading to volume overload, such as massive intravenous infusions of saline, especially if accompanied by a low level of plasma protein, will also result in pulmonary edema. Intra-alveolar edema fluid does not accumulate until the lymphatic drainage capacity is exceeded. Chronic pulmonary congestion, as occurs in mitral stenosis, is reflected by numerous hemosiderin-laden macrophages. Pulmonary edema may also result from any condition that increases alveolar capillary permeability, such as pneumonia, chemical agents, and toxic gases and fumes.

   b. A model of acute alveolar injury, with pulmonary edema and respiratory failure, is acute **adult respiratory distress syndrome (ARDS).** This syndrome is recognized in many situations where poor vascular perfusion of the lungs exists, such as in postoperative surgical patients and with septicemia, pancreatitis, from severe thermal burns, severe pulmonary infections, oxygen toxicity, alveolar damage by inhalation of chemical irritants, drug overdoses, anaphylactic and hypersensitivity reactions, and major tissue trauma other than that to the thorax. Important in the pathogenesis is hypoperfusion of the distal pulmonary microvasculature. There is direct pulmonary vascular endothelial damage, often accompanied by platelet microthrombi with sludging of capillary red blood cells and sequestration of neutrophils, resulting in pulmonary microvascular constriction from platelet-derived serotonin, physiologic shunting of blood away from atelectatic areas, and local tissue acidosis. Morphologically, there is alveolar wall damage, pulmonary edema, hyaline membrane formation, and proliferative type II pneumonocytes. Common to many of the above conditions is the use of high concentrations of oxygen as supportive therapy. Oxygen-derived free radicals (superoxide and hydroxyl ions) may cause necrosis of alveolar epithelium by affecting the cell membrane lipids. There is focal atelectasis and alveolar collapse because of altered surface tension. The ultimate cause of the syndrome is, however, unknown.

4. **Pulmonary veno-occlusive disease** occurs predominantly in children below the age of 15

years, but it may involve adults as well. Clinical signs include severe pulmonary hypertension, accompanied by right ventricular hypertrophy and enlarged central pulmonary arteries. There is congestion, edema, interstitial fibrosis, hemosiderosis, and arterial hypertensive changes with lymphatic dilatation. There are thromboses in small veins, with or without recanalization.

5. Pulmonary vasculitis exists in Wegener's granulomatosis and polyarteritis nodosa.

III. CONGENITAL PULMONARY ABNORMALITIES

A. **CONGENITAL LOBAR EMPHYSEMA AND PULMONARY SEQUESTRATIONS.** Congenital lobar emphysema occurs in infants and young children and is due to bronchial obstruction because of either a congenital absence of or hypoplasia of bronchial mucosa. Hyperinflation of one lobe occurs during the expiratory phase due to bronchial collapse. Extralobar sequestrated lung occurs as isolated lung tissue with alveoli and bronchi behind the lung proper and in or below the diaphragm. Blood supply is aberrant from the aorta or subclavian, intercostal, or diaphragmatic arteries.

B. **CONGENITAL ADENOMATOID MALFORMATION** is frequently associated with hydrops and polyhydramnios, respiratory distress of the newborn, and recurrent infections in the older child. There are variable degrees of cystic change, which consists of microscopic tubular malformations lined by cuboidal epithelium and admixed broad bands of smooth muscle.

C. **BRONCHOGENIC CYSTS** occur singly or in multiples and may be associated with cysts of the pancreas, liver, and kidney.

D. **BRONCHOPULMONARY DYSPLASIA** is seen in the lungs of neonates and likely is organization of antecedent diffuse alveolar damage, such as occurs in oxygen toxicity. The nucleoprotein hyaline membrane lining the damaged alveolar surfaces resembles that seen in ARDS.

IV. INFLAMMATORY CONDITIONS OF THE LUNG

A. **ACUTE LARYNGOTRACHEITIS** mainly affects young children and is characterized by a hoarse, high-pitched cough and is caused by streptococcus, hemophilus, and certain viruses. The mucosa is hyperemic and edematous and may be covered by a fibrinous membrane. Hemophilus-induced epiglottitis-tracheitis in the pediatric patient may have a fulminating course with rapid death.

B. **BRONCHITIS** is inflammation at all levels of the bronchial tree.

1. **Acute bronchitis** is acute inflammation in the larger bronchi and is associated with irritant gas inhalation, complicated by bacteria such as *Staphylococcus aureus*, *Hemophilus* species, and *Streptococcus* species. Influenza viruses are also known etiologic agents. The pathologic spectrum includes an exudative infiltrate of neutrophils and fibrin, vascular congestion, and occasionally severe ulceration.

2. **Chronic bronchitis** is due to alterations in smaller airways, such as bronchioles, as well as in the larger bronchi. Cigarette smokers commonly have the changes associated with chronic bronchitis, including squamous metaplasia of the bronchial mucosa, submucosal edema, fibrosis, and varying amounts of lymphocytes. Some degree of intra-alveolar fibrosis (chronic obstructive pulmonary disease) often accompanies chronic bronchitis.

C. **EXTRINSIC (REAGINIC) AND INTRINSIC ASTHMA** are the result of hypersensitivity, which may be complicated by bacterial infections. In atopic, extrinsic asthma, levels of immunoglobulin E (IgE) are usually elevated. Hypersensitivity may be due to bacterial proteins, aspirin, or various organic and inorganic industrial-occupational materials. The bronchi have thickened walls with narrowed lumina and generally are filled with plugs of mucus in the acute attack. They undergo spasms, with edema of the bronchial wall and release of viscid mucus. The subepithelial basement membrane is markedly hyalinized, and goblet cells are accentuated. Bronchial smooth muscle is hypertrophic, and there may be infiltrations of eosinophils. Charcot-Leyden crystals and Curschmann's spirals are found within the sputum and emanate from the eosinophils. Intrinsic asthma differs from extrinsic asthma, which is triggered by an environmental allergen, through factors relating to an internal pathophysiologic derangement. While the pathophysiology of intrinsic asthma is more complex than that initiated by an inhaled allergen (mold), the pathologic derangements found in the lungs are similar to those associated with extrinsic asthma.

D. **INFECTIOUS PNEUMONIA** is inflammation of the lungs; it is characterized by early congestion, leukocyte infiltration, consolidation, and eventual resolution. The infection and inflammation may be complicated by other conditions of the lungs, such as passive congestive heart
failure, poor ventilation, as occurs in bedridden patients, and reduced vascular perfusion, as in
shock lung (ARDS). Pneumonitis may result from aspiration of gastric contents, such as occurs
with vomiting.

1. **Bacterial pneumonia** may secondarily complicate pulmonary damage due to other causes
such as trauma, hemorrhage, neoplastic obstruction of large bronchi, and pulmonary infarction and as a consequence of aspiration of gastric contents or chemical pneumonitis due to
toxic fume inhalation. If bacterial pneumonitis occurs as a primary event, it may involve one
lobe (as in pneumococcal pneumonia due to *Streptococcus pneumoniae*). This form of infection characteristically occurs in alcoholics or malnourished, debilitated individuals. In the
acute phase, the alveolar sacs are filled with an exudate of red cells, neutrophilic leukocytes,
and fibrin. The exudate is eventually removed by an ingress of macrophages and lymphocytes, with eventual resolution.

2. **Bronchopneumonia** consists of changes similar to those of bacterial pneumonia but involves
purulent bronchitis as well. It may be caused by *Staphylococcus, Pseudomonas, Klebsiella,
Proteus,* and other gram-negative coliform bacteria. Some of the latter organisms may be acquired within the hospital setting (a nosocomial infection). Bronchopneumonia, especially
that caused by pathogenic (coagulase-positive) staphylococci, may be complicated by
abscesses, empyema, pneumatocele, and pyopneumothorax.

3. **Interstitial pneumonia** is usually associated with the viral pneumonias, especially influenza.
Atelectasis may be present in the inner lobule while the septa become prominent and
edematous. The predominant inflammatory infiltrate is composed of lymphocytes, plasma
cells, and histiocytes, and it extends into the interstitium and the septum. Viruses directly attack the lower respiratory tract epithelium, which results in cell necrosis.
a. **Adenovirus** may cause necrotizing bronchitis and terminal bronchiolitis. Severe cases of
all types may be associated with the formation of hyaline membranes lining the alveoli.
b. Cytomegalovirus, herpesvirus, measles, pneumonitis, and respiratory syncytial virus are
especially important in pneumonitis in immunosuppressed patients.

4. **Primary atypical pneumonia** refers to interstitial inflammation with or without alveolar
hyaline membrane formation and is caused by mycoplasmas (pleuropneumonia-like
organisms). This form of pneumonitis is associated with a rising titer of red blood
cell–agglutinating antibodies, which react at 4° to 6° C (cold agglutinins). Very high titers (in
excess of 1:10,000) of circulating mycoplasma-associated cold agglutinins often correlate with
red cell clumping seen in microscopic examination of a blood smear.

E. **NONINFECTIOUS PNEUMONIAS** may be complicated by opportunistic, secondary invading
bacteria.

1. **Aspiration and chemical pneumonitis** occur secondary to aspiration of liquid vomitus or any
chemical irritant. Bloody sputum may result secondary to an acute tracheobronchitis with
edema and hyperemia of airways and eventual necrosis of the bronchial mucosa with consequent peribronchiolar hemorrhages. Other pathologic changes include pulmonary edema,
congestion, and acute infiltration of inflammatory cells, which becomes extensive. Complications include abscesses, bronchiectasis, and extensive necrosis.

2. **Lipid pneumonia** is due to the use of laxatives, nose drops, and mineral oil and results from
aspiration of small oil droplets, which produces peribronchial consolidation. Lipid-laden
macrophages are found within the alveolar spaces as are moderate inflammatory infiltrates.

3. **Hemorrhagic pneumonitis** is associated with interstitial pneumonitis as well as glomerulonephritis (Goodpasture's syndrome). Pathologically, there is acute necrotizing alveolitis with
marked hemorrhages.

4. **Eosinophilic pneumonia** may occur as a component of Löffler's syndrome, which is
characterized by marked peripheral blood eosinophilia and infiltration of the lungs by
eosinophils in addition to bronchopneumonia and variable degrees of pulmonary edema,
necrotizing arteritis, granuloma formation, and lymphoid interstitial inflammation. Other
causes of eosinophilic pneumonia are *Ascaris* infestations, hypersensitivity states, and
polyarteritis nodosa.

F. **SUPPURATIVE DISORDERS**

1. **Bronchiectasis** refers to a permanent bronchial dilatation associated with suppuration. The

lower lobes are involved in many cases. The cause of bronchiectasis appears to involve an interplay between peribronchial fibrosis and overdistention of distensible bronchi. Concurrent bronchial inflammation appears to weaken the bronchial walls, allowing further dilatation. There is also a component of bronchial obstruction with distal accumulation of retained mucus and superimposed bacterial infection. Bronchiectasis occurs commonly with situs inversus viscerum (Kartagener's syndrome) and cystic fibrosis. Pathologically, the bronchi are dilated and filled with mucus and numerous neutrophils. There may be chronic inflammation in the surrounding parenchyma as well as alveolar fibrosis.

2. **Pulmonary abscess** consists of a confined area of suppuration within the parenchyma itself and can result from bronchiectasis, lobar pneumonia, bronchopneumonia, aspiration of gastric contents and foreign objects, septic embolism resulting from osteomyelitis, cavernous sinus thrombosis, or postpartum endometritis, and pulmonary embolism.

G. INFECTIOUS GRANULOMATOUS DISORDERS

1. **Primary pulmonary tuberculosis** continues to be an important cause of death in the United States, although the death rate has improved since the last century. Commonly, the apices of the lungs are involved, but the lower lobes or any other site may be affected. The initial tuberculous lesion (Ghon's lesion) is subpleural in location and occurs either in the lower portion of the upper lobe or in the superior segments of the lower lobe. The Ghon complex consists of the initial primary lesion plus involved lymph nodes. The granulomas characteristically have gross visible necrosis and a cheesy, crumbly (caseous) character. Tuberculosis may spread to distant organs by lymphatics or, as in the case of miliary tuberculosis, may spread via the bloodstream to involve all of the lungs as well as distant body sites.

2. **Histoplasmosis**, more commonly seen in the large river valleys of the midwest and eastern United States, is caused by a small yeast, *Histoplasma capsulatum*. Infection by this organism may be asymptomatic and subclinical; scarred calcified granulomas are the usual result in immunologically intact individuals.

3. **Coccidioidomycosis** occurs in the San Joaquin Valley and arid desert regions of the southwestern United States. It is usually a mild infection in its primary form in the lungs but may be severe and become disseminated in immunosuppressed individuals.

4. **Aspergillosis and phycomycosis** occur less commonly than other suppurative disorders but are important in the presence of immunosuppression and malignancy. Branching hyphae are seen microscopically.

H. PNEUMOCONIOSIS is a pathologic state of the lung, resulting from direct inhalation of particulate material, which is generally of occupational (mining and mill working) origin.

1. **Anthracosis** is the common deposition of carbon dust, grossly visible as blackened pigment on the pleural surfaces as well as in the lymph nodes and the parenchyma. It is caused by inhalation of coal dust, cigarette smoking, and inhalation of the polluted air of congested, urban environments. Anthracotic pigment is commonly seen in most city dwellers, and unless it is inhaled with silica, is not generally associated with disease.

2. **Silicosis** is caused by the deposition in the lungs of silica, which has been directly inhaled as a result of occupational exposure by miners, metal grinders and polishers, sand blasters, and cement workers. Silica particles are quite small and may be less than 2 μ in diameter. Alveolar macrophages phagocytose the silica dust and die after rupture of the silica-laden phagolysosomes. The released material is engulfed by the macrophages with eventual drainage by lymphatics to the lymph nodes where silicotic fibrotic nodules result. If severe, marked fibrotic changes in the lungs occur as a result of the presence of numerous silicotic nodules. Silica dust is remarkably fibrogenic. Pulmonary tuberculosis and rheumatoid lung may supervene in some patients with silicosis.

3. **Asbestosis** is an important form of pneumoconiosis that affects shipyard, roofing, and insulation workers who are exposed to asbestos. Asbestos fibers find their way to the pleural surfaces and are visualized as pigmented, ferruginous bodies. The pleura becomes thickened with fibrous adhesions, which encase the lungs; after a long period of exposure, malignant mesothelioma may form. In addition, asbestosis patients carry a high risk for the development of bronchogenic carcinoma. Cancer of the lung may ensue as long as 18 years after exposure to asbestos.

4. **Berylliosis** is caused by exposure to beryllium fumes, dust, or any of its compounds, such as beryllium oxide, sulfate, and fluoride. Granulomas in the lung may form as well as a mononuclear inflammatory infiltrate within the alveolar spaces. Over time, the lungs become

very heavy, with fibrosis and the formation of many granulomas. Beryllium granulomas are similar in some cases to tuberculous granulomas.

5. **Farmer's lung**, an example of hypersensitivity pneumonitis, is an immunologically mediated inflammation due to antigens of the mold *Micropolyspora faeni*, which grows on improperly stored hay, corn, tobacco, and barley. In the early stages, focal peribronchiolar granulomas are seen as well as an interstitial infiltrate of giant cells, lymphocytes, and macrophages. Eventual pulmonary fibrosis and emphysema may ensue.

V. CHRONIC OBSTRUCTIVE PULMONARY DISEASE (EMPHYSEMA)

A. **GENERAL CONSIDERATIONS.** Emphysema is one of the most common causes of chronic obstructive pulmonary disease in the United States and is characterized by overdistended alveoli that are distal to the terminal bronchioles, with consequent alveolar septal wall destruction. There is an association with urban living, air pollution, and cigarette smoking. Possible pathogenesis includes chronic bronchiolitis with damage to smooth muscle and elastic tissue; consequent obstruction of the bronchioles by inflammatory cells and mucus occurs, which leads to alveolar sac distention and rupture. Loss of elasticity of bronchi and bronchioles as a result of bronchial asthma, bronchitis, or even particulate deposition may play an important role during the expiratory phase of respiration. There is a high association of increased pulmonary artery pressure and eventual cor pulmonale. In diffuse emphysema, the lungs become markedly increased in volume; the pleural cavities are filled, producing a barrel-chested configuration of the thorax. Focal emphysema includes the large bullae and subpleural cystic changes that are found adjacent to scars and areas of healed tuberculosis or anthracosis.

B. **TYPES**

1. **Centrilobular emphysema** is the most common subtype of emphysema, predominantly occurring in men and associated with cigarette smoking. It primarily involves the secondary lobules and begins in the upper lobes. The central portions of the acini are involved, but the distal alveoli are uninvolved.

2. **Panlobular (panacinar) emphysema** tends to begin in the lower lobes in older individuals and may be associated with scoliosis, silicosis, and Marfan's syndrome. All of the pulmonary acini are involved, including the distal alveoli.

3. **Alpha₁-antitrypsin deficiency** occurs in families as an autosomal dominant trait, which may be either homozygous or heterozygous. Deficiency of the serum enzyme α_1-antitrypsin is associated with severe panacinar emphysema and is manifested early in life compared to the other forms of emphysema. Cigarette smoking is particularly hazardous to individuals with this condition because alveolar macrophages are stimulated to secrete elastases and other proteolytic enzymes that damage pulmonary parenchyma and may lead to more severe forms of emphysema.

VI. **INTERSTITIAL LUNG DISEASE** includes a large category of disorders that produce a marked decrease in pulmonary compliance (stiff lungs). Ventilation perfusion disruption occurs with consequent hypoxemia in most patients. Since the interstitium becomes generally thickened, in most cases, there is a decrease in diffusing capacity.

A. **DIFFUSE ALVEOLAR INJURY** (acute interstitial pneumonitis) is due to a variety of causes, including oxygen toxicity, prolonged treatment with mechanical respirators, ARDS, uremia, aspiration pneumonitis, neonatal hyaline membrane disease, fat embolism, toxic inhalates, drugs, thermal burn inhalation, radiation damage, and viral pneumonitis. The lungs are remarkably heavy and stiff due to inflammation and edema, with formation of alveolar lining hyaline membranes. Interstitial fibrosis and inflammation are also present.

B. **CHRONIC INTERSTITIAL PNEUMONIA** results from many of the acute forms of pneumonia and is characterized by the organization of the interstitial infiltrate, which may extend over a period of years, resulting in pulmonary fibrosis. This yields a honeycomb appearance to the lungs, both microscopically and radiologically. The causes of the condition include pneumoconiosis, chronic passive congestion, nitric oxide inhalation, lupus erythematosus, rheumatoid arthritis, progressive systemic sclerosis (scleroderma), radiation, viral pneumonia, and those unknown (idiopathic).

1. **Usual interstitial pneumonitis (UIP)** is the most common type of chronic interstitial pneumonia (Fig. 6-1). It may be caused by multiple conditions, but it is idiopathic in at least one-half of the cases. Idiopathic pulmonary fibrosis (Hamman-Rich syndrome) and fibrosing alveolitis are synonyms for UIP. Many of the collagen vascular diseases are associated with it.

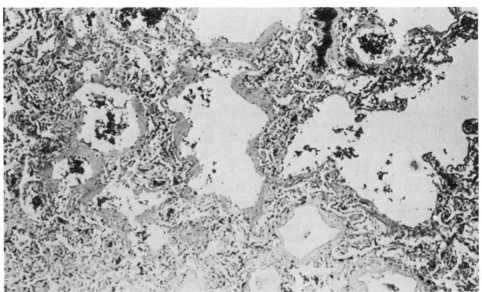

Figure 6-1. Usual interstitial pneumonitis (UIP). The interstitium is widened from fibrosis and infiltration of sparse mononuclear inflammatory cells. Note the patent alveolar spaces.

Microscopically, the alveolar spaces are still intact, although the walls become markedly widened by fibrosis and mononuclear cell infiltration.

2. **Desquamative interstitial pneumonitis [DIP]** (Fig. 6-2) is characterized by a marked proliferation and desquamation of the alveolar lining cells, which fill the alveolar spaces. These cells are alveolar macrophages (phagocytic pneumonocytes) admixed with type II pneumonocytes.

3. **Lymphoid interstitial pneumonitis (LIP)** may occur in association with Sjögren's syndrome and is characterized by an interstitial infiltration of aggregates of lymphoid cells, which may be severe enough to suggest lymphoma.

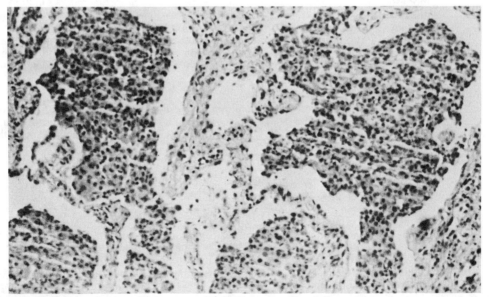

Figure 6-2. Desquamative interstitial pneumonitis (DIP). Mononuclear inflammatory cells, desquamated alveolar lining cells, and alveolar macrophages fill the alveolar spaces. Compare these with the patent air spaces of usual interstitial pneumonitis (UIP).

VII. MISCELLANEOUS PULMONARY DISORDERS

A. PULMONARY ALVEOLAR PROTEINOSIS is a chronic lung disease associated with progressive dyspnea, expectoration of thick yellow sputum, chest pains, and marked fatigue. It occurs in adults with a slight male preponderance. The cause is unknown, but it results in the filling of the alveolar spaces by proteinaceous and lipid material, which is markedly eosinophilic and granular, with needle-shaped, doubly refractile crystals and laminated bodies. There is a slight association with concomitant nocardiosis.

B. SARCOIDOSIS is characterized by the presence of non-necrotizing epithelioid granulomas occurring in the subpleural lung, parenchyma, interstitium, and peribronchial lymph nodes. The central hilar lymph nodes may be especially involved. Granulomas characteristically are non-caseating, as can be seen in tuberculosis. No organism has ever been clearly identified with this disease.

C. ALVEOLAR MICROLITHIASIS is a rare chronic disorder, which is occasionally found in families, and has a possible associated abnormality of the carbonic anhydrase system. Calcium salts are precipitated in the alveoli as a result of an increase in pH. The result is the diffuse formation of calcific bodies within both lungs. The bodies are laminated concretions lying within the alveolar spaces and are composed of calcium phosphate, calcium carbonate, and magnesium carbonate. Marked fibrosis and cardiac hypertrophy result.

VIII. PULMONARY NEOPLASIA.
Most tumors of the lung are malignant, and the majority (95 percent) originate in or around the larger airways (first- and second-order bronchi) and are epithelial in character (bronchogenic carcinoma is so-called because it arises from bronchial epithelium). The risk of developing lung cancer is 20 times higher in heavy cigarette smokers, but just living in urban, industrial areas also plays a role. Cancer deaths in men are predominantly due to lung cancer. While breast carcinoma causes the most cancer deaths in women, the incidence of lung cancer in women is increasing rapidly. Benzopyrene in cigarette tar can initiate carcinoma, but many other contaminants, such as radioactive substances and heavy metals, are also present.

A. BENIGN TUMORS occur infrequently in the lung but include hamartoma, which is a benign growth involving lobular masses of hyaline cartilage with a component of myxoid connective tissue, adipose cells, smooth muscle cells, and clefts lined by respiratory epithelium, as well as lipoma, leiomyoma, and rare neural tumors.

B. MALIGNANT TUMORS

1. **Squamous cell carcinoma** is a tumor of the smaller bronchi within the pulmonary parenchyma and is the tumor most closely associated with cigarette smoking in men. It is also the tumor associated with hypercalcemia. Often present in the bronchial mucosa in the vicinity of the tumor is squamous carcinoma in situ as well as squamous dysplasia and metaplasia. It frequently is associated with narrowing of the bronchi, collapse of the parenchyma with obstruction, and consequent pneumonia distal to the obstruction. Metastasis occurs via lymphatic and hematogenous routes. Depending on the degree of keratin and intercellular bridge formation, grades of differentiation occur, which vary from well to moderate to poor (Fig. 6-3).

2. **Adenocarcinoma.**
   a. **General Considerations.** Adenocarcinoma also arises in association with first- and second-order bronchi but also tends to occur more peripherally than the central squamous cell carcinoma and is found equally in both sexes. It is said to occur in association with old trauma, tuberculosis, and infarctions and hence has been connected with the development of scars. This is controversial because some tumors have the ability to form their own fibrous stroma. The association of adenocarcinoma with cigarette smoking is not as tight as that of squamous cell carcinoma. Adenocarcinoma may be well, moderately, or poorly differentiated, but most contain epithelial mucin that stains positive with mucicarmine. Adenocarcinoma grows slower than squamous cell and undifferentiated carcinomas and tends to have a better prognosis.
   b. **Bronchioalveolar carcinoma** is a special form of adenocarcinoma and has a pneumonia-like picture both grossly and radiologically. Uniformly tall and columnar cells line the alveolar spaces, appear to reproduce terminal bronchial cell architecture, and grow in a diffuse pattern throughout the lung, but they maintain an air space in the alveolar sacs. Mitoses are rarely seen.

3. **Undifferentiated (anaplastic) carcinomas** do not demonstrate distinguishing features that enable them to be characterized as squamous cell or adenocarcinoma. The prognosis is poor.

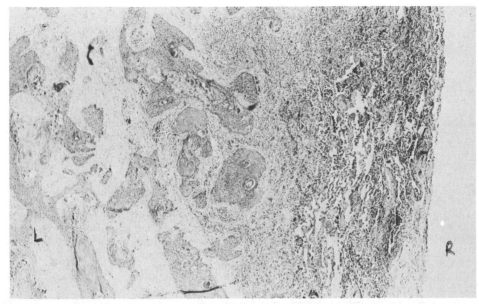

Figure 6-3. Well-differentiated squamous cell carcinoma. The nests of malignant squamous epithelium contain keratin pearls in the *left side* of the photomicrograph. Note the compressed (atelectatic) lung tissue in the *right side* of the photomicrograph.

a. **Large cell undifferentiated carcinoma** is composed of sheets of large round to polygonal malignant cells, and, in some cases, it may be related to a poorly differentiated adenocarcinoma. Prognosis is poor, and if the giant cell carcinoma form is present, it is then practically hopeless.

b. **Small cell carcinoma** is divided into two types: **oat cell**, which resembles lymphocytes, and **intermediate cell**, which is fusiform in appearance (Fig. 6-4). The tumor contains dense core granules similar to the argentaffin cell granules of the gastrointestinal tract and is active in the secretion of hormones and hormone-like products. These granules are thought to be identical to APUD secretory granules. The hormonal substances produce a

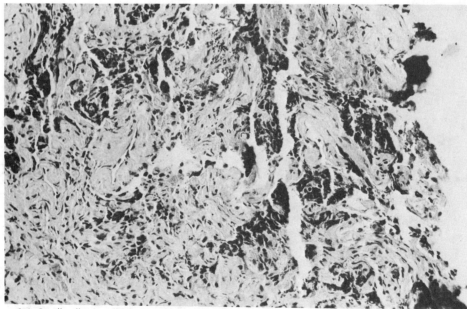

Figure 6-4. Small cell (oat cell) carcinoma. Note the crush artifact of the hyperchromatic undifferentiated malignant cells, which is commonly seen in biopsies of this form of lung cancer. Close inspection reveals the lymphocyte-like character of some of the tumor cells.

variety of paraneoplastic syndromes such as Cushing's syndrome [connected with adreno-corticotropic hormone (ACTH) secretion], a syndrome of inappropriate antidiuretic hormone (ADH) production, and myasthenic (Eaton-Lambert) syndrome. Digital nail clubbing, pulmonary osteoarthropathy, and Horner's syndrome (ptosis and miosis) are also peripheral clinical signs of lung cancer found in all types, including small cell carcinoma.

4. **Bronchial gland neoplasms** are thought to arise from the sub-bronchial seromucous glands and were once erroneously classified as bronchial adenomas.
   a. **Mucoepidermoid carcinoma** consists of nests and cords of malignant squamous cells with areas of mucopolysaccharides. Both low- and high-grade forms of the tumor exist.
   b. **Adenoid cystic carcinoma** is thought to arise from the larger bronchial mucous glands and morphologically resembles the adenoid cystic carcinoma that is found within the salivary glands. It grows slowly initially but eventually metastasizes to regional lymph nodes and shows a propensity for perineural growth patterns.

5. **Carcinoid tumor**, previously and erroneously called a bronchial adenoma, consists of a group of malignant tumors demonstrating an endocrinoid microscopic pattern with nests of uniform circular to polygonal cells, which abut blood vessels (Fig. 6-5). The tumor usually involves large bronchi in patients less than 45 years of age and has an endobronchial growth pattern, which fills the bronchial lumina. This tumor secretes a variety of biogenic amines, especially serotonin. It can invade locally and is capable of metastasis. The carcinoid syndrome of diarrhea, facial flushing and cyanosis, and wheezing rarely occurs in disease confined to the lung but may occur if there is metastasis to the liver. The prognosis is generally good, with an 80 percent 5-year survival rate.

   Carcinoid belongs to the amine precursor uptake and decarboxylation (APUD) group of tumors by virtue of its ultrastructural dense core of argentaffin granules.
   a. The **spindle cell variant** of carcinoid tumor has a more aggressive course with a high incidence of metastasis and more mitoses and spindle cells than the classic carcinoid tumor and is referred to as **atypical carcinoid.**
   b. Another special variety of carcinoid tumor is the **tumorlet**, which consists of small round or spindle cells and is small in diameter and found around the peribronchial arteries. The malignant potential of these carcinoids is very low.

IX. PATHOLOGY OF THE PLEURA. The visceral pleural surface of lungs is the site of secondary involvement by underlying conditions such as pneumonia, collagen vascular disease, rheumatoid disease, congestive heart failure, and tumor metastases. Pleural mesothelial cells readily react with the fluid effusing into the potential space between the visceral and parietal pleurae.

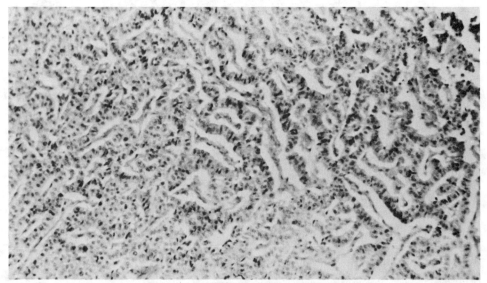

Figure 6-5. Bronchial carcinoid tumor. The tumor cells are arranged in tubular glands and ribbons. This pattern resembles those of carcinoids arising from the small intestine and appendix.

A. EFFUSIONS

1. **Hydrothorax** is the accumulation of clear serous (nonexudate) fluid in the pleural cavity and commonly results from congestive heart failure, renal failure, and cirrhosis.

2. **Chylothorax** is the accumulation of milky (chylous) lymph, usually in the left pleural cavity, as a result of duct obstruction by tumors as well as trauma.

3. **Hemothorax** is hemorrhage into the spaces from damage to any large vessel but especially occurs as a result of ruptured aortic aneurysms or trauma to the ascending aorta.

B. INFLAMMATIONS (PLEURITIS)

1. **Infectious pleuritis** is caused by organisms (bacterial, viral, and fungal). Bronchopleural fistula and empyema result from pathogenic staphylococcus infection of the lung.

2. **Noninfectious pleuritis** is a result of pulmonary infarction, rheumatoid lung disease, lupus erythematosus, and uremia.

C. PLEURAL TUMORS are mainly the result of metastasis from other sites such as the breast, but any visceral carcinoma may reach the pleural surfaces by lymphatic routes. Pleural effusion results from metastatic carcinoma and can be easily demonstrated by cytologic study of the aspirated fluid.

1. **Benign pleural tumors** are uncommon and are usually local fibrous mesotheliomas.

2. **Malignant mesotheliomas** (Fig. 6-6) are identified today with occupational exposure to asbestos. These tumors spread diffusely over the surfaces of both lungs, eventually completely encasing them in a thick rind of fibrous stroma, which contains the infiltrating nests and ducts of malignant mesothelial cells. The prognosis is very poor.

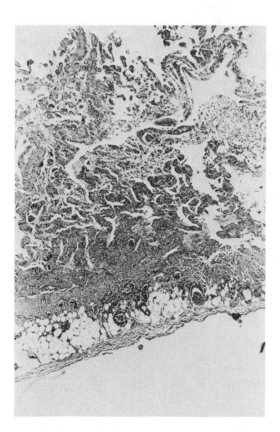

Figure 6-6. Malignant mesothelioma of the pleura. There is a papillary-like configuration of the small cords and glands, accompanied by a fibrous stromal reaction.

STUDY QUESTIONS

Directions: Each question below contains five suggested answers. Choose the **one best** response to each question.

1. Which of the following infections is often the cause of interstitial pneumonia?

(A) Gram-positive bacterial
(B) Gram-negative bacterial
(C) Viral
(D) Fungal
(E) Parasitic

2. Which form of chronic interstitial pneumonia listed below is characterized by marked proliferation and desquamation of alveolar lining cells?

(A) Usual interstitial pneumonitis
(B) Idiopathic pulmonary fibrosis
(C) Desquamative interstitial pneumonitis
(D) Lymphoid interstitial pneumonitis
(E) Hamman-Rich syndrome

3. Of the lung tumors listed below, which type belongs to the amine precursor uptake and decarboxylation (APUD) group of tumors?

(A) Hamartoma
(B) Mucoepidermoid carcinoma
(C) Adenoid cystic carcinoma
(D) Bronchial carcinoid
(E) Squamous cell carcinoma

4. Which of the following tumors is associated with occupational exposure to asbestos?

(A) Bronchioalveolar carcinoma
(B) Oat cell carcinoma
(C) Mesothelioma
(D) Squamous cell carcinoma
(E) Adenocarcinoma

ANSWERS AND EXPLANATIONS

1. The answer is C. (*IV D 3*) Interstitial pneumonia is usually caused by viral infections, including influenza, adenovirus, cytomegalovirus, herpesvirus, measles, and respiratory syncytial virus. These viruses produce alveolar cell necrosis and may be associated with deposition of hyaline membranes along the alveoli.

2. The answer is C. (*VI B 2*) Desquamative interstitial pneumonia is characterized by proliferation of desquamated alveolar lining cells within the alveolar spaces. These hyperplastic cells have the features of macrophages and are mixed with type II pneumonocytes. The causes of this disorder are thought to include viral, immunologic, and toxic injury to the lungs, which induce the cellular proliferation and the pneumonia.

3. The answer is D. (*VIII B 5*) Bronchial carcinoid is included in the group of malignant tumors that have varying microscopic patterns. In electron micrographs, these tumor cells have dense cores of argyrophilic granules and numerous mitochondria. Most bronchial carcinoids do not produce the typical carcinoid syndrome. Although bronchial carcinoid is a relatively rare tumor, making up less than 5 percent of bronchial neoplasms, it is potentially curable by surgical resection in most cases.

4. The answer is C. (*IV H 3*) It is now estimated that nearly two-thirds of all malignant mesotheliomas are associated with a history of industrial exposure to asbestos. However, asbestos is so widespread in our environment that nearly one-half of all individuals now autopsied in the United States have asbestos bodies in their lungs. There are two histologic forms of malignant mesothelioma—fibrous and epithelial. The prognosis is poor for both; however, individuals with the fibrous type have a slightly better survival rate than do those with the epithelial type.

7

The Mediastinum

I. ANATOMY. The mediastinum is the area of the thorax that is located between the pleural cavities; it is bounded by the thoracic inlet above and the diaphragm below and extends anteriorly to posteriorly from the sternum to the spine. It is divided into four compartments.

   A. SUPERIOR MEDIASTINUM is located above the pericardium and contains the aortic arch, thymus, great vessels, trachea, the upper esophagus, and thoracic duct.

   B. ANTERIOR MEDIASTINUM is the space between the pericardium and the sternum. It contains lymph nodes, vessels, and fat.

   C. MIDDLE MEDIASTINUM contains the heart, pericardium, tracheal bifurcation, pulmonary arteries, and pulmonary veins.

   D. POSTERIOR MEDIASTINUM is located behind the trachea and pericardium and in front of the vertebral column. It contains the descending aorta, esophagus, thoracic duct, greater and lesser azygos veins, intercostal veins, the vagal nerves, and the great splanchnic nerves.

II. INFLAMMATIONS

   A. ACUTE MEDIASTINITIS is a serious inflammation caused by traumatic rupture and perforation of the esophagus, infiltration of the esophagus and trachea by carcinoma, and descending infections. As a consequence, there is an abscess formation that usually requires surgical drainage.

   B. CHRONIC MEDIASTINITIS occurs frequently in the anterior mediastinum in front of the tracheal bifurcation and is generally a manifestation of granulomatous diseases such as tuberculosis and histoplasmosis.

   1. Histologically, there is diffuse fibrosis in which caseating or noncaseating epithelioid granulomas can be identified. Cultures and special stains may be helpful in the identification of the causative organisms. The major complications are due to constriction of the superior vena cava, but obstruction may be apparent in the tracheobronchial tree, pulmonary veins, and esophagus.

   2. Cases of **idiopathic fibrous mediastinitis** have been reported.

III. MEDIASTINAL CYSTS are rare but can occur in locations such as the pericardium and the lymphatic, tracheal, bronchial, and gastroenteric systems. They are probably formed as defects during embryonic life and may reach different sizes. Surgical resection of the cysts is curative.

   A. BENIGN CYSTS are largely asymptomatic and arise in the anterior and middle mediastinum.

   B. BRONCHOGENIC CYSTS arise commonly in the middle mediastinum and in the tracheal area. They are filled with liquid, and upon communication of the cysts with the trachea or bronchus, the liquid may empty into the air passages. Infection leads to abscess formation.

   C. ENTERIC CYSTS occur along the esophagus and are lined with intestinal or gastric epithelium. Abscess formation and, if the cysts contain acid-secreting cells, perforation, ulceration, and hemorrhage may occur.

   D. PERICARDIAL CYSTS are benign and are located usually in the middle mediastinum next to the pericardium.

IV. TUMORS

A. **GERM CELL TUMORS.** The histogenesis of these tumors is unclear, but they are believed to arise from misplaced germ cells during embryonic life.

   1. The most common malignant tumors of this type are **seminomas**, which arise in the anterior mediastinum and which are histologically identical to the seminomas of the testis.

   2. **Teratomas** can occur in both the anterior and middle mediastinum.
      a. **Mature (benign cystic) teratomas** are the most common of the benign germ cell neoplasms. They present during adult life as growths of different sizes that may adhere to and perforate adjacent structures. They are histologically identical to the benign cystic teratomas of the ovary. Surgical resection is curative.
      b. **Malignant teratomas** comprise less than 5 percent of the mediastinal teratomas and predominantly affect males; they are characterized by rapid growth.
         (1) **Grossly**, they appear as solid masses with extensive areas of hemorrhage and necrosis.
         (2) **Histologically**, the malignant components are usually squamous or undifferentiated carcinomas and rarely sarcomas.
         (3) The **prognosis** of these tumors is poor, with less than 1-year survival.

   3. **Choriocarcinomas** are highly malignant tumors of the anterior mediastinum, which occur predominantly in males and present as friable hemorrhagic soft masses. They are histologically identical to the choriocarcinomas of the uterus or testis. When the diagnosis is made, a primary testicular tumor should always be excluded first.

   4. Other types of germ cell tumors, such as endodermal sinus tumors and embryonal cell carcinomas, are known to occur in the mediastinum but are rare.

B. **THYMOMAS** arise in the superior mediastinum and are tumors of the thymus, which is essentially an epithelial organ that is composed of lymphocytes and other mesenchymal cells and is covered by a thin fibrous capsule. Prominent during infancy and puberty, the thymus physiologically disappears or involutes in the adult.

   1. **Incidence.** Thymomas are the most common neoplasms of the mediastinum. They occur in either sex and at any age, although the average age of the patients is 49 years.

   2. **Clinical Data.** The majority of thymomas are slow-growing well-encapsulated tumors with benign clinical behavior. One-third of the patients are asymptomatic, and the tumor is found incidentally on routine chest x-ray. Other patients, however, present with an anterior mediastinal mass, cough, dysphagia, dyspnea, and retrosternal pain. Some thymomas are manifested through the appearance of a systemic disease such as myasthenia gravis, red cell hypoplasia, and hypogammaglobulinemia.

   3. **Pathology.**
      a. **Grossly**, most thymic tumors are lobulated or multinodular and appear enclosed by a fibrous capsule of variable thickness, although some tumors are nonencapsulated and appear to extend by local invasion. Cut surface shows colors varying from pink to yellow. Cystic changes are encountered in up to 40 percent of the neoplasms.
      b. **Histologically**, the majority of thymomas are composed of an admixture of lymphocytes and epithelial cells.
         (1) The epithelial cells are characterized by eosinophilic cytoplasm and large vesicular nuclei and are believed to be the neoplastic cells. Ultrastructurally, they are characterized by the presence of branching tonofilaments, elongated cell processes, and basal laminae. Occasionally, the epithelial tumor cells are arranged in whorls, parallel bundles, or in cartwheel patterns. Hassall's corpuscles may be present, but are usually rare.
         (2) The lymphocytes are found in close association with the epithelial cells and may have a reactive appearance.
         (3) Differing amounts of fibrous septa, which divides the tumor into nodules, may be present.
         (4) **Malignant thymomas** are characterized by extensive infiltration and invasion of the capsule and adjacent structures. They are also manifested by the presence of pleural implants or distant metastases. Nuclear pleomorphism, mitosis, and necrosis are not reliable signs of malignancy.

   4. **Prognosis.**
      a. The most important factor determining the prognosis of patients with thymomas is the growth behavior and the extent of the tumors. **Well-encapsulated thymomas** are cured

by surgical excision and rarely recur; the 10-year survival for patients with these tumors approaches 100 percent. Surgical resection of **malignant thymomas** is difficult due to the extensive infiltration and invasion of the capsule and adjacent structures. The 10-year survival for patients with malignant thymomas is usually nil.

    b. The histologic type of thymoma has no value in predicting prognosis. Various syndromes, especially myasthenia gravis and red cell hypoplasia, affect survival to a greater extent than do the direct effects of the tumor.

  5. Treatment. The primary form of therapy for these lesions is surgical excision. The role of postoperative radiation is debatable for tumors that are well-encapsulated and have been completely resected.

C. MALIGNANT LYMPHOMAS are one of the most common types of neoplasms of the mediastinum. They occur in all compartments. They may present as primary mediastinal disease or as a manifestation of a disseminated process. Most mediastinal malignant lymphomas originate in one or more of the lymph nodes that are normally present in this location. The most common type is Hodgkin's disease (60 percent); other types such as follicular center cell lymphomas are also encountered. These tumors are histologically identical to those found in the hematopoietic system.

D. TUMORS OF NEURAL ORIGIN are found almost exclusively in the posterior mediastinum.

  1. Neurofibromas present as large, nonencapsulated, tan masses. Histologically, they show a myxoid background in which wavy collagen bands and mast cells are found. Surgical resection of the lesion is curative.

  2. Neurilemomas also present as encapsulated tumor masses, but histologically the Antoni A and Antoni B fibers are characteristic. Surgical resection is curative.

E. MESENCHYMAL TUMORS, such as lipomas, lymphangiomas, and hemangiomas, can occur anywhere in the mediastinum. These lesions are histologically identical to those found in the soft tissue.

F. METASTATIC TUMORS. Metastatic malignant tumors frequently involve the mediastinum and simulate primary tumors in this area.

  1. Bronchogenic carcinoma is the most common malignant neoplasm to involve secondarily the mediastinum, and it indicates extension of the tumor outside of the lungs, worsening the prognosis of the patients.

  2. Other tumors known to metastasize to the mediastinum are germ cell tumors of the testis, melanoma, and breast and kidney cancers.

STUDY QUESTIONS

Directions: Each question below contains five suggested answers. Choose the **one best** response to each question.

1. Which of the following germ cell tumors is the most common malignant tumor of the anterior mediastinum?

(A) Cystic teratoma
(B) Embryonal cell carcinoma
(C) Choriocarcinoma
(D) Seminoma
(E) Endodermal sinus tumor

2. What is the most common tumor of the mediastinal tissues?

(A) Benign cystic teratoma
(B) Choriocarcinoma
(C) Seminoma
(D) Neurofibroma
(E) Thymoma

ANSWERS AND EXPLANATIONS

1. The answer is D. (*IV A 1–4*) The most common malignant germ cell tumor occurring in the mediastinum is the seminoma. This tumor is believed to arise from germ cells that do not locate normally during embryonic development. Although this tumor arises in the mediastinum, its histologic appearance is identical to the seminoma arising in the testes.

2. The answer is E. (*IV B*) Thymomas are tumors of the thymus—an organ composed of epithelial and lymphoid tissue. The normal thymus decreases in size from infancy to adulthood. Any prolonged enlargement of the thymus in an adult must be evaluated to exclude the presence of a thymoma. Most thymomas are well-encapsulated, relatively slow-growing tumors. They usually present clinical problems because of encroachment on adjacent mediastinal structures such as the trachea and esophagus or because of related systemic diseases such as myasthenia gravis.

I. ESOPHAGUS

A. ANATOMY. The esophagus is a muscular tube about 25 cm long, which extends from the pharynx to the cardia at the gastroesophageal junction. It is covered by stratified nonkeratinized squamous epithelium.

B. CONGENITAL ANOMALIES

1. **Atresia.** Pure atresia is rare, but when it occurs, it is frequently found in association with tracheal fistula. It is associated with hydramnios in the last 3 months of pregnancy.

2. **Tracheoesophageal Fistula.**
   a. Tracheoesophageal fistula is a common congenital anomaly with an incidence of 1 in 800 live births. It is not predominant in either sex, and it is associated with hydramnios.
   b. In the most common type, the upper esophagus ends in a blind pouch and the anterior wall of the pouch tends to fuse with the posterior wall of the trachea.

3. **Heterotopia** is the presence of islands of ectopic gastric, pancreatic, or intestinal epithelium in the esophagus; it may be the cause of esophagitis.

4. **Hernias** are produced by congenital maldevelopment of the diaphragm.

5. **Diverticula** occur as either **traction** diverticula, which result from pull of the external surface of the esophageal wall due to inflammatory adhesions, or **pulsion** diverticula, which result from an increase in the extraluminal pressure.

C. INFLAMMATIONS

1. **Esophagitis** is an inflammatory condition that predominantly affects the lower half of the esophagus.
   a. **Clinical Data.** The cardinal symptom is heartburn or a burning sensation behind the sternum. Associated regurgitation, mild anemia, and dysphagia may occur. Endoscopic examination shows a red, friable, and erosive mucosal lesion, which bleeds easily. However, occasionally no gross abnormality is noted.
   b. **Types of Esophagitis.**
      (1) **Reflux esophagitis** is the most common type of esophagitis; it is caused by incompetency of the lower esophageal sphincter, which then permits reflux of gastric content into the lower esophagus. The sphincter incompetence is usually idiopathic, but may be secondary to prolonged intubation, surgery, or protracted vomiting. The acidic content, which is regurgitated, is the injurious agent.
      (2) **Viral esophagitis,** usually herpetic in type, causes ulcerative lesions. It occurs in patients with compromised host defenses and is frequently asymptomatic.
      (3) **Fungal esophagitis** is caused most commonly by *Candida albicans*. Microscopically, white, irregular patches can be seen in the mucosa or ulcerative lesions that conform to the mucosa and submucosa, with considerable tissue necrosis. It is common in patients with compromised host defenses.
      (4) **Acute corrosive esophagitis** occurs most commonly in children under the age of 6 years and is the result of the accidental ingestion of commercial corrosive products. In adults, it occurs as the result of suicide attempts. It is most common at the level of the tracheal bifurcation.
      (5) **Chronic granulomatous disease** can occur in association with processes such as Crohn's disease, tuberculosis, and sarcoidosis.

(6) Esophagitis can occur secondarily to **radiation**. Pathologically, the early microscopic changes consist of mucosal inflammation and epithelial hyperplasia. Eventually, there is increased height of lamina propria papillae and increased thickness of the basal layer. Dilated and congested vessels are seen in the top of the papillae.

2. Peptic ulcer is associated with the presence of columnar (gastric) epithelium in the distal esophagus, which is known as **Barrett's epithelium**. The origin of this epithelium is still debated, but it is generally believed to be an acquired phenomenon, the result of re-epithelialization of the squamous mucosa. The gross and microscopic changes of this type of lesion are identical to those seen in peptic ulcers of the stomach.

3. Varices. The venous drainage of the esophagus is composed of a submucosal venous plexus and a serosal plexus, both of which drain into the portosystemic venous system. In portal hypertension, the plexuses dilate and form the esophageal varices, which are prone to bleeding and ulceration.

D. MOTOR DISORDERS. The transportation of food from the mouth to the stomach requires the coordination of two physiological mechanisms: esophageal peristalsis and relaxation of the low esophageal sphincter, both of which are initiated by swallowing. Disorders may result from relaxation of the esophageal sphincter or decreased progression of peristalsis.

1. Achalasia. Achalasia is the lack of relaxation of the esophagus due to increased resting tone of the lower esophageal sphincter and the uncoordinated, nonprogressive peristaltic contractions of swallowing. Food does not pass from the esophagus to the stomach at the cardia level.
   a. Clinical Data. It may affect all ages, but achalasia usually starts in the third or fourth decade and presents as dysphagia of both solids and liquids. Regurgitation and aspiration occur in one-third of the patients, and chest pain while resting is a common complaint.
   b. Pathology. There is a loss of autonomic (Auerbach's) ganglia in the body of the esophagus and lower esophageal sphincter area, and there can be degeneration of the vagal fibers going to the esophagus. The definite diagnosis of this condition is made by x-ray and by the positive Mecholyl test, which indicates increased sensitivity to cholinergic stimulation, causing marked esophageal contraction.

2. Scleroderma. Scleroderma is a collagenous vascular disease, which causes sclerosis of the subcutaneous tissue of the skin and of the cardiorespiratory and gastrointestinal systems.
   a. Clinical Data. Approximately 70 percent of patients with scleroderma have abnormalities of the esophageal junction; they may also complain of dysphagia and heartburn.
   b. Pathology. The basic abnormality is due to the atrophy of the smooth muscle of the gut wall rather than to excessive collagen deposition, as was thought previously. This may result from primary muscle disease or secondarily to a neurogenic disorder. The muscle fibers are replaced by deposits of fibrous tissue, leading to stenosis. Later, the arteries and arterioles are compressed by the deposition of fibrous tissue, producing anoxia and ischemia, with subsequent mucosal ulceration.

E. CARCINOMA

1. Incidence. In most countries, esophageal carcinoma accounts for approximately 2 percent to 5 percent of deaths due to malignant neoplasms. It is seen most frequently in patients who are over the age of 50 years and is four times more common in men than in women.

2. Etiology. Although the etiology of this cancer is not known, it is associated with certain elements.
   a. Genetic. There is a possible association with blood type A.
   b. Environmental. Alcohol consumption, smoking, and ingestion of hot spicy foods have been connected with esophageal carcinoma. Cancer also has been associated with conditions such as esophageal stricture due to lye ingestion, achalasia, Plummer-Vinson syndrome, and Barrett's epithelium in the esophagus.

3. Clinical Data. Most cases present as progressive dysphagia, first of solid foods and then of liquids, which leads to malnutrition. Retrosternal pain may occur in the back or neck; anemia and regurgitation may also occur. Endoscopic examination and x-ray show evidence of a stenotic lesion. The diagnosis is confirmed by cytology and biopsy of the lesion.

4. Pathology.
   a. The cancer occurs most frequently in the distal third of the esophagus. **Grossly,** the lesions may be polypoid but most frequently are stenotic and grow along the axis of the esophagus (Fig. 8-1). On cut section, the gray-white tumor usually replaces the entire esophageal wall.
   b. Histologically, the majority (90 percent) of the tumors are squamous cell carcinomas, which arise from the squamous epithelium. All grades of differentiation may be dem-

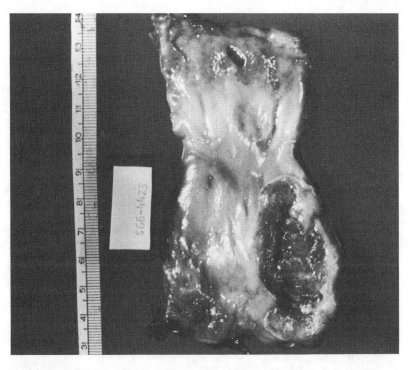

Figure 8-1. Gross view of a carcinoma involving the distal segment of the esophagus.

onstrated—from the well-differentiated tumors, characterized by nests of keratinizing cells to growths without keratin formation, which are composed of poorly differentiated anaplastic cells. Adenocarcinomas, which arise from gastric epithelium, paraesophageal mucous glands, or Barrett's epithelium, can also occur but are rare.

5. **Prognosis and Treatment.** About 75 percent of the patients have liver and lung involvement when first seen, but only 5 percent have palpable lymphadenopathy. Direct invasion occurs frequently to the mediastinal tissues, the trachea, and the bronchi. The prognosis of patients with these tumors is usually very poor, with a 5-year survival rate of 0 percent to 7 percent. Palliation is achieved with surgery and radiation, and cures have occasionally been reported.

F. **OTHER TUMORS**, such as leiomyomas, leiomyosarcomas, and granular cell tumors, can occur in the esophagus.

II. STOMACH

A. **ANATOMY.** The stomach develops as an unequal dilatation of the foregut and is anatomically divisible into three parts: the **fundus**, part of which is close to the gastroesophageal junction, is covered by a surface epithelium, which dips down to form crypts (foveolae lined by tall mucin-secreting cells); the **body**, two-thirds of the proximal remainder, is lined by epithelium similar to that lining the fundus; and the **pyloric antrum**, which makes up the distal third of the stomach and extends up to the pyloric sphincter, is lined by a columnar surface epithelium.

B. **CONGENITAL ANOMALIES**

1. **Pyloric stenosis** occurs in approximately 0.4 percent of all live births and is more common in firstborn males. There is a concentric bulbous thickening, due to hypertrophy and spasm of the muscular coat, of the pylorus, which terminates abruptly at the first (thin-walled) portion of the duodenum. The primary defect is probably in the myenteric plexus.

2. **Heterotopia.** The presence of heterotopic tissue (small intestine epithelium or pancreatic tissue) is not uncommon and is clinically associated with gastritis and peptic ulcer.

3. **Hiatal Hernia.** There are two types of hiatal hernia: the **sliding hernia** results when traction of the stomach pulls a portion of it into the thorax; the **rolling** type occurs when a portion of the stomach dissects along the esophagus through a defect in the diaphragmatic wall. Reflux of gastric contents produces esophagitis.

C. INFLAMMATIONS

1. Gastritis.

a. Acute.

(1) **Etiology.** Acute gastritis is the acute inflammation of the gastric mucosa. It may be the manifestation of certain conditions such as duodenal ulcer, sensitivity to aspirin, steroid therapy, ingestion of noxious substances, alcoholism, and anemia.

(2) **Clinical Data.** It is characterized by upper central abdominal discomfort, heartburn, gastric pain, and occasional nausea and vomiting. Endoscopically, patchy areas of congested erythematous mucosa may be identified.

(3) **Gross examination** of the stomach shows congestion of the gastric mucosa, which appears covered by large amounts of mucus. Small petechiae, erosion, and ulcers may be present.

(4) **Histologically**, the predominant lesion is an acute, patchy, superficial inflammation, with focal necrosis and exfoliation of the epithelium.

b. Chronic (Atrophic).

(1) **Etiology.** Chronic gastritis has been associated with chronic alcohol ingestion, pernicious anemia, cigarette smoking, and long-term ingestion of salicylates (aspirin). It occurs in elderly people, in males of blood group A, and in individuals of low socioeconomic status.

(2) **Clinical Data.** Patients may be asymptomatic or complain of dyspepsia, discomfort, or pain.

(3) **Grossly**, atrophic gastritis produces a thin, smooth mucosa with prominence of the submucosal vessels.

(4) **Histologically**, the main features of this disease are atrophy of the glandular epithelium and infiltration of the lamina propria by chronic inflammatory cells—predominantly lymphocytes and plasma cells but eosinophils and neutrophils may also be present. Marked degrees of atrophy are commonly associated with cystic dilatation of the glands, atypia of the crypt, epithelium, and intestinal metaplasia.

   (a) **Intestinal metaplasia** is the most common and important epithelial change.

   (b) The epithelium assumes the morphological and histochemical characteristics of intestinal mucosa, with the appearance of goblet and Paneth's cells. This epithelial change is considered by many authors to be a precancerous lesion.

   (c) In cases of pernicious anemia, biopsies may show chronic gastritis with severe atrophy, decreased mucous glands, and extensive cystic dilatation.

(5) **Prognosis.** Patients with pernicious anemia and atrophic gastritis have a higher tendency to develop carcinoma.

c. Hypertrophic (Menetrier's Disease).

(1) **Incidence.** This is a rare process of unknown etiology that radiologically and clinically can mimic primary malignant lymphoma and carcinoma of the stomach. It occurs most frequently in men who are 40 to 60 years of age.

(2) **Clinical Data.** Some patients present with edema, protein-losing enteropathy, and frequent achlorhydria due to the loss of plasma and glandular atrophy.

(3) **Pathology.**

   (a) **Grossly**, the process is characterized by thickened mucosal folds (about 7 mm compared to the normal 1 mm) and folds resembling cerebral convolutions. Some of the gastric pits are cystically dilated and filled with mucus. The greater curvature is most often involved.

   (b) **Histologically**, the oxyphilic glands are atrophic, containing only rare parietal cells and showing extensive pyloric metaplasia. The glands are markedly elongated. The lamina propria is edematous and shows a moderate and mixed inflammatory infiltrate. Eosinophils are prominent. Smooth muscle fibers and bundles are seen extending upward into the lamina propria from the muscularis mucosa.

(4) **Prognosis.** Carcinoma may develop, but the incidence is very low in patients with Menetrier's disease.

d. Peptic ulcers occur in the lowest part of the esophagus, in the anterior portion of the stomach, and in the anterior and posterior walls of the first portion of the duodenum.

(1) **Etiology.** Several factors are known to predispose to peptic ulcers.

   (a) **Aspirin Ingestion.** Acute ulcers caused by aspirin ingestion may evolve into chronic ulcers and be the source of bleeding.

   (b) **Hyperacidity** is due to increased acid output.

   (c) **Hormones**, such as glucagon, stimulate the acid-secreting cells. In **Zollinger-Ellison syndrome**, there is increased secretion of glucagon by the pancreatic cells, with ulceration of the duodenum and jejunum.

   (d) Inheritance. Individuals with blood type O are more liable than individuals with other blood types to develop stomach and duodenal ulcers.

   (e) Stress, tobacco use, diet, and congenital defects such as Meckel's diverticulum have also been associated with peptic ulcers.

(2) Incidence. Peptic ulcers occur in all age groups, but they are more common in adults and predominate in men.

(3) Pathogenesis. Several factors have been implicated in the pathogenesis of duodenal ulcers, but in general the cause of the ulcers is believed to be hypersecretion of peptic acid and a decrease in protective mechanisms, such as mucus production by the gastric cells.

(4) Pathology.

   (a) Grossly, the ulcers may be single or multiple and appear as circumscribed lesions characterized by the loss of the mucosa and variable amounts of underlying tissue. In the chronic stage, the ulcers penetrate the muscle, leading to fibrosis and thickening of the overlying serosa, which appears whitish and opaque.

   (b) Histologically, the earliest stages are characterized by destruction and necrosis of the mucosa, submucosa, and sometimes the muscle coat. The surrounding tissue initially shows acute inflammatory cells and later lymphocytes, plasma cells, and macrophages. In chronic ulcers, there is extensive deposition of collagen and a dense scar replaces the granulation tissue. The normal muscle fibers appear interrupted by fibrosis, and there is diffuse vein and arterial thrombosis.

(5) Complications.

   (a) Perforation is a common complication of acute peptic ulcers, particularly of those located on the anterior wall of the stomach and duodenum. Patients present with diffuse abdominal pain, shock, and peritonitis (Fig 8-2).

   (b) Hemorrhage. Since the vessels of the stomach and duodenum are thin, they can be eroded by acute or chronic ulcers, leading to severe hematemesis. If the bleeding is not very severe, the ulcers may be asymptomatic and only manifested by the presence of blood in the stools.

   (c) Fibrosis may involve the peritoneal surface and cause adhesion to the neighboring structures.

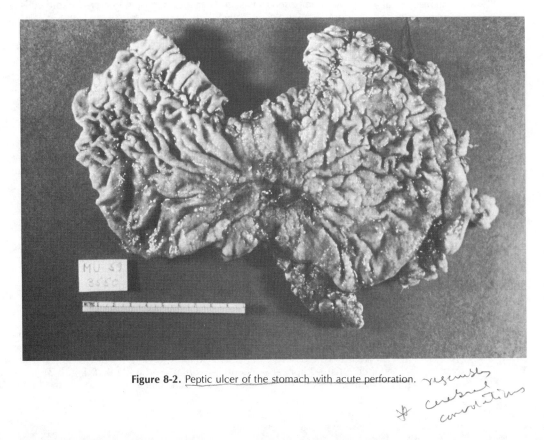

Figure 8-2. Peptic ulcer of the stomach with acute perforation.

(d) **Carcinoma.** The development of carcinomas from preexisting ulcers is still in debate.

(e) **Treatment.** If the ulcer is large or any of the above complications occur, surgery (partial gastrectomy) is recommended. Conservative therapy (antacids) is used in small, asymptomatic lesions.

D. BENIGN TUMORS

1. **Leiomyoma** is the most common benign neoplasm of the stomach and is frequently an incidental finding at autopsy. Patients between the ages of 30 and 70 years present with hemorrhage of the ulcerated mucosa over the tumor, iron deficiency anemia, or abdominal pain, but generally a tumor smaller than 3 cm does not produce symptoms. The tumors are often multiple; the regions of the pars media and antrum are the most common locations. The tumor originates from the longitudinal or circular muscle or from the muscularis mucosa and projects into the gastric lumen as a nodule or polyp. The histologic appearance is identical to that of smooth muscle tumors elsewhere.

2. **Gastric Polyps.**
   a. **Clinical Data.** Gastric polyps are unusual benign neoplasms, which occur in patients between 55 and 70 years of age, with equal predominance in men and women. These polyps fall into three categories: hamartomas, regenerative or inflammatory polyps, and true neoplasms (adenomas and papillomas).
   b. **Grossly**, they appear as sessile or finger-like, pedunculated projections in the lumen of the stomach. The tumors are usually single and tend to arise in the pyloric antrum or along the lesser curvature.
   c. **Microscopically**, the tumors can adopt a villous growth pattern and an adenomatous appearance or have mixed features. The cells can resemble those in the superficial zone of the stomach, with variations of nuclear hyperchromatism or may arise from metaplastic intestinal epithelium, reproducing goblet and Paneth's cells.
   d. **Prognosis.** There is some association between these tumors and carcinoma, which seems to relate to the tumor size. Adenomas can be found alone or in association with a separate focus of cancer. Gastric polyps are sometimes seen in patients with familial colonic polyposis or Peutz-Jeghers syndrome.

3. **Glomus tumors** are well-circumscribed, and although rare, they can occur in the stomach, where they lie within the muscle coat at the pylorus and may project into the gastric lumen. Microscopically, they are composed of vascular spaces lined by round epithelioid cells with large nuclei and eosinophilic cytoplasm. They follow a benign course, and surgery is usually curative.

4. **Other tumors**, such as schwannomas, carcinoid tumors, and lipomas, can occur in the stomach. Their histologic appearance and prognosis are identical to these tumors elsewhere.

E. MALIGNANT TUMORS

1. **Carcinoma.**
   a. **Incidence.** Carcinoma of the stomach is a common neoplasia in certain countries, such as Japan, the Scandinavian countries, and Iceland. In the United States, it is the fifth cause of all cancer deaths, with an apparent decline in incidence. It affects men more commonly than women in a ratio of 2:1, and most patients are over 50 years of age.
   b. The etiology of this tumor is not known, but there are certain predisposing conditions.
      (1) Genetics (a higher incidence in patients with blood type A)
      (2) Gastric atrophy
      (3) Achlorhydria or hypochlorhydria
      (4) Gastric polyps
      (5) Pernicious anemia
   c. **Clinical Data.** In the early stages, the tumors are usually asymptomatic but eventually anorexia, epigastric distress, weight loss, anemia, and melena occur. An epigastric mass and evidence of metastases are characteristic of the late stages. Endoscopy, cytology, and biopsy are helpful tools in confirming the diagnoses.
   d. **Pathology.** Carcinoma of the stomach is most common in the prepyloric region, in the pyloric antrum, and on the lesser curvature.
      (1) **Grossly**, there are five principal types.
         (a) **Nodular.** The tumor consists of raised but not polypoid nodules of growth, which may become confluent and ulcerated.
         (b) **Ulcerated.** The tumor presents as a shallow ulcer with raised edges. The surrounding tissues appear thickened, nodular, and infiltrated (Fig. 8-3).
         (c) **Fungating.** This is a protuberant carcinoma, which projects into the lumen as

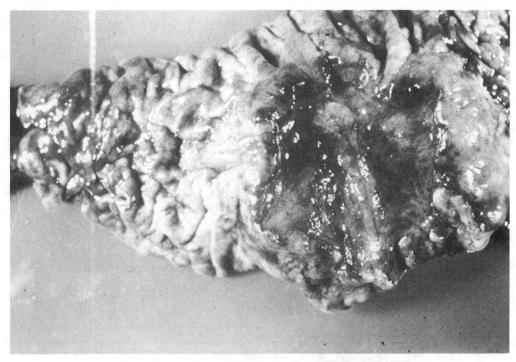

Figure 8-3. Gross view of a large ulcerated gastric carcinoma.

a solid polypoid, partly ulcerated mass, commonly involving the deep tissues.
- **(d) Superficially spreading** cancer grows in the mucosa and submucosa and does not initially involve the deep tissues. It may be difficult to detect, presenting as a thickening of the mucosa, which eventually ulcerates.
- **(e) Linitis plastica** ("leather bottle") stomach shows a deep spreading pattern of growth in which the tumor cells excite an extensive fibrosis, converting the stomach into a thick narrow tube.

(2) Histology.
- **(a)** Most carcinomas arise from the mucus-secreting cells of the superficial zone of the mucosa of the stomach and are, therefore, adenocarcinomas with a tendency to form glandular structures. Varying degrees of differentiation, atypia, pleomorphism, and mitosis may be present.
- **(b)** In the linitis plastica tumor type, however, glandular formation is rare and most tumor cells grow individually. These cells are rich in mucin, which displaces the nuclei towards the periphery of the cells. These cells are known as **signet ring** cells (Fig. 8-4).
- **(c)** A small proportion of gastric cancer (0.6 percent) are tumors of mixed epithelial elements, such as adenocarcinomas with focal squamous differentiation (adenosquamous carcinomas).

e. Prognosis and Treatment. Gastric cancer is often incurable because it is diagnosed at a late stage. The overall 5-year survival in all cases is approximately 10 percent, but for patients who do not have lymph node involvement, the 5-year survival approaches 40 percent. The tumor spreads via lymphatics, and bilateral ovarian metastasis (Krukenberg's tumor) is common in female patients. Surgical resection (hemigastrectomy or total gastrectomy) is recommended according to the location and extension of the tumor.

2. Leiomyosarcoma.
- **a. Incidence.** This gastric neoplasm is rare and represents about 1 percent of the primary malignant tumors of the stomach.
- **b. Clinical Data.** The tumor is often asymptomatic, but abdominal pain, hematemesis, or a gastric mass may be present. It occurs predominantly in those individuals 50 to 70 years old.
- **c. Pathology.**
  - **(1) Grossly,** leiomyosarcoma is identical to that occurring in the uterus and soft tissues.

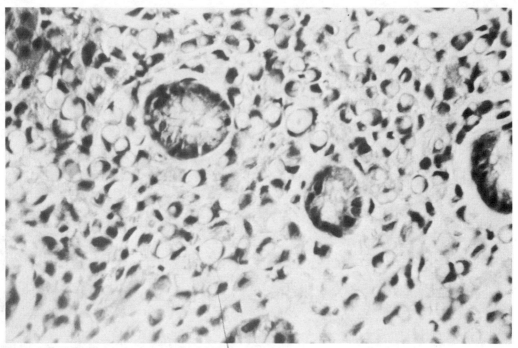

Figure 8-4. Characteristic signet ring cells of the linitis type of gastric cancer [hematoxylin and eosin (H and E) stain, x 400].

(2) **Histologically**, it is very important to distinguish a leiomyosarcoma from its benign counterpart. Necrosis, hemorrhage, increased cellularity, pleomorphism, and large tumor masses are features that suggest malignancy. It is also believed that a tumor with more than five mitoses per ten high-power fields behaves in an aggressive fashion.

   d. **Prognosis and Treatment.** Leiomyosarcoma spreads via hematogenous dissemination, especially to the lungs and liver. Surgical resection of the tumor followed by radiation therapy is the modality of treatment.

3. **Malignant Lymphoma.** The stomach may be the site of primary lymphoma or may be involved secondarily. The most common primary lymphoma of the stomach is a diffuse histiocytic lymphoma or follicular center cell, large, noncleaved type. It is histologically identical to that occurring primarily in the lymph nodes. The prognosis of patients with gastric lymphoma is better than that of patients with epithelial tumors or carcinoma.

III. SMALL BOWEL

A. **ANATOMY.** The small bowel varies in length between 600 cm and 900 cm and is composed of the duodenum, jejunum, and ileum. The normal mucosa consists of a basal layer from which finger-like villi project into the lumen. Between the villi, crypts of Lieberkühn extend into the basal layer and reach the muscularis mucosae.

B. **CONGENITAL ANOMALIES**

1. **Heterotopic Tissue.** Islands of heterotopic pancreatic tissue may be found in the duodenum and in other segments of the small bowel. Histologically, they are composed primarily of ducts and acini; islets usually are absent.

2. **Meckel's diverticulum** originates when the vitelline duct is unobliterated.
   a. There is persistence of a fibrous cord, which extends from the diverticulum to the umbilicus, adjacent bowel, or the mesentery. It arises within approximately 80 cm of the ileocecal valve from the antimesenteric border of the bowel.
   b. Heterotopic tissues such as gastric, duodenal, and colonic mucosa are commonly present. Ulceration with perforation or inflammation may occur if the diverticulum is not surgically excised. In children, Meckel's diverticulum may be the cause of massive intra-abdominal hemorrhages.
   c. It occurs in 2 percent of the adult population, predominantly in men.

3. **Omphalocele.** There is persistence of the amniotic sac, which contains a variable length of ileum, cecum, colon, and occasionally liver and stomach. The bowel is adherent to the sac, and at some point the sac impedes the normal return of the intestines to the abdominal cavity. Omphalocele is commonly associated with abdominal muscle defects and malformations of the alimentary tract.

C. INFLAMMATIONS

1. **Giardiasis** is the infestation of the small intestine by the parasite *Giardia lamblia*, which infects principally the duodenum and jejunum. Heavy infestation is necessary to produce symptomatology. Giardiasis is the most prevalent intestinal parasitic disease in the United States. Approximately 13 percent of those infected become asymptomatic carriers.
   a. **Clinical Data.** The most common symptoms are lassitude, abdominal pain, diarrhea, and anemia. Some patients develop steatorrhea similar to that seen in sprue syndrome. Rarely, giardiasis causes cholecystitis and cholangitis.
   b. **Histologically**, the changes in the small intestinal mucosa are generally nonspecific. There is acute focal inflammation in the crypts, which is associated with a polymorphonuclear infiltration of the mucosa and adjacent lamina propria.
   c. The **diagnosis** is made by identification of the organism in the duodenal secretion by duodenal biopsies, by culture of duodenal secretions, or by demonstrating cysts and trophozoites in stools.

2. **Whipple's Disease (Intestinal Lipodystrophy).**
   a. Whipple's disease is a condition that affects mainly adult males, and it is considered familial. The symptoms are predominantly diarrhea, weight loss, and migratory polyarthritis. The process is believed to be of infectious etiology since bacilliform organisms [e.g., *Brucella* and *Escherichia coli (E. coli)*] have been detected in the cells.
   b. **Histology.** The lamina propria of the intestinal mucosa and mesenteric lymph nodes shows granular yellow patches, which correspond to aggregates of macrophages containing inclusions in the cytoplasm. Deposits of macrophages with the same histologic characteristics may occur anywhere in the body, especially in the liver, spleen, heart, brain, and joints (Fig. 8-5).
   c. **Treatment.** The disease responds favorably to antibiotic therapy.

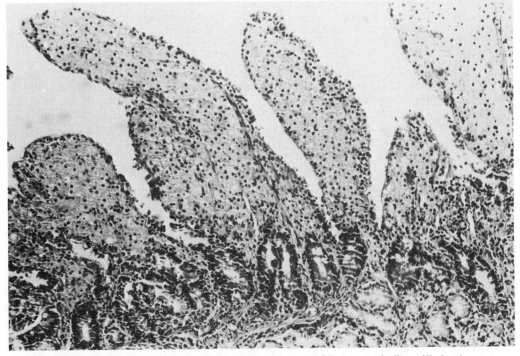

Figure 8-5. Whipple's disease of the small bowel. The lamina propria of the intestinal villi are filled with aggregates of macrophages [hematoxylin and eosin (H and E) stain, x 100].

D. MALABSORPTION. The malabsorption syndrome is characterized by impaired intestinal absorption of nutrients, especially fats. This phenomenon can be the result of a variety of organic and functional disorders.

1. **Clinical Data.** Malabsorption is manifested by diarrhea, bulky foul stools, abdominal distention, and malnutrition, with associated vitamin deficiencies.

2. **Types.**
   a. **Primary malabsorption** or steatorrhea comprises a group of disorders, including celiac disease and tropical sprue.
      (1) **Celiac disease** (nontropical sprue) is caused by a genetically controlled enzymatic or metabolic defect, which is characterized by sensitivity to or intolerance of gluten. The pathogenesis of the disease is not known, but some authors believe it results from a shortened life span of the epithelial cells.
         (a) Histologically, the small intestine shows shortening and flattening of the villi, which may be fused. In severe cases there is a flat mucosa with thickening of the basal layer and crowding of the enterocytes. The surface epithelial cells are low, cuboidal, and have irregular nuclei. These changes are more intense in the upper part of the jejunum.
         (b) **Treatment.** The symptoms usually disappear after gluten is eliminated from the diet. A rare but well-known complication of celiac disease is the development of malignant lymphoma, which should be suspected in patients with a long history of celiac disease who do not respond to a gluten-free diet.
      (2) **Tropical sprue** is similar to nontropical sprue clinically and histologically. The process, however, does not respond to elimination of gluten from the diet, but is reversible with folic acid, vitamin B_{12}, and tetracycline supplementation. This disease has an unknown etiology and occurs mainly in the tropics.
   b. **Secondary malabsorption** may be the complication of conditions such as cystic fibrosis, surgical resection of segments of the gastrointestinal tract, biliary tract disease, regional enteritis, and administration of antibiotics.

E. MECHANICAL DISORDERS

1. **Intussusception.**
   a. Intussusception is the invagination during life of a variable length of bowel into the part immediately below it. The condition is most common in children from 6 months to 2 years of age.
   b. Although a definite cause has not been identified, some cases have occurred due to bezoars, Meckel's diverticulum, and lymphoid hyperplasia. The ileocecal valve is the most common location of intussusception. The symptoms are the same as those of intestinal obstruction and acute abdomen. Surgery is curative.

2. **Volvulus** is twisting of the bowel, causing obstruction of the blood supply and ischemia of the twisted segment. The most common cause of volvulus is an abnormally long mesentery, but fibrous adhesions and Meckel's diverticulum may be associated.

F. TUMORS

1. **Carcinoid Tumor.**
   a. **Incidence.** Carcinoids are a type of the most common tumors to occur in the small intestine. The last portion of the ileum is the most common location. They arise from the neuroendocrine Kulchitzky's cells.
   b. **Clinical Data.** Most small tumors are asymptomatic, and only about 10 percent of intestinal carcinoids are accompanied by the carcinoid syndrome. Diarrhea, abdominal pain, episodes of blushing, cyanosis, dyspnea, and valvular lesions of the heart are the major clinical symptoms of the syndrome, which is seen only in patients with liver metastases and who produce potent humoral agents such as serotonin.
   c. **Pathology.**
      (1) **Grossly**, the tumor presents as a yellow, nodular mucosal elevation that is 1 or 2 cm in diameter.
      (2) **Histologically**, the tumor is usually composed of a nest of cells with uniform round to oval nuclei and abundant eosinophilic cytoplasm. The cells may also be arranged in cords or rosettes.
   d. **Treatment.** Resection of the lesion is curative if distant metastases have not occurred and if there is no evidence of carcinoid syndrome.

2. **Other Tumors.** The benign and malignant neoplasms of the small bowel are identical to those of the colon and will be discussed in the large bowel section (V).

IV. APPENDIX. The appendix is a vestigial organ with no specific function.

A. INFLAMMATIONS

1. **Acute appendicitis** is one of the most common acute surgical emergencies treated at any hospital. It is seen most frequently in young people, but it can occur at any age and in either sex.
   a. **Clinical Data.** Exquisite pain in the right lower quadrant, which extends to the periumbilical area, fever, vomiting, and leukocytosis are the most common symptoms.
   b. **Pathology.**
      (1) **Grossly**, the appendix is edematous and swollen, with a fibrinous and purulent exudate covering the serosal surface. The mucosa is often necrotic and ulcerated. A fecalith may occlude the lumen.
      (2) **Histologically**, acute inflammation varies from mild to severe, with necrosis and complete destruction of the appendiceal wall. Polymorphonuclear leukocytes are predominant, and microabscesses are scattered through the different appendiceal layers, but lymphocytes may also be present. Secondary thrombosis of the appendiceal vessels is common. Acute inflammation may extend into the periappendiceal fat and in severe cases produce periappendiceal abscesses.
   c. **Treatment.** Surgical excision of the appendix is curative. If a periappendiceal abscess forms, antibiotics may be required.

2. **Chronic appendicitis** is not believed to be an existing condition by pathologists and clinicians because most of the appendices that are surgically removed under this diagnosis are essentially normal when studied histologically.

B. PARASITES

1. *Oxyuris vermicularis* is a pinworm, which is the cause of about 3 percent of cases of appendicitis in the United States. It affects children between 7 and 11 years of age but rarely produces acute appendicitis. The organism is identified histologically in the lumen of the appendix. Occasionally, there may be a granulomatous reaction with the presence of epithelioid histiocytes.

2. Severe infestations by *Schistosoma mansoni* may occur in the appendix. In some cases, granulomas containing schistosomes may be present in the appendiceal wall.

C. TUMORS

1. **Mucocele** refers to the obstruction of the appendiceal lumen through inflammatory scarring or by fecaliths, with accumulation of mucus.
   a. **Histologically**, the mucosa may be flattened and atrophic, with pools of mucus penetrating the layers of the appendix. In other cases, the mucosa may show areas of hyperplasia and a papillary configuration, which are identical to those seen in hyperplastic polyps of the colon. Secondary changes include thinning of the appendiceal wall, extensive ulceration, and calcification.
   b. **Treatment.** Surgical resection of the tumor is usually curative if the appendix is not perforated and the mucoid material does not spill into the abdomen. Pseudomyxoma peritonei is a common complication if the tumor ruptures in situ in the abdomen.

2. **Carcinoid tumor** is the most common tumor of the appendix and is usually an incidental finding. It generally occurs in the third and fourth decades of life, but it may also be present in children.
   a. **Pathology.**
      (1) **Grossly**, the tumor is small, has a characteristic fine, yellow appearance, and is well circumscribed. The most common location is the tip of the appendix.
      (2) **Histologically**, the classic carcinoid tumor is formed of solid nests of homogeneous cells with abundant eosinophilic cytoplasm and uniform round nuclei. Rosette formation may be seen in some cases. The cells stain strongly positive with Grimelius, Fontana, and Masson stains. Mitosis and necrosis are virtually absent.
   b. **Treatment.** Surgical resection of the appendix is curative. Metastatic spread and development of carcinoid syndrome are quite unusual when the tumor occurs in the tip of the appendix.

3. **Adenocarcinoma.** Primary adenocarcinoma of the appendix is quite rare. It may produce enlargement of the organ. Frequently, the symptoms are identical to those of acute appendicitis. **Histologically**, it is identical to colonic adenocarcinoma. Right hemicolectomy is the treatment of choice.

V. LARGE BOWEL

A. The large intestine from the cecum to the anus is about 150 cm long. The colon is divided into the cecum, ascending colon, transverse colon, and descending colon. The wall of the colon consists of the mucosa, which is composed of epithelial tubules embedded in a connective tissue framework, muscularis mucosa, submucosa, muscularis propria, the serosa, and peritoneum.

B. CONGENITAL ANOMALIES

1. **Atresia and Stenosis**. Atresia of the bowel is a condition in which there is discontinuity of the lumen of the bowel. Stenosis of the bowel is narrowing without complete luminal obstruction. In the rectum, these abnormalities may include different types: imperforate anus, blind rectal end, imperforate anus with separation of anus and rectum, and anal stenosis. These abnormalities can be corrected surgically. The lower anatomically that the process occurs, the better the prognosis because it is possible that the sphincter muscles will remain intact.

2. **Hirschsprung's Disease.**
   a. **Incidence.** This congenital condition predominantly affects infant males with a male to female ratio of 6:1.
   b. **Clinical Data.** The infants present with constipation, gaseous abdominal distention, and repeated episodes of intestinal obstruction. Radiologically, the upper rectum and colon appear markedly dilated, and the rectosigmoid area is narrowed.
   c. **Pathogenesis.** The disease results from a localized absence of ganglion cells in the lower part of the rectum, which results in inadequate muscular relaxation to allow passage of stool.
   d. **Diagnosis.** The diagnosis is made through a biopsy of the abnormally constricted part of the rectum. If ganglion cells are not found, a transmural, or full-thickness, biopsy is recommended for evaluation of the submucosal myenteric plexuses. Diagnosis of Hirschsprung's disease is confirmed if there is a proliferation of nerves, vessels, and muscle bundles but no ganglia.
   e. **Treatment.** Surgical resection of the dilated aganglionic segment is curative.

C. BENIGN CONDITIONS

1. **Melanosis coli** refers to the brown pigmented appearance of the colonic mucosa, which is commonly seen in older individuals. The color is due to deposits of brown pigment (lipofucsin) in the macrophages that are present in the lamina propria. The condition is due to the habitual use of cascara laxatives.

2. **Diverticulosis.**
   a. Diverticulosis is the presence of multiple blind end orifices in the colonic wall. It affects predominantly the lower descending and rectosigmoid colon and is a common finding in autopsies of the aged.
   b. In addition to aging, a diet low in fiber and roughage as well as other conditions that cause weakening of the muscularis mucosa and lamina propria, such as hemorrhoids and ovarian atrophy, are believed to promote the formation of diverticula.
   c. The pathogenesis of diverticula appears to be increased intraluminal pressure with herniation of the mucosa and submucosa through the bowel wall.
   d. Occasionally the diverticula become inflamed, perforate, and form fistulas, which extend to the serosa, causing peritonitis.

3. **Pneumatosis Intestinalis.**
   a. Radiologic studies reveal gas-filled cystic spaces of varying sizes along the perivascular structures of the bowel wall. The lesions may be either submucosal or subserosal. This condition occurs frequently in individuals with pulmonary emphysema. Patients may be asymptomatic.
   b. **Histologically**, there may be no evidence of mucosal disease, but in cases in which pneumatosis is associated with vascular disease or other intestinal disorders, the biopsy reveals empty spaces in the submucosa, serosa, or both with giant cells and clusters of bacteria at their edges.

4. **Endometriosis.** Foci of ectopic endometrial tissue may be found in the bowel wall, which appears thickened due to proliferation of fibrous tissue. This type of fibrosis may cause stenosis and mimic diverticular disease.

5. **Colitis Cystica Profunda.**
   a. This process is characterized by the extension of mature epithelium into the submucosa

or deeper portions of the bowel wall. The most common form occurs in the rectum. It is believed to be the result of a defective anal sphincter, which causes prolapse of and mucosal ulcerations predominantly on the anterior wall.

   b. Histologically, the mucosa shows a prominent villose surface and an increase of fibrous and smooth muscle cells in the lamina propria. As the condition progresses, the cystic changes in the mucosa increase and extend into the submucosa. The epithelial elements appear completely benign, and no evidence of atypia, pleomorphism, or necrosis is seen.

D. INFLAMMATIONS. Colonic inflammations are one of the most common conditions to be diagnosed by colorectal biopsies. These inflammatory lesions may develop in the course of viral infections and motor and vascular disorders.

   1. Bacterial Colitis.
   a. The most common bacteria implicated in infectious colitis and proctitis are pathogenic strains of *Shigella, Salmonella, E. coli,* and *Campylobacter.*
   b. The organisms invade the mucosa directly, and it becomes necrotic and shows a marked acute inflammatory reaction. The **earliest changes** are those of vascular congestion and edema of the lamina propria. Later there is damage to the surface epithelium and upper crypts.
   c. In the **late stages** of most infections, a more diffuse colitis develops, which is impossible to distinguish from other causes of active inflammatory disease.

   2. Parasitic Colitis.
   a. Amebiasis.
      (1) Amebiasis is caused by a common protozoan, *Entamoeba histolytica,* and involves the large bowel, predominantly the cecal region. Diarrhea, pain, and cramps are the most common symptoms. The disease is normally spread through contaminated food and water, although venereal transmission occurs between male homosexuals due to fecal-oral contamination.
      (2) Characteristically small, round mucosal ulcers are found with sigmoidoscopy. **Histologically**, biopsies show the typical liquefaction, inflammation, and mucosal ulcerations known as "collar button" ulcers because of a broad base and narrow neck. The ameba can be found in the exudate, where round trophozoites with large nuclei and ingested erythrocytes are identified. Special stains such as periodic acid–Schiff (PAS) are helpful in recognizing the organism.
      (3) The most serious complication is invasion of veins with subsequent metastasis to the liver, where an abscess may form. Sometimes these abscesses penetrate the diaphragm and cause empyema and lung abscess.
   b. Schistosomiasis.
      (1) When schistosomiasis is caused by the blood fluke, *Schistosoma mansoni,* it is one of the most important parasitic infestations, occurring in Africa, North and South America, and Europe.
      (2) The parasite lays its eggs in the abdominal venules. The ova then perforate the different layers of the bowel, where they produce a marked eosinophilic reaction and epithelioid granulomas. The organisms can sometimes be found in the center of the granulomas (Fig. 8-6).
      (3) In severe infestations, vasculitis, formation of rectal fistulas, and abscess formation can complicate the condition.
   c. Cryptosporidiosis.
      (1) Recently, the protozoan, *Cryptosporidium,* has been recognized as a frequent cause of colitis, gastroenteritis, and malabsorption. It occurs in both immunocompromised and normal individuals who complain of a gastrointestinal influenza-like syndrome.
      (2) Identification of concentrations of oocytes from the feces is the most useful tool for diagnosis.

   3. Antibiotic-Associated Colitis.
   a. Some individuals may develop colitis following the use of various antibiotics. Originally colitis was seen as a complication resulting from use of clindamycin and ampicillin, but now it has been noted after the use of almost all antimicrobial agents. It is believed that the treatment favors the proliferation of *Clostridium difficile,* which is normally present in the bowel, leading to increased production of the species toxin.
   b. Clinical Data. Diarrhea and abdominal pain are common symptoms. The finding of pseudomembranes through sigmoidoscopy and a positive assay for the toxin are diagnostic.
   c. Histologically, mucosal biopsies show areas of crypt injury with marked intraluminal acute inflammation and a surface membrane. In the later stages, there is more diffuse colitis with necrosis of the mucosa.

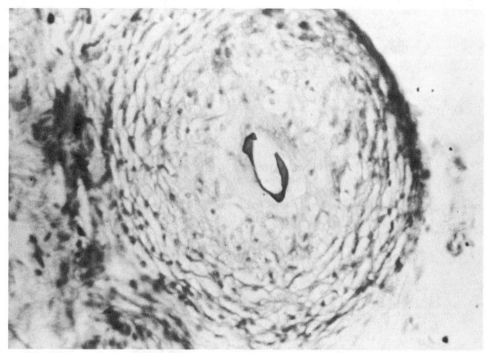

Figure 8-6. High-power view of an epithelioid granuloma containing the ova of a schistosome (acid-fast bacilli, x 400).

4. Crohn's Disease (Regional Enteritis).
  a. Incidence. Crohn's disease is a chronic inflammatory disease of unknown etiology that occurs in patients of both sexes (although slightly predominantly in men) who range in age from 20 to 30 years. About 5 percent of the cases are familial, and individuals of Jewish lineage are affected more often than are those of nonJewish lineage.
  b. Clinical Data. Some symptoms are shared with ulcerative colitis and include right lower quadrant pain associated with cramps and constipation, diarrhea, nausea, vomiting, and weight loss. Bleeding occurs less frequently than in ulcerative colitis.
  c. Pathology.
    (1) Crohn's disease is distinguished by segmental areas of involvement and involves the terminal ileum and cecum predominantly but may affect the entire alimentary tract. The ileum is narrowed and partially obstructed. All coats of the bowel are thickened by extensive fibrosis and muscular hypertrophy.
    (2) Histologically, the characteristic features are the transmural inflammation of the bowel, the presence of lymphoid aggregates scattered throughout the different layers of the bowel wall, and the development of epithelioid granulomas of the sarcoid type.
    (3) The mucosal surface is reddened and has a nodular cobblestone-like appearance and multiple linear ulcerations. In chronic cases, deep ulcers may give origin to fistula formation and perforations. In the preserved mucosa, the glands appear dilated with a decreased number of goblet cells. The muscularis mucosa is hypertrophied, and the nerves in the involved segment become prominent and increase in number. Regional lymph nodes are reactively enlarged and may contain granulomas.
  d. Treatment and Prognosis. Surgery, with resection of the affected segment of bowel, may be necessary if there is perforation and formation of fistulous tracts with development of adhesive peritonitis. Supportive treatment with steroid therapy is given to the patients, but recurrence of the disease is frequent.

5. Ulcerative Colitis.
  a. Incidence. Ulcerative colitis is a disease of unknown etiology that affects individuals of any age but predominates in young adults. Both sexes are affected equally. It is believed that ulcerative colitis is caused by a deranged immunologic mechanism. Psychogenic causes have also been suggested.

b. **Clinical Data.** The patients present with relapsing bloody mucoid diarrhea, which may last for days or weeks and may lead to dehydration and electrolyte imbalance. Although the colon is the primary organ affected, ulcerative colitis has been associated with systemic symptoms such as arthritis, skin lesions, and uveitis.

c. **Pathology.**

   (1) **Grossly**, ulcerative colitis predominantly affects the large bowel in the rectosigmoid area, but with progression of the disease, the entire colon becomes involved. The mucosa is reddish and edematous, and linear ulcers are present along the axis of the colon. There is shortening of the bowel and narrowing of the lumen due to thickening of the muscle. Occasionally the bowel is very friable and bleeds easily.

   (2) **Histologically**, the changes of ulcerative colitis are predominantly mucosal. There is accumulation of polymorphonuclear cells in Lieberkühn's crypts, with rupture of the crypt wall and eventual microabscess formation (Fig. 8-7). The lamina propria shows edema and an increased number of acute and chronic inflammatory cells. Ulcerations with areas of mucosal generation and pseudopolyp formation are common findings as well.

d. **Prognosis and Treatment.** There is an increased incidence of carcinoma of the colon in patients with long-standing ulcerative colitis. Treatment consists of antibiotics, steroids, and conservative therapy, but surgery is eventually necessary in the majority of the cases.

E. VASCULAR DISORDERS

1. **Ischemic Disease.**

a. The bowel receives blood from the superior and inferior mesenteric arteries, rectal arteries, and branches of the internal iliac and pudendal arteries. In intestinal ischemia, the bowel receives less blood than is necessary to maintain its structure and function. The three main causes are **vascular occlusion** due to formation of atheromas, **thrombi**, or emboli, **hypotension** (as seen in shock and ventricular failure), and **mechanical venous compression**.

b. The effect of ischemic disease on the bowel is extensive hemorrhagic necrosis and infarction.

c. **Grossly**, the bowel is dilated with congested and reddish mucosa. The wall is friable and thinner than normal, and linear ulcers are seen on the mucosal surface. Bloody matter fills the lumen.

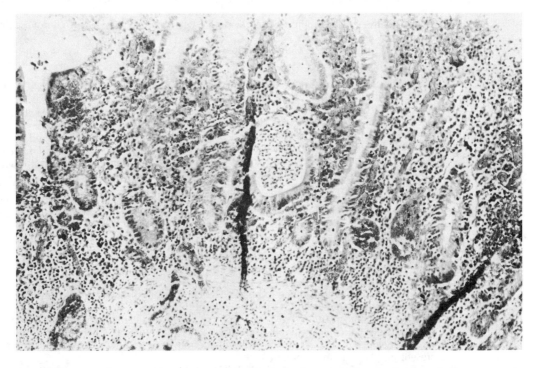

Figure 8-7. High-power view of bowel mucosa showing microabscesses in the glands. These findings are seen in ulcerative colitis [hematoxylin and eosin (H and E) stain, x 250].

d. Histologically, the early signs of disease consist of patchy or diffuse areas of hemorrhagic necrosis of the mucosa without associated inflammation. At this stage, the changes are reversible if the blood flow is restored. Later, the disease is characterized by complete necrosis of the mucosa and secondary bacterial involvement, leading to ulceration, fibrosis, and stricture. Perforation can occur in late stages with associated peritonitis.

e. Treatment. Resection of the involved segment of bowel may be necessary if the ischemia persists.

2. Vasculitis.

a. Inflammation of blood vessels affects the bowel as part of a variety of systemic disorders such as polyarteritis nodosa, lupus erythematosus, and rheumatoid arthritis.

b. Involvement of small arteries and veins is common, with patchy necrosis and inflammation of the overlying mucosa.

3. Vascular Ectasia (Angiodysplasia).

a. Vascular ectasia is an acquired condition that is probably due to elevated transmural pressure. This causes muscular compression of intramural veins, which leads to excessive arteriovenous connections that extend into the mucosa, where they rupture and cause hemorrhage.

b. Once the bleeding area is identified by special techniques and x-ray studies, resection of the affected area can be performed.

4. Hemorrhoids.

a. Hemorrhoids are variceal dilations of the anal and perianal venous plexuses and are secondary to various conditions that increase the intra-abdominal venous pressure.

b. Histologically, ectatic veins are covered by either rectal or anal mucosa. Thrombosis, inflammation, and recanalization of the occluded vessels are common findings.

F. COLONIC POLYPS. By definition, any mucosal protrusion is considered a polyp.

1. Hyperplastic Polyps.

a. Hyperplastic polyps are non-neoplastic protrusions of the colonic mucosa, composed of elongated glands that are made up of an overgrowth of mature goblet and columnar epithelial cells.

b. They are the most common type, accounting for 90 percent of all colorectal polyps. They appear grossly as discrete, smooth, rounded mucosal elevations of 1 to 5 mm in size. They frequently occur in the rectosigmoid area, but can involve any part of the bowel.

c. Histologically, they are composed of sawtooth crypts arranged regularly in a fibrovascular stroma (Fig. 8-8).

d. Hyperplastic polyps are not precancerous.

2. Adenomatous Polyps.

a. Adenomas can occur at any age, but predominate in individuals over the age of 40 years. Multiple lesions are noted in more than 10 percent of the cases.

b. Grossly, adenomas are pedunculated or sessile polypoid lesions, which occur in all sizes and shapes and have a characteristic raspberry- or cauliflower-like appearance.

c. Histologically, adenomas are composed of glands, the cells of which are lined by an eosinophilic epithelium with elongated nuclei arranged in a palisade or stratified manner. Different amounts of mucous and goblet cells are present within the glands, but mucin production by the cells is usually decreased. Mitoses are present along the crypt lengths and the surface of the glands.

d. When a polyp is examined, it is necessary to evaluate its stalk to ascertain the benign nature of the polyp and to rule out the presence of an invasive tumor. Resection of the lesion is curative.

3. Villous Adenomas.

a. Villous polyps are sessile lesions composed of multiple papillary projections or villi. They occur predominantly in the rectum and are larger in size than either hyperplastic or adenomatous polyps.

b. This type of polyp is considered to be a precancerous condition with areas of carcinoma that have been identified in up to 40 percent of the polyps.

c. Grossly, the polyps vary in size from 1 to 8 cm and have a cauliflower-like appearance.

d. Histologically, thin delicate papillae are covered by tall columnar epithelial cells showing variable degrees of nuclear atypia. Areas of adenomatous and tubular differentiation are present in a large number of cases.

e. Pure villous adenomas and mixed tubulovillous adenomas are considered to be precancerous lesions of adenocarcinomas. Surgery, with proper evaluation of the stalk, should be performed.

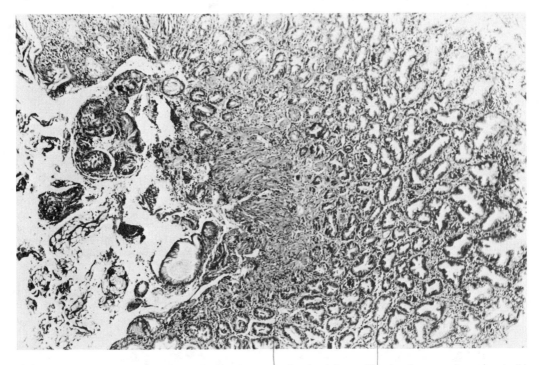

Figure 8-8. Low-power view of a hyperplastic polyp. Note the glandular proliferation [hematoxylin and eosin (H and E) stain, x 100].

Fibrous tissue   *saw-tooth crypts*

4. Juvenile (Retention) Polyps.
   a. These polyps are common in children, but they can occur at any age. The etiology is not known, but it is believed that the polyps either represent hamartomas or are the result of crypt plugging with retention of mucus and secondary inflammation. They occur in the colon and rectum.
   b. Histologically, they are characterized by the presence of cystic glands embedded in an inflamed fibrous stroma. The surfaces of the polyps may be focally ulcerated.
   c. Generalized juvenile polyposis is an autosomal dominant syndrome of uncertain cancer risk. Multiple (20 to 80) polyps are found in the colon.

5. Peutz-Jeghers Syndrome.
   a. A familial polyposis syndrome, Peutz-Jeghers syndrome is characterized by areas of hyperpigmentation, with melanin deposition in the buccal mucosa, lips, and fingertips and by polyps in the gastrointestinal tract.
   b. Colonic polyps are present in about 40 percent of the cases. The lesions reveal a mixture of both small and large intestinal-type glands, with broad bands of smooth muscle present in the lamina propria.
   c. The polyps can affect the stomach, small intestine, jejunum, ileum, and colon.

6. Cronkhite-Canada Syndrome.
   a. This syndrome is characterized by generalized gastrointestinal polyposis, alopecia areata, skin pigmentation of the oral region, and thick split nails.
   b. The polyps are cystic and resemble those in colitis cystica superficialis.

7. Familial Multiple Polyposis.
   a. In this disease, the entire colon is studded with polyps of variable sizes, generally of the adenomatous type. The appendix and, rarely, the ileum are also involved.
   b. Familial polyposis is inherited as an autosomal dominant trait and affects one-half of those at risk. The process is usually recognized during childhood or adolescence.
   c. The incidence of carcinoma in this disease is so high and cancers occurs so often in young adults that total colectomy is recommended once the diagnosis is established.

8. Carcinoma.
   a. Incidence. Colorectal carcinoma is one of the most common cancers in both sexes in the United States and predominates in individuals who are over 50 years of age.

    b. Etiology. It is believed that most carcinomas evolve from preexisting adenomas, but they are known to occur in association with other processes, such as chronic colitis, familial polyposis syndromes, schistosomiasis, and diverticulitis.

    c. Clinical Data. Most patients complain of constipation, but occult bleeding is common as are generalized weakness and anemia. The tumor can be demonstrated radiographically or by sigmoidoscopy, by which large necrotic ulcerated masses can be seen.

    d. Pathology.

        (1) Grossly, the tumor has an appearance that differs according to the side of the colon involved. A tumor that is present in the right side is usually <u>bulky and cauliflower-like</u>, with areas of hemorrhage and necrosis (Fig. 8-9). In the more distal portions of the colon, the tumor has a napkin-ring configuration (Fig. 8-10).

        (2) Histologically, most of the tumors are well to moderately differentiated adenocarcinomas, which resemble normal colonic mucosa (Fig. 8-11). Mucin production by the tumor is variable. A signet-ring cell tumor, similar to that found primarily in the stomach, may occur and carry a poor prognosis.

    e. Prognosis and Treatment. Carcinoma of the bowel spreads predominantly through lymphatics, but vascular invasion can also occur. The lymph nodes, peritoneum, liver, and lungs are the most common sites of metastases. Surgical resection of the tumor with viable margins is the recommended treatment, and cures may be obtained in 40 percent of the cases.

G. Other benign and malignant tumors such as leiomyomas, leiomyosarcomas, and lymphomas can occur in the colon. Their histology is identical to the same tumors occurring elsewhere.

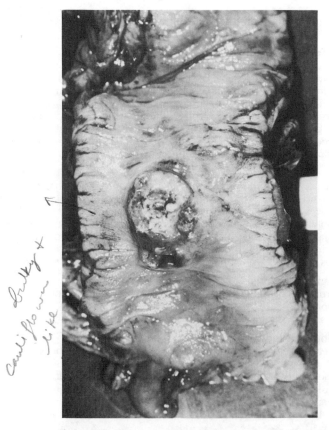

Figure 8-9. Gross appearance of a <u>carcinoma of the cecum</u>.

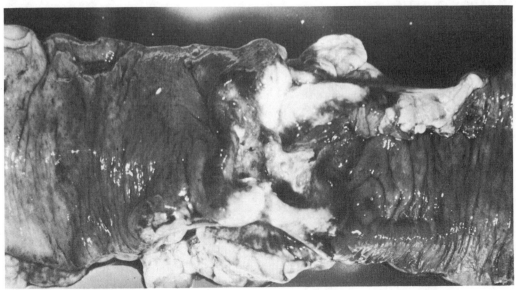

Figure 8-10. A carcinoma of the rectosigmoid, as characterized by a napkin-ring configuration.

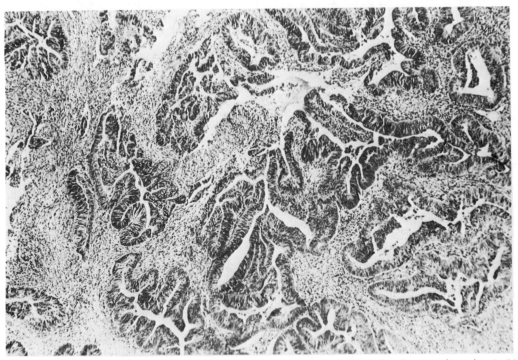

Figure 8-11. Medium-power view of a well-differentiated adenocarcinoma of the colon [hematoxylin and eosin (H and E) stain, x 200].

STUDY QUESTIONS

Directions: Each question below contains five suggested answers. Choose the **one best** response to each question.

1. What is the name given to a persistent vitelline duct remnant?

(A) Omphalocele
(B) Heister's diverticulum
(C) Rokitansky's diverticulum
(D) Meckel's diverticulum
(E) Nuck's diverticulum

2. Hirschsprung's disease is usually caused by the congenital absence of ganglion cells in the myenteric plexus of which segment of the large intestine?

(A) Cecum
(B) Ascending colon
(C) Transverse colon
(D) Descending colon
(E) Rectum & sigmoid colon

Directions: Each question below contains four suggested answers of which **one or more** is correct. Choose the answer

A   if **1, 2, and 3** are correct
B   if **1 and 3** are correct
C   if **2 and 4** are correct
D   if **4** is correct
E   if **1, 2, 3, and 4** are correct

3. True statements concerning Menetrier's disease (hypertrophic gastritis) include which of the following?

(1) It mimics gastric lymphoma in radiographs
(2) There is hypoproteinemia and plasma protein loss
(3) The gastric mucosa folds are thicker than 1 mm
(4) There is cystic dilatation of the gastric glands

4. Which of the following signs help to distinguish ulcerative colitis from Crohn's disease?

(1) Granulomatous inflammatory reaction
(2) Nontransmural involvement
(3) Predominant involvement of rectosigmoid colon
(4) Melanotic diarrhea

ANSWERS AND EXPLANATIONS

1. The answer is D. (*III B 2*) Meckel's diverticulum is a persistent remnant of the vitelline (also known as the omphalomesenteric) duct, and it can cause significant clinical problems. In about 50 percent of cases of Meckel's diverticulum there are heterotopic nests of functioning gastric mucosa. Peptic ulcers caused by this tissue can result in intestinal bleeding and produce a confusing clinical picture, which often resembles acute appendicitis.

2. The answer is E. (*V B 2*) Hirschsprung's disease, or congenital megacolon, results from a failure in the development of the myenteric plexuses of Meissner and Auerbach in the colon. Innervation of the colon occurs during embryogenesis and proceeds from the cecum to the anus. Interruption of this sequential development leaves the more distal segments of the colon aganglionic. In all cases of Hirschsprung's disease the internal anal sphincter is aganglionic, and in most cases the rectum and part of the sigmoid colon are abnormal. It is very rare that the more proximal colonic segments are affected.

3. The answer is E (all). (*II C 1 c*) Chronic hypertrophic gastritis (Menetrier's disease) is characterized by marked enlargement of the gastric mucosal folds well beyond the normal 1 mm thickness. These thickened folds produce radiographic signs that can mimic those of gastric lymphomas and some carcinomas. Hypertrophic gastritis can lead to excessive leakage of plasma proteins. There is cystic dilatation of the glands in histologic sections of affected stomach tissues, sometimes with glandular epithelial hyperplasia.

4. The answer is A (1, 2, 3). (*V D 4, 5*) Both Crohn's disease and ulcerative colitis are considered to be inflammatory bowel diseases, and, although there are many similarities between the two, certain diagnostic signs exist. Crohn's disease causes formation of granulomas in about three-fourths of affected individuals; however, granulomas are not found typically in individuals with ulcerative colitis. The ulcers and inflammation of ulcerative colitis are predominantly mucosal and submucosal in contrast to the more typical transmural inflammation of Crohn's disease. Occasionally, ulcerative colitis arises in the cecum or ascending colon, but it is more typically a disease of the rectosigmoid and descending colon. The diarrhea of ulcerative colitis is usually a mixture of blood, mucus, and fecal material, but at least one-half of the patients with Crohn's disease may also have melanotic stools; therefore, this particular sign is not a good discriminator.

The Biliary Tract and Exocrine Pancreas

I. INTRODUCTION. The conditions that involve the biliary tract include **gallstones** (cholelithiasis), **inflammations**, and benign and malignant **neoplasms**.

II. THE GALLBLADDER

A. ANATOMY. The normal gallbladder is a thin-walled sac with a capacity of about 50 cc. It consists of a fundus, body, and neck, and it is connected via the cystic duct to the common bile duct.

B. PHYSIOLOGY

1. The gallbladder performs two functions.
   a. The mucosa absorbs water and electrolytes from dilute hepatic bile, thereby concentrating it. The gallbladder epithelium apparently is anatomically suited to **concentrate bile**.
   b. During meals, the muscle of the gallbladder contracts, **propelling bile** into the small intestine where it actively participates in fat absorption. Two controlling factors in this process have been described.
      (1) The autonomic nervous system plays a minor role in the process.
      (2) Hormones, which are produced in the small intestine, perform a major role.

2. Entry of amino acids and fats into the intestinal lumen stimulates production and release of the **cholecystokinins** (CCKs), which make the gallbladder contract and the sphincter of Oddi relax, allowing entry of bile into the gut. Once bile enters the intestine, it acts via a negative feedback mechanism to inhibit further release of CCK. The sphincter of Oddi then contracts, the gallbladder muscle relaxes, and hepatic bile flows into the gallbladder once again.

C. CONGENITAL ABNORMALITIES

1. **Abnormal forms** include a bilobate or hourglass gallbladder.

2. **Abnormal position** of the gallbladder may lead to problems at surgery.

3. The **variability of the cystic duct** in length and course also can lead to surgical difficulties, especially when the area is inflamed.

D. GALLSTONES (CHOLELITHIASIS)

1. **Incidence.** Gallstones affect approximately 20 million Americans and account for about $1 billion in medical expenses annually. Gallstones are common in affluent countries, in which their frequency increases inexorably with age.

2. **Etiology.** Cholesterol-rich gallstones, which account for 95 percent of cases of cholelithiasis, are the result of a disorder in which the liver fails to provide enough bile salts or the proper combination of bile salts to keep cholesterol in solution in bile. The alterations in biliary lipid composition may result from genetic abnormalities in hepatic metabolism or from an extrahepatic abnormality (abnormal gallbladder contractility) that leads to a small bile acid pool. The association of gallstones with obesity suggests that gallstones may be produced by overconsumption of calories, especially of refined carbohydrates.

    a. In all Western countries, the majority of carbohydrates eaten is in refined form, as in sugar and white flour. In contrast, Africans ingest most if not all of their carbohydrates in unrefined form and are largely free of gallstones. The Eskimos have only become prone to cholelithiasis since they recently adopted Western eating habits.

    b. Cholesterol-rich gallstones can be induced in experimental animals by feeding them a diet with a high content of refined carbohydrates. Such diets are known to cause suppression of bile salt production by the liver and consequently result in a small bile pool.

    c. Gallstones are far more frequent in women than in men, and recent studies have shown that women have significantly smaller bile acid pools.

  3. Clinical Data. Clinical conditions commonly associated with the presence of gallstones are shown in Table 9-1. The mnemonic, fair, fat, fertile, female, and forty, as used to describe the typical patient who has gallstones, is only moderately correct.

  4. Types of Gallstones.

    a. Mixed stones comprise about 80 percent of all stones. They are multifaceted, laminated, have a crystalline appearance on cut surface, and are usually multiple. Varying combinations of cholesterol, calcium carbonate, and calcium bilirubinate comprise these stones; the specific composition determines the color, which ranges from yellow to green through brown. Mixed stones are associated with chronically inflamed gallbladder (chronic cholecystitis).

    b. Combined stones make up 10 percent of gallstones and are composed of a "pure" nucleus with a mixed stone shell or vice versa. These are the largest stones, and often a single one will fill the entire gallbladder. They are barrel-shaped, usually solitary, and also are associated with chronic cholecystitis.

    c. Pure pigment stones comprise 5 percent of all stones. They are dark brown to black, rough, sharp, pointed, small, and always multiple. Such stones predominate in Oriental countries and are seen in patients with cirrhosis. Bile duct obstruction, bile stasis, and hemolysis are common clinical associations. The bile in affected individuals shows normal or near normal levels of bile salts, cholesterol, and phospholipids but increased unconjugated bilirubin. The combination of elevated bilirubin and increased calcium content in the bile (secondary to stasis or an unknown mechanism) leads to precipitation of the relatively insoluble unconjugated bilirubin. The gallbladder itself may appear normal or show minimal evidence of chronic inflammation.

    d. Pure cholesterol stones comprise 3 to 5 percent of all stones and occur singly. They are oval, crystalline bodies, white to pale yellow in color. The gallbladder may show cholesterosis.

E. CHOLECYSTITIS

  1. Acute Cholecystitis.

    a. Pathogenesis. The inflammation is usually sterile at the onset. The cystic duct then becomes blocked by a stone or mucus, and the bile in the gallbladder becomes increasingly concentrated until it acts as a chemical irritant. At this point, an inflammatory response develops in the gallbladder wall. Secondary bacterial invasion then occurs unless

---

Table 9-1. Conditions Associated with a High Incidence of Gallstones

Cholesterol Stones
    Racial background: American Indian (>white>black)
    Demographic location: Europe (>North America>Asia)
    Obesity
    Certain drugs: oral contraceptives, estrogenic compounds
    Intestinal bypass surgery
    Increasing age
    Pregnancy (?)
    Diabetes mellitus (?)
    Hyperparathyroidism (?)

Pigment Stones
    Racial background: Oriental (>Occidental)
    Hemolytic anemias of various types, especially hereditary
    Cirrhosis of the liver

the cystic duct obstruction is relieved (e.g., by the stone falling back into the gallbladder). The organisms involved probably reach the gallbladder either via the lymphatics from the gut or via the portal venous system to the liver and gallbladder. In patients operated on within 24 hours of the onset of acute cholecystitis, culture of the gallbladder yields a positive result in only about 30 percent of cases; in patients operated on after 72 hours, the incidence of positive culture rises as high as 80 percent. The most common organism found is *Escherichia coli* (*E. coli*), but *Salmonella typhi* also may be observed.

   b. Clinical Data. Acute cholecystitis may develop in patients without gallstones, usually as a result of bacteremia from another site. It also may be seen following major trauma, in association with tumors of the bile ducts (obstruction), and in vasculitides. Acute cholecystitis is, however, nearly always associated with stones. Common symptoms are right upper quadrant pain, nausea, vomiting, fever, and slight jaundice, the last often indicating that stones are present in the common bile duct as well as in the gallbladder.

   c. Pathology. The pathology is that of acute inflammation with vascular congestion, edema, and polymorphonuclear leukocytic infiltration of the mucosa and the gallbladder wall. Mucosal erosion, ulceration, and foci of necrosis may be found.

   d. Course. Acute cholecystitis usually resolves, but it may become suppurative or chronic. Resolution is thought to result either when obstruction to the cystic duct is relieved by a stone falling back or when the pressure within the gallbladder forces the contents past the obstruction in the cystic duct.

   e. Complications. If acute inflammation progresses, the blood vessels running in the wall may become thrombosed secondarily, leading to gangrene and perforation of the gallbladder with spreading peritonitis.

2. Chronic Cholecystitis.

   a. Clinical Data. Chronic cholecystitis almost always develops in association with gallstones. It usually comes to clinical attention because of recurrent bouts of biliary colic or repeated bouts of acute inflammation. Other symptoms such as belching, fullness after food, nausea, heartburn, and inability to eat normal-sized meals also have been attributed to cholecystitis. Such symptoms usually are aggravated by fatty foods. Sometimes the complications of gallstones (e.g., acute pancreatitis, carcinoma of the gallbladder, gallstone ileus, or obstructive jaundice), rather than the stones themselves, are responsible for the initial symptoms.

   b. Pathology (Fig. 9-1). In chronic cholecystitis, stones are present in the lumen of the gallbladder and may be single or multiple; the multiple ones usually are faceted. Two or

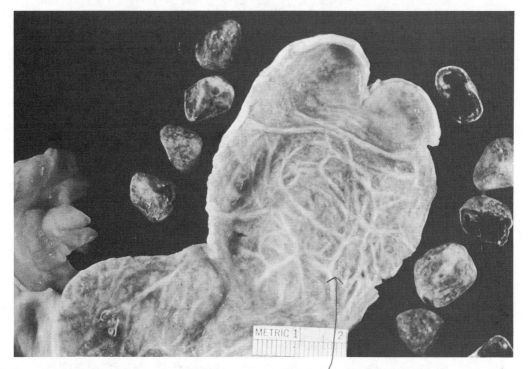

Figure 9-1. Opened gallbladder showing thickened walls with fibrous bands crisscrossing the mucosa. Numerous gallstones that were originally in the gallbladder lumen have been removed.

three different generations of stones, each generation being of comparable size, may be present. The wall of the gallbladder becomes thickened and opacified by each bout of inflammation and may become so thick that it occludes the lumen. Sometimes the gallbladder becomes grossly shrunken by repeated bouts of inflammation and is difficult to find at operation.

c. The **histologic features** of chronic cholecystitis confirm the presence of fibrous tissue as the cause of thickening in the wall. Often areas of mucosal ulceration result from trauma by stones in the lumen. Evidence of mucosal alteration (Rokitansky-Aschoff sinuses) may be noted. Although carcinoma of the gallbladder is rare, when it does develop, it almost invariably is in the presence of gallstones and chronic cholecystitis (Fig. 9-2).

F. TUMORS OF THE GALLBLADDER

1. **Benign tumors** (polyps and papillomas) may occur but are rare.
   a. **Polyps.**
      (1) Most of these are cholesterol polyps, which are not neoplasms. They appear as yellow excrescences arising on a small pedicle from a mucosa that is usually otherwise normal. Rarely, there is an associated diffuse speckling of the mucosa with small lipid accumulations, the ''strawberry gallbladder'' of cholesterosis. Cholesterol polyps may be found floating freely in bile having become detached from their site of origin. Under these circumstances, it is conceivable that they could provide nuclei for the formation of gallstones.
      (2) **Histologically**, the polyps consist of collections of foamy histiocytes containing cholesterol esters with a covering layer of columnar epithelium.
   b. **Adenomyomatosis** is characterized by hyperplasia of all the elements of the gallbladder wall. Although usually localized to the fundus of the gallbladder, it may sometimes occur as a more generalized process.
      (1) **Grossly**, the localized form, referred to as an adenomyoma, consists of a nodular protuberance, commonly with an umbilicated center. The cut surface is gray and cystic in appearance.
      (2) **Microscopically**, there is hyperplasia of the muscle layer and the mucosa. The mucosa forms branched tubular structures (Rokitanksy-Aschoff sinuses), which project into the muscle, simulating gland formation. Because of the resemblance to glandular tissue, adenomyomatosis often has been considered to be a neoplasm. Furthermore, the apparent invasion of the muscle layer by glands has led some to believe that the lesion is an adenocarcinoma. Both of these ideas are false. **The process is not neoplastic** but an exaggerated inflammatory and fibrous process; good evidence from the literature that malignant change has ever taken place in an area of adenomyomatosis does not exist.
   c. **Papillomas** (true benign epithelial neoplasms) are very rare in the gallbladder, although such lesions can been seen at the edge of carcinomas.

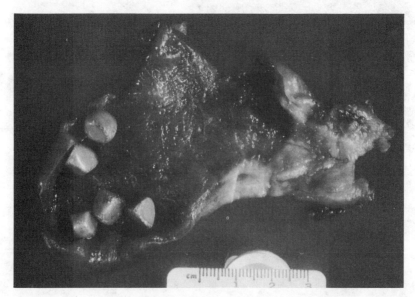

Figure 9-2. Gallbladder, surgically removed for chronic cholecystitis and cholelithiasis, containing an area of thickened wall in the lower end. Metastatic tumor was found in the liver as well as in the gallbladder.

2. Malignant Tumors: Carcinoma.
   a. Clinical Data.
      (1) Carcinoma of the gallbladder accounts for 1 percent to 3 percent of all gastrointestinal cancers.
      (2) It occurs most frequently in women (male to female ratio is 1:4), usually after the age of 50 years.
      (3) Gallstones are found in 80 percent to 100 percent of gallbladders containing carcinoma (Fig. 9-2). Although some physicians have postulated that gallstones occur as a result of the cancer, with fragments of necrotic tumor acting as stone nidi, clinical, pathologic, and experimental evidence opposes this view. Symptoms of biliary tract disease usually have been present for many years before the discovery of the neoplasm, suggesting that infection and gallstone formation are the primary events, not secondary changes, induced by the tumor. Other authorities have postulated that mechanical irritation caused by gallstones and infection leads to neoplastic change. Another possibility is that some carcinogen in bile induces cancer formation. Induction of gallbladder tumors in animals requires introduction of foreign bodies into the gallbladder lumen.
   b. Pathology.
      (1) Approximately 90 percent of carcinomas are adenocarcinomas. Pure squamous cell carcinoma is rare, but adenoacanthomas containing elements of both adeno- and squamous cell carcinoma are more common.
      (2) The majority of tumors are well-differentiated, with anaplastic growths accounting for fewer than 10 percent of cases.
      (3) Two-thirds of carcinomas occur in the fundus of the gallbladder; the rest are found mainly in the neck area.
      (4) Adenocarcinomas are usually of the scirrhous variety; the remainder are either papillary or mucoid in type. The scirrhous form spreads mainly by direct local invasion into the surrounding organs (i.e., the liver, duodenum, colon, stomach, and abdominal wall). Lymphatic spread may occur to the cystic duct node, then along the lymphatics in the sheath of the common bile duct to the pancreatoduodenal nodes. Extension along nerve fibers is common.
   c. The **prognosis** is miserable: the tumor typically is not diagnosed until late in its course, probably because the early symptoms resemble those of chronic cholecystitis and cholelithiasis, which patients may have had for years. By the time a new distinctive symptom (e.g., jaundice or severe pain) develops and the disease is diagnosed, extensive disease, liver metastases, or both usually are present. The only survivors of gallbladder cancer are those patients who have small tumors, found incidentally in specimens removed surgically for chronic cholecystitis and stones.

III. BILIARY TRACT

A. BILIARY ATRESIA is the most common fatal liver disorder in children in the United States.

   1. Pathogenesis. This condition results from a developmental anomaly of extrahepatic bile ducts, intrahepatic ducts, or both. The pathogenesis remains debated, but many physicians believe that the disorder results not from genetic abnormalities but from an intrauterine viral infection of the liver. Furthermore, they believe that the time during fetal development at which the infection occurs determines which portions of the duct system are affected. If infection occurs late in intrauterine life, an affected child may manifest neonatal hepatitis, which often resolves, and may have a normal duct system.

   2. Clinical Data. Infants with extrahepatic biliary atresia must be diagnosed and surgically treated early in life; if untreated, they develop fatal biliary cirrhosis by 2 to 3 months of age. Jaundice is the most common symptom. Intrahepatic biliary atresia is usually untreatable.

B. STRICTURES OF THE BILE DUCTS

   1. Whether congenital (rare), acquired (rarer), or surgically induced (unfortunately common), strictures (narrowing and fibrosis) of the extrahepatic bile ducts may lead to biliary cirrhosis.

   2. Clinical Data. The anatomy of the extrahepatic biliary tree is complex, with up to 20 percent of the population showing significant normal variations in the bile ducts, gallbladder, and arterial or venous structures. Thus, no cholecystectomy should be considered routine because the procedure can lead to serious bile duct strictures and eventual mortality. One-third of patients with strictures have lesions affecting the common bile duct or its major branches, and they often develop biliary cirrhosis and die as a result. Another group of patients with strictures die as a result of attempts at surgical correction.

C. STONES

1. Stones rarely may actually form in the extrahepatic large bile ducts but are more frequently a result of gallbladder calculi that have entered the common duct through the cystic duct. Gallstones in the gallbladder are associated with stones in the ducts in 15 percent of patients, and duct stones are thought to be left behind in 3 percent to 4 percent of cholecystectomies.

2. **Clinical Data.** If stones cause obstruction, there is a risk of infection and liver abscess. Unrelieved obstruction leads to secondary biliary cirrhosis. The common bile duct is narrowest just above the papilla of Vater, and it is at this location that stones collect, not at the actual opening. Pain, jaundice, and fever follow in 90, 50, and 33 percent of patients, respectively. With recurrent attacks of obstruction, fibrosis and stenosis may occur in the area of the sphincter of Oddi and cause acute or chronic pancreatitis. Stones rarely occur in intrahepatic ducts.

D. TUMORS OF THE BILE DUCTS

1. Benign tumors are rare, and most represent mesenchymal lesions (leiomyomas) rather than epithelial lesions. Carcinomas may occur at any point along the extrahepatic ducts; but most carcinomas arise in the distal common bile duct, with the next most frequent site of origin being the bifurcation of the left and right hepatic ducts. Both malignant and benign tumors are rare in intrahepatic ducts.

2. **Clinical Data.** Adenocarcinomas are the most common tumors. They are frequently well-differentiated, occur in elderly patients (in the fifth to seventh decade of life), and cause jaundice, pain, and weight loss. Carcinoma of the bile ducts is 10 times more common in patients with long-standing ulcerative colitis than in the general population, although the reasons for this are not known. Because of anatomy, curative procedures often cannot be attempted.

E. LESIONS OF THE AMPULLA

1. Stones may become impacted in the ampullary region and cause inflammation, fibrosis, and stenosis of the sphincter of Oddi.

2. Carcinoma (adenocarcinoma) of the ampullary area (Fig. 9-3) can cause symptoms by obstructing the flow of bile. The Whipple procedure (radical pancreatoduodenectomy) produces a 5-year survival rate of 40 percent.

3. Other lesions, such as papillomas, may cause biliary symptoms and jaundice by indirect pressure on the lower end of the bile duct.

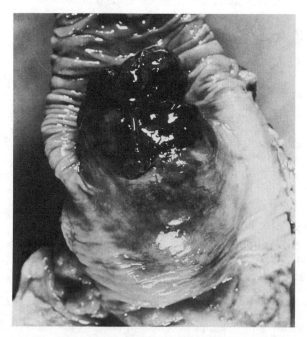

Figure 9-3. Polypoid, hemorrhagic tumor projecting into the duodenal lumen. It proved to be an adenocarcinoma of the ampulla.

F. SCLEROSING CHOLANGITIS is a rare disorder that is characterized by diffuse fibrous narrowing of the extrahepatic bile ducts; the intrahepatic ducts and gallbladder are usually involved to a lesser extent.

1. **Clinical Data.** The disorder manifests as obstructive jaundice. Males are affected more often than females, and the age at onset is variable. Onset is insidious, with nausea and abdominal pain followed by jaundice and pruritus.

2. **Definitive diagnosis** requires laparotomy. Criteria for the diagnosis include
   a. Diffuse thickening and stenosis of the extrahepatic bile ducts
   b. The absence of previous biliary surgery
   c. The absence of biliary tract calculi
   d. The exclusion of sclerosing carcinoma of the bile duct

3. The association of sclerosing cholangitis with other disorders has been noted.
   a. Inflammatory bowel disease (most often chronic ulcerative colitis but rarely Crohn's disease) is found in some patients. The etiologic significance of the bowel disease is uncertain, but the age at onset of sclerosing cholangitis is lower in those patients with bowel disease than in those without.
   b. Diffuse retroperitoneal fibrosis and fibrosing lesions in other areas (e.g., the neck and mediastinum) occur in some patients with sclerosing cholangitis. In such cases, a general disturbance of collagen or fibrous tissue may be responsible for the lesions; the origin of the fibrosis is unknown but may be immunologically mediated.

4. **Pathology.**
   a. **Grossly**, the bile duct is thickened and cord-like, and the involvement may be diffuse or segmental. Sclerosing cholangitis is always more widespread than carcinoma of the hepatic duct junction, but it cannot be distinguished grossly from carcinoma. The duct lumen is narrow and the wall grossly thickened in cross section. Gallstones are not found in the duct or gallbladder. The gallbladder may be involved in the fibrotic process.
   b. **Histologically**, the duct mucosa is intact, and inflammation and fibrosis involve mainly the inner and outer part of the wall. On rare occasions, hypertrophic changes in the mucosa have been recorded. Differentiation from carcinoma of the bile duct may be difficult, particularly when the carcinoma is of a sclerosing variety. When the periluminal system of glands that is present in the normal bile duct is distorted by fibrosis and inflammation, histologic distinction from adenocarcinoma is extremely difficult, especially when biopsy material comes from the ampullary area. The liver also shows obstructive changes.

IV. EXOCRINE PANCREAS

A. CONGENITAL/GENETIC ABNORMALITIES. Congenital malformations or abnormal locations of pancreatic tissue may not become clinically apparent until adult life or may remain asymptomatic throughout life.

1. **Ectopic Pancreas.**
   a. **Location.** Ectopic pancreatic tissue may be found in various parts of the upper intestinal tract, the most frequent sites being the mucosa of the stomach, the duodenum, the ileum, and the jejunum. Accessory pancreatic tissue is found in approximately 3 percent of autopsies.
   b. **Clinical Data.** If symptoms occur, they result from gastrointestinal obstruction by the ectopic tissue. Gastrointestinal bleeding and intussusception are other complications.

2. **Annular Pancreas.**
   a. In this congenital anomaly, a ring of pancreatic tissue originating from the head of the pancreas encircles the descending part of the duodenum.
   b. **Clinical Data.** Annular pancreas has more clinical relevance than ectopic pancreas because in a small infant its existence produces intermittent or permanent duodenal stenosis, with vomiting and failure to thrive as the first symptoms.

3. **Cystic Fibrosis.**
   a. **Clinical Data.** This is the most common cause of childhood pancreatic disease, although the degree of pancreatic involvement is variable. Eighty percent of affected children have overt pancreatic insufficiency manifested by steatorrhea or malabsorption. A sweat test confirms the diagnosis.
   b. **Pathology.** Cystic fibrosis is a systemic disorder, affecting all exocrine glands, in which a chemical abnormality in exocrine secretion results in impaction of secretions in the exocrine ducts. The resulting inflammation and scarring lead to atrophy of ductal and acinar tissue with consequent insufficiency of exocrine function.

c. The **prognosis** of the condition is variable, depending primarily on the extent of pulmonary involvement. The pancreatic enzyme deficiencies can be reversed easily by oral supplements.

B. INFLAMMATORY DISORDERS

1. Acute Pancreatitis.

a. **Etiology.** The exact cause of acute pancreatitis is unknown, but a variety of clinical conditions, the most important of which are biliary tract stones and alcoholism, have been associated (Table 9-2). The incidence of the associated lesions depends on the specific population studied; thus, series from large urban hospitals show a higher percentage of cases of acute pancreatitis associated with alcohol than with gallstones.

b. **Pathogenesis.** There are three theories.

   (1) **Reflux of bile and duodenal contents** into the pancreas **secondary to ampullary obstruction** (e.g., by a stone) causes pancreatic damage, with release of trypsinogen and trypsin initiation of a destructive cycle. Although an ampullary stone rarely is found in patients with acute pancreatitis, supporters of this theory argue that the causative stone gets dislodged.

   (2) Pressure in the pancreatic duct is higher than pressure in the biliary tree because of a spasm of the sphincter of Oddi. The spasm is attributed to increased intestinal secretions following an overindulgence in alcohol or food. The **pressure differences cause reflux** of enzymes into the pancreatic parenchyma from the duct system, initiating pancreatitis. Hypertriglyceridemia has been found in many patients with pancreatitis, including those seen after alcoholic binges; triglycerides may cause an increase in pancreatic secretions and thus raise duct pressure, starting the process. On the other hand, hydrolysis of the triglycerides by pancreatic lipase may release free fatty acids that are directly toxic to tissues.

   (3) Following some as yet disputed or **unknown initiating vascular event,** pancreatic enzyme leakage ensues and an inflammatory process begins. Increased blood flow, edema, and further enzymatic digestion begins a vicious circle of increasing vascular damage, stasis, and microthrombus formation. The greater this process, the more severe the pancreatitis.

c. **Clinical Data.**

   (1) **Signs and symptoms** include pain (mild to marked), nausea, vomiting, occasional jaundice, and fever.

   (2) **Laboratory data** may show leukocytosis, increased serum amylase and lipase levels, transient diabetes, and hypocalcemia (the latter is a grim prognostic sign).

   (3) **Complications.** Discoloration of the loin (Grey Turner's sign) and discoloration around the umbilicus (Cullen's sign) occur rarely but always indicate severe and extensive autodigestion. The appearance of an abdominal mass heralds the development of abscess formation, pseudocyst, or an area of fat necrosis in the omentum and is also of serious portent. (Cysts and pseudocysts as complications are discussed in IV B 2 d.)

d. **Pathology.**

   (1) Acute pancreatitis is an **autodigestive disease;** the gland is "cannibalized" by its own enzymes. The fundamental lesion is tissue destruction (from chemical inflammation) caused by various proteolytic enzymes, some as yet unidentified. These enzymes are released into the pancreas and surrounding tissues following an initial insult to the gland. The nature of the initial insult in general determines the severity of the resulting pancreatitis.

Table 9-2. Conditions Associated with Pancreatitis

Condition	Proposed Mechanism
Gallstones	Blockage of "common" channel
Alcoholism	Duodenitis and spasm of the sphincter of Oddi
Trauma	Liberation of pancreatic enzymes
Idiopathy	Unknown
Infection (mumps)	Inflammatory response
Drugs	Unknown
Hyperparathyroidism	Unknown
Pancreatic carcinoma	Ductal obstruction
Vasculitis	Ischemia

(2) If the insult is mild, cellular edema alone occurs, and the pancreas grossly appears edematous, with the changes fully reversible. If the cell envelope is breached or if there is arteriolar damage with ischemia and bleeding, hemorrhagic changes are seen grossly. If the insult is more severe, areas of necrosis develop, and, later still, there is frank sloughing of tissue with the inevitable sequelae of infection and abscess formation. Generally, the gross appearance of the pancreas is dependent upon the duration and severity of the illness when the gland is inspected.

(3) Secondary changes follow severe damage to the pancreas. There is an immediate **extravasation of extracellular fluid** (up to 30 percent of the total blood volume in severe cases) into the pancreas and surrounding tissues. Some fluid also may escape into the peritoneal cavity, but most collects in the retroperitoneal space. This is also evidence that the release of enzymes may have a **systemic vasoactive effect** and hence be responsible for the apparently irreversible changes seen in some patients.

e. Prognosis. Over 50 percent of cases resolve with treatment. Mortality increases in the presence of old age (over 60 years), cardiovascular disease, diabetes, or hemorrhagic pancreatitis. Clinical and biological restitution of the pancreas takes place if the primary cause or factors are eliminated. Should the cause of the disease persist (essentially gallstones in the main duct), acute pancreatitis may recur. Even here, complete recovery is generally observed if the cause is dealt with adequately.

2. Chronic pancreatitis (or relapsing chronic pancreatitis if the clinical evolution is marked by acute exacerbations) is characterized by residual pancreatic damage, either anatomical or functional, which persists even if the primary causes or factors are eliminated. Very often the course of the disease is inexorably progressive.

a. Etiology. Some authors believe that recurrent episodes of acute pancreatitis lead to chronic pancreatitis. However, in some series, acute pancreatitis has been shown to occur at a mean age of 50.7 years, 13 years later than the mean age of onset of chronic pancreatitis (37.7 years). Thus, other authorities feel that the acute condition may be superimposed on the chronic but that rarely does the acute form cause chronic pancreatitis.

b. Clinical Data. Pain of varying degrees is very common. Weight loss, hypoglycemia, and fever may occur. The fever is usually secondary to infection of a cyst or pseudocyst.

c. Pathology.

(1) The lesions in chronic pancreatitis, characterized by an irregular sclerosis with destruction and loss of exocrine parenchyma, may be either focal, segmental, or diffuse.

(2) Typically, early in the course of the disease, the lesions are discrete (affected lobules lie side by side with normal lobules). The fundamental pathologic changes include protein plugs in the ducts, some of which are calcified, a decrease in the number of acinar cells, which are replaced by dilated ducts, and sclerosis. At this stage, the duct of Wirsung is normal, but pseudocysts and acute lesions (more frequently edema than necrosis or hemorrhage) accompanying recurrent attacks of pain often are present.

(3) In later stages, the pancreatic duct is dilated and partially obstructed either by stenosis, generally at the level of the head, or by stones. The lesions become more diffuse, but until complete destruction of the gland (which is rare) occurs, it is always possible to find some fairly normal lobules revealing the irregularly distributed lesions. Perineural cellular infiltration and lesions of the nerves are a regular feature. Calcification is always located near the ducts.

d. Complications of Chronic Pancreatitis.

(1) Cysts. Pancreatic cysts can be neoplastic (see IV C 2) or non-neoplastic (unilocular). When pancreatolithiasis is present, the ducts dilate, producing intrapancreatic cysts **(retention cysts)**. These cysts occur frequently and may or may not communicate with a duct. All stages of development are found between the microscopic dilation of the small ducts frequently seen in calcifying chronic pancreatitis and these intrapancreatic cysts. A wide range of transition also exists among small intrapancreatic cysts, bigger cysts, partially intrapancreatic cysts, and large extrapancreatic pseudocysts, which have originated in the pancreas.

(2) Pseudocysts.

(a) A pseudocyst may develop, usually ventral to the anterior surface of the pancreas, following a single episode of acute pancreatitis or in association with chronic relapsing pancreatitis. Following acute pancreatitis, serosanguineous fluid from the pancreas can flow into the lesser sac, causing a peritoneal reaction and a cyst to be formed. This cyst is called a pseudocyst because it actually is an encapsulated hematoma. It may or may not communicate with a pancreatic duct. Pancreatitis is the cause of pseudocysts in 72 percent of cases; trauma accounts for 20 percent of cases. Sometimes pseudocysts penetrate through the diaphragm into the posterior mediastinum and are responsible for the manifestations of the disease, followed some years later by calcifying chronic pancreatitis (Fig. 9-4). Three elements appear necessary for the creation of a pseudocyst.

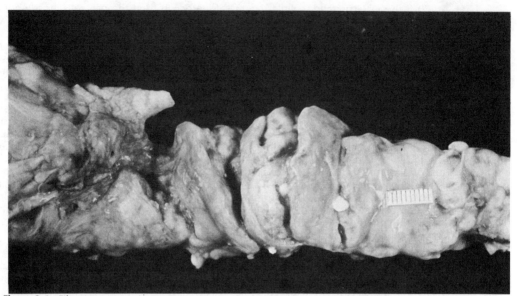

Figure 9-4. Fibrotic, narrowed pancreas with numerous calcified stones involving the main duct system. The patient was a 38-year-old man with a long history of alcoholism who died of complications of cirrhosis.

        (i) Ductal rupture communicating with a potential sac (e.g., the lesser sac)
        (ii) An actively secreting pancreas
        (iii) Interference with normal ductal drainage
    (b) Surgery is always indicated for pseudocysts because complications, including hemorrhage leading to a rapid increase in size, compression or thrombosis of the splenic vein, persistent jaundice, and infection leading to abscess formation and rupture into the stomach, are frequent. In contrast to acute pancreatitis, however, true necrotic pseudocysts are rare in chronic pancreatitis.
  (3) Some authors believe chronic pancreatitis may predispose to **cancer of the pancreas** (see IV C).
  (4) **Bile duct strictures** may occur, leading to biliary cirrhosis.
  (5) Subcutaneous **fat necrosis** may be noted.

C. NEOPLASMS

  1. Carcinoma (Figs. 9-5 and 9-6). Most pancreatic malignancies are adenocarcinomas, arising from ductal epithelium.
    a. Clinical Data. The incidence of cancer of the pancreas appears to be increasing in all age groups, with about 25,000 new cases now diagnosed yearly in the United States. Different symptoms are associated with tumors located in the head of the pancreas versus the body and tail.
      (1) Head of the Pancreas. Although a carcinoma here is usually painless, **jaundice** is a common symptom. (Courvoisier's law: painless jaundice associated with a palpable gallbladder is diagnostic of cancer of the head of the pancreas. The rationale is that neoplastic obstruction of the common bile duct leads to dilatation of the gallbladder in the face of continued bile production.) If the tumor invades the gut, weight loss and melena become additional symptoms.
      (2) Body and Tail of the Pancreas. Possible symptoms are **migratory thrombophlebitis**, weight loss, back pain, diarrhea, and an epigastric mass. Additional signs are lymphadenopathy, pulmonary symptoms (due to metastasis), and ascites.
    b. Pathology. The cancer, most frequently located in the head or body of the pancreas, spreads directly or by invasion of lymphatic, perineural, or vascular pathways to involve contiguous viscera (such as the liver). It also may involve other vital structures such as the superior mesenteric vessels and portal vein, or the tumor may metastasize to the para-aortic lymph nodes, retroperitoneal tissues, and peritoneum before symptoms appear.
    c. Prognosis. Although improved methods of diagnosing pancreatic carcinoma have led in some cases to earlier diagnosis, little success has been achieved in significant extirpation of the disease, and definitive resection still can be offered to only a small portion of patients.

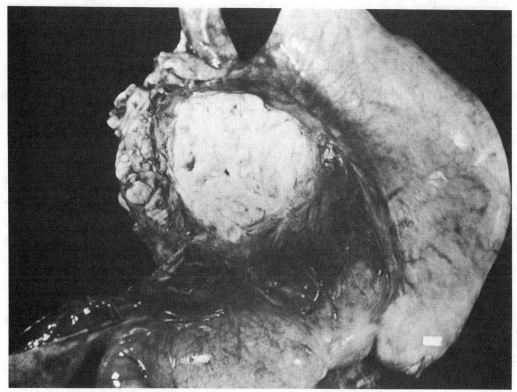

Figure 9-5. Large adenocarcinoma occupying the tail and a portion of the body of the pancreas and protruding into the lesser curvature of the stomach.

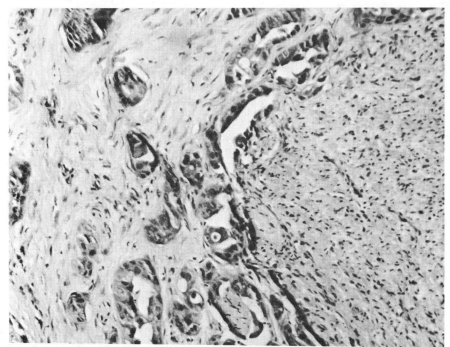

Figure 9-6. Common histologic pattern of adenocarcinoma of the pancreas, moderately differentiated (high power). Invasion of a large nerve trunk (as shown on the *right*) is a common finding in pancreatic carcinoma.

If the tumor is resectable (Whipple's procedure), patients with tumors of the pancreatic head have a 5-year survival rate of 5 percent, while there is a 0 percent survival rate for those with lesions of the pancreatic body or tail. In contrast, surgical excision of tumors of the ampulla or distal bile duct (which cause jaundice while the tumors are small) is associated with a 5-year survival rate of about 40 percent.

2. **Cystadenomas** are rare neoplasms and can be divided into two major groups.
   a. Microcystic, glycogen-rich, **nonmucinous cystadenoma** is a benign lesion usually found in older patients (seventh decade of life). It shows no sex predilection and may either cause abdominal pain or be discovered incidentally.
   b. **Mucinous cystadenoma** occurs chiefly in middle-aged women and attains a large size. It contains cytologically atypical or frankly malignant foci and is regarded as actually or potentially malignant. Sixteen percent of patients with this tumor are diabetic, but whether diabetes is related directly to the lesion or is coincidental is unknown.

STUDY QUESTIONS

Directions: Each question below contains five suggested answers. Choose the **one best** response to each question.

1. All of the following statements concerning gallbladder cancer are false EXCEPT

(A) it only can be cured by cholecystectomy

(B) it is found in 20 percent of patients over 65 years of age who are operated on for chronic cholecystitis

(C) most of the tumors are squamous cell carcinomas

(D) abdominal pain is a rare symptom

(E) men are affected more often than women

2. The criteria for a diagnosis of primary sclerosing cholangitis include

(A) demonstration of cholelithiasis

(B) the absence of previous biliary tract surgery

(C) the finding of vascular thrombosis involving the common bile duct and gallbladder

(D) discovery of carcinoma of the ampulla

(E) a history of ulcerative colitis

3. A 16-year-old girl with a family history of congenital spherocytosis enters the hospital for splenectomy as primary therapy for her disease. Surgery discloses

(A) chronic pancreatitis

(B) duodenal ulcer

(C) cholelithiasis

(D) chronic cholecystitis

(E) none of the above

4. A 67-year-old man presents with weakness and a 25-pound weight loss over a 6-month period. A history of vague upper abdominal pain, back pain, and intermittent diarrhea is obtained. Physical examination discloses a wasted appearance, pallor, and slight scleral icterus. Laboratory data include a hematocrit of 28 percent (the normal range is 38 percent to 45 percent), bilirubin of 3.0 mg/dl, and elevated phosphorus. The major diagnostic consideration is

(A) chronic cholecystitis with bile duct stone

(B) carcinoma of the body of the pancreas

(C) duodenal ulcer with penetration into the pancreas

(D) carcinoma of the transverse colon with hepatic metastases

(E) not enough information is given for diagnosis

5. Adenocarcinoma of the pancreas is associated with each of the following conditions EXCEPT

(A) a locally invasive neoplasm

(B) liver metastases

(C) jaundice

(D) back pain

(E) thrombophlebitis

6. Which of the following patients is most likely to develop carcinoma of the gallbladder?

(A) A 57-year-old man with an allergy to chocolate

(B) A 72-year-old woman with fatty food intolerance

(C) A 40-year-old American Indian woman with diabetes

(D) A 29-year-old pregnant woman

(E) A 47-year-old alcoholic man with multiple episodes of pancreatitis

7. All of the pathologic features listed below are found in pancreatic pseudocysts EXCEPT

(A) hemorrhage
(B) continuity with the pancreas
(C) location in the foramen of Winslow
(D) mucinous epithelial lining
(E) fibrous tissue in its wall

8. Complications of acute cholecystitis include each of the following conditions EXCEPT

(A) liver abscess
(B) bile peritonitis
(C) perforation of the gallbladder
(D) gallstone ileus
(E) empyema

Directions: The group of questions below consists of lettered choices followed by several numbered items. For each numbered item select the **one** lettered choice with which it is **most** closely associated. Each lettered choice may be used once, more than once, or not at all.

Questions 9–13

For each disease listed below, select the condition of the biliary tract with which it is most likely to be associated.

(A) Ulcerative colitis
(B) Sickle cell anemia
(C) Diabetes
(D) Alcoholism ∝ gall stones
(E) None of the above

C 9. Cystic fibrosis of the pancreas
E 10. Bile duct stricture
A 11. Sclerosing cholangitis
D 12. Acute pancreatitis
B 13. Salmonella cholecystitis

ANSWERS AND EXPLANATIONS

1. The answer is A. (*II F 2*) The only gallbladder cancers that can be cured are those that are found incidentally in specimens removed by means of cholecystectomy for treatment of cholecystitis. These tumors are uncommon, occurring as only 1 percent to 3 percent of all gastrointestinal cancers. For the most part they are adenocarcinomas, accompanied by abdominal pain similar to that experienced in cholecystitis and cholelithiasis. Women are affected more frequently than men.

2. The answer is B. (*III F 2*) Primary sclerosing cholangitis must be a diagnosis of exclusion. For the diagnosis, gallstones cannot be present, prior surgery cannot have been performed in the area, and carcinoma cannot be present in the region. Although fibrosis is found, vascular thrombosis is not. Inflammatory bowel disease, usually of the ulcerative colitis type, is common in patients with sclerosing cholangitis, but it is not found universally and is not required for diagnosis.

3. The answer is C. (*II D*) Patients with congenital hemolytic anemias such as spherocytosis form bilirubinate stones (cholelithiasis). They rarely have significant inflammation as is found in cholecystitis. Neither pancreatitis nor ulcers would be expected findings.

4. The answer is B. (*IV C 1*) Overall, pancreatic carcinoma is the most likely diagnosis. The relatively short duration of symptoms and significant weight loss argue against a chronic condition; therefore, chronic cholecystitis is not a consideration. A penetrating ulcer would present more acutely, and weight loss as evidenced in this case would be unusual. Although metastatic colon cancer is a possibility since the symptoms indicate malignancy, back pain would normally not be present.

5. The answer is A. (*IV C 1 a*) Pancreatic carcinoma of the exocrine type is an aggressive metastasizing tumor, unlike carcinomas of endocrine (islet cell) type, which can be only locally invasive. Liver metastasis is common in adenocarcinoma of the pancreas. Jaundice, back pain, and thrombophlebitis are widespread clinical findings in such cancers.

6. The answer is B. (*II F 2 a*) Cancer of the gallbladder is a disease that mainly affects elderly women with gallstones. Fatty food intolerance is the symptom of the gallstones and associated cholecystitis. A history of many years of gallbladder disease symptoms is often obtained in patients with gallbladder cancer.

7. The answer is D. (*IV B 2 d*) A pseudocyst represents an encapsulated hematoma resulting from the ravages of pancreatitis; no epithelium is present in it. Hemorrhage and a fibrous tissue lining are found. The location in the foramen of Winslow is characteristic. Since a pseudocyst results from pancreatitis, continuity with the pancreas would be expected.

8. The answer is D. (*II E 1*) Acute cholecystitis, which may begin as a sterile (uninfected) process, may eventually become an infectious lesion. Hence, empyema and liver abscess can result. The inflammation of the gallbladder wall may lead to its necrosis and subsequent perforation. Release of bile into the peritoneal cavity can produce bile (chemical) peritonitis. Gallstone ileus is a rare complication of chronic cholecystitis.

9-13. The answers are: 9-C, 10-E, 11-A, 12-D, 13-B. (*III*) The destruction of the exocrine pancreas in patients with cystic fibrosis may in some cases (10 percent to 15 percent) extend to the islet cells, and diabetes may result. Bile duct stricture most commonly results from operative mishaps during cholecystectomy (i.e., suturing or transection of the bile duct). In some patients with inflammatory bowel disease (especially ulcerative colitis), sclerosing cholangitis is found. In many patients with sclerosing cholangitis, however, ulcerative colitis is or has been present. The meaning of this association has not yet been identified. Acute pancreatitis may have many causes, but the major identifiable causes are gallstones and alcoholism. The exact mechanism whereby alcohol abuse produces pancreatitis remains unclear, but the strong association of the two conditions is a clinical fact. Patients with sickle cell anemia are prone to unusual infections, including salmonellosis. Salmonellosis may produce bone infections (osteomyelitis) or acute cholecystitis in these individuals.

I. INTRODUCTION. The disorders that often affect the liver are congenital, cirrhotic, infectious, neoplastic, and metastatic.

    A. EMBRYOLOGY. In the third week of fetal development, a shallow groove in the entodermal epithelial floor of the foregut gives origin to the liver parenchyma and the epithelial lining of the intrahepatic and extrahepatic duct systems.

    B. HISTOLOGY. The liver is composed of polygonal cells (hepatocytes) with granular eosinophilic cytoplasms and centrally located nuclei. The hepatocytes are rich in glycogen and lipofuscin. Lining the hepatocytes is a system of narrow channels, or **sinusoids**, represented by flat elongated cells in which the plumper cells (Kupffer's cells) of the reticuloendothelial system can be identified. The portal triad contains bile ducts, a portal vein branch, a branch of the hepatic artery, and lymphatic channels. A few lymphocytes may be present in this area.

II. CONGENITAL ABNORMALITIES

    A. AGENESIS or absence of the liver is incompatible with life.

    B. ACCESSORY LOBES (supernumerary hepatic lobes) are relatively frequent findings, particularly on the inferior surface of the liver.

    C. SITUS INVERSUS. The liver is present in the left hypochondrium.

    D. CONGENITAL CYSTIC DISEASE of the liver is associated with congenital polycystic kidneys and is caused by a developmental defect in the formation of the bile ducts. The cysts are asymptomatic, filled with clear fluid, and histologically lined by cuboidal epithelium.

    E. CONGENITAL HEPATIC FIBROSIS

        1. Clinical Data. This condition occurs in children and adolescents who present with hepatosplenomegaly and bleeding from gastrointestinal varices secondary to portal hypertension. A positive familial history is obtained in half of the cases because hepatic fibrosis is inherited as an autosomal recessive trait. Routine liver function tests are usually normal.

        2. Pathology. Grossly the liver is enlarged and firm in consistency. Gross cysts are usually absent. Microscopically there is diffuse periportal fibrosis in which islands of hepatic tissue are trapped. A large number of bile ducts may be either collapsed or markedly dilated.

        3. Treatment and Prognosis. Affected patients are good candidates for portosystemic surgical shunts, although the mortality rate is approximately 50 percent, due to complications such as renal failure and hemorrhage.

    F. EXTRAHEPATIC BILIARY ATRESIA

        1. Clinical Data. Most affected infants are chemically jaundiced from birth but may remain anicteric for several weeks. They have dark urine, pale stools, and hepatomegaly. Later, progressive cirrhosis leads to portal hypertension.

        2. Pathology.
            a. The **macroscopic appearance** of the liver varies according to the stage of the disease. At first, the liver enlarges, is dark green in color due to bile pigment retention, and becomes finely nodular as cirrhosis develops.

    b. Histologically there is cholestasis, periportal ductular proliferation, and bile plugs in the cholangioles and interlobular bile ducts. Eventually there is fibrosis with linkage of the portal areas and cirrhosis. In these late stages, bile lakes are present. Atresia of the extrahepatic biliary tree may be total, or the atresia may involve only proximal or distal segments.

  3. Prognosis and Treatment. Surgery to establish and sustain bile drainage can be performed but only in patients who have patent hepatic ducts. One-third of the surgically treated patients develop progressive disease with fibrosis and cirrhosis; in the remaining patients, death occurs within the first year of life due to hepatic insufficiency.

G. INTRAHEPATIC BILIARY ATRESIA

  1. Clinical Data. Affected infants present with pruritus, cholestasis, elevated serum lipids, growth retardation, and occasionally, mental retardation.

  3. Pathology. The hallmark of the disease is a decrease in the number of bile ducts, with less than one bile duct per portal triad. The entity is associated with α_1-antitrypsin deficiency.

  3. Prognosis and Treatment. Some affected patients respond to a treatment of diet and cholestyramine therapy to lower the serum bile acid levels to normal. In others, the disease progresses to cirrhosis and death results from hepatic failure.

H. CONGENITAL DEFECTS OF BILIRUBIN METABOLISM

  1. Gilbert's Syndrome.
    a. Patients present with intermittent and chronic jaundice, but the disease follows a benign clinical course.
    b. This disorder is characterized by unconjugated hyperbilirubinemia, attributed to compensated hemolysis and abnormal bilirubin uptake by the hepatocytes.
    c. The liver appears histologically normal.

  2. Crigler-Najjar syndrome is a disorder produced by the congenital absence of the hepatic enzyme glucuronide transferase, which leads to unconjugated hyperbilirubinemia. Clinically there are two forms.
    a. Severe. There is a total lack of glucuronide transferase, and clinically it is manifested by bilirubin encephalopathy (kernicterus), which results in death at an early age.
    b. Moderate. The hepatocytes have some levels of the enzyme present. Cerebral disease is uncommon, and survival is longer than that in the severe form.

  3. Dubin-Johnson syndrome is a process characterized by conjugated and unconjugated hyperbilirubinemia and is the result of a defect in the capacity of the hepatocyte to excrete organic anions. The basic liver architecture is preserved, but the liver has a characteristic black color due to a pigment, probably lipofuscin, present in the hepatocytes.

  4. Rotor's syndrome has the same features as the Dubin-Johnson syndrome, but there are no pigment deposits in the liver.

III. CIRRHOSIS

  A. INTRODUCTION. Cirrhosis is a diffuse fibrotic process that involves the entire liver, destroying its normal architecture. It is associated with nodular hepatic regeneration and necrosis of the hepatocytes.

  1. Clinical Data. Cirrhosis is manifested by portal hypertension, splenomegaly, esophageal varices, ascites, jaundice, and in the late stages by encephalopathy, defective coagulation with bleeding, endotoxemia, and renal failure.

  2. Morphological Data. The morphological division of cirrhosis is based upon the sizes of the nodules. If micronodular, the nodules are fairly even and about 3 mm or less in diameter (Fig. 10-1); if macronodular, the nodules are irregular, larger than 3 mm in diameter and surrounded by bands of fibrous tissue. If mixed, the sizes of the micro- and macronodules are seen in about equal proportions.

  B. CLASSIFICATION ACCORDING TO ETIOLOGY AND PATHOGENESIS

  1. Alcoholic Cirrhosis (Laennec's Cirrhosis).
    a. Etiology and Incidence. The relationship between hepatic lesions and alcohol intake has been known for centuries, and the incidence of cirrhosis in alcoholic patients is at least six times higher than it is in nonalcoholic patients. About 1 in 5 alcoholics develop

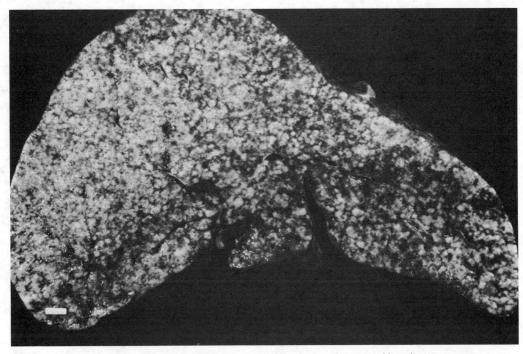

Figure 10-1. Micronodular cirrhosis. Most nodules have a diameter of less than 3 mm.

cirrhosis. The role and mechanism of ethanol in the pathogenesis of cirrhosis are still under investigation.

b. Clinical Data. There are ascites, jaundice, portal hypertension with esophageal varices and bleeding, hepatosplenomegaly, skin angiomas, and liver failure.

c. Pathology. Alcoholic liver disease can be divided into three types according to the histologic findings.

  (1) Fatty liver (fatty metamorphosis) is the most common. The accumulation of fat in the liver is caused by an increase in fat deposits and a decrease in the capacity of the liver to remove fat. The changes can be mild, moderate, or severe. The hepatocytes are distended by large droplets of fat, which may fill the entire cytoplasm. These droplets may coalesce to form large fatty cysts that produce an inflammatory reaction and cause the formation of granulomas (lipogranulomas). The number of lipogranulomas present varies in each case.

  (2) Alcoholic hepatitis can occur with a fatty liver, cirrhosis, or in a previously normal organ (Fig. 10-2). The hepatocytes are swollen and have indistinct boundaries, and the nuclei show degenerative changes. The affected cells are surrounded by or infiltrated with neutrophils. **Mallory's bodies** (hyaline bodies) or eosinophilic masses may be present in the cytoplasm of the hepatocytes. It has been suggested that these bodies represent elements of the contractile system of the liver cells. The combination of neutrophils, Mallory's bodies, and parenchymal fibrosis in the form of fine collagen fibers around centrilobular liver cells is almost always diagnostic of alcoholic hepatitis. This process is considered to be the major pathway of liver injury to cirrhosis, but it can be reversible in patients who stop drinking.

  (3) Cirrhosis is characterized by widespread alteration of the normal liver architecture with the parenchyma dissected by connective tissue that divides the lobule into segments. In each segment, the liver cells regenerate to compensate for the necrosis and then parenchymal nodules are formed. Often alcoholic cirrhosis is originally micronodular in type, but eventually the nodules increase in size and become macronodular.

  (4) Prognosis. Patients with alcoholic liver disease are prone to infections, malnutrition, and a relatively high risk of developing liver cell carcinomas. Once cirrhosis is established, the damage is irreversible and progresses to portal hypertension.

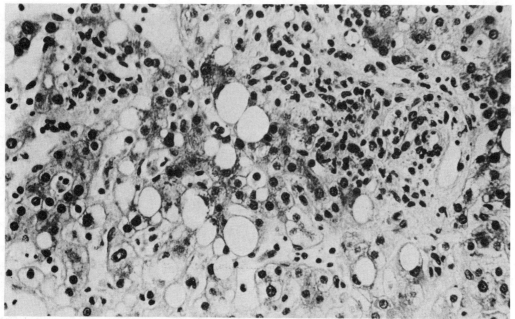

Figure 10-2. Alcoholic hepatitis with acute inflammation surrounding the hepatocytes and mild fatty changes (x 250).

2. Vascular Cirrhosis.

    a. Chronic venous congestion (cardiac cirrhosis) usually follows severe and prolonged right-sided heart failure and produces a firm liver with a characteristic **"nutmeg"** pattern on a cut section. Histologically, dark, congested, and hemorrhagic centrilobular areas alternate with paler midzonal areas that have a yellowish tinge from fatty changes. There is a loss of hepatocytes and fibrosis between the central and portal areas. The fibrous septa contain few inflammatory cells, and there is occasional bile duct proliferation.

    b. Budd-Chiari syndrome is a very rare disorder that affects men and women between the ages of 20 and 40 years with equal frequency. The etiology is not known.

        (1) Clinical Data. Patients present with ascites, abdominal pain, hepatomegaly, and mild jaundice. The condition should be suspected in individuals who have a tendency to thrombosis or tumors near the liver.

        (2) Pathology. The major feature is occlusion as the result of thrombosis in either the intrahepatic portion of the vena cava or in the large hepatic veins near their entrances into the vena cava. Microscopic changes include sinusoidal congestion with atrophy or destruction of the parenchyma in the perivenular areas and thrombi in medium-sized veins. When the lesion becomes chronic, there is centrilobular fibrosis with prominent periportal regeneration.

        (3) Prognosis. Most cases are fatal.

3. Metabolic Cirrhosis.

    a. Hemochromatosis (hemosiderosis) refers to an increase of hemosiderin in the parenchymal cells of the liver and other organs. The combination of cirrhosis and iron overload is the result of a variety of disorders.

        (1) Classification.

            (a) Primary (idiopathic) hemochromatosis is an inherited defect in iron metabolism, which leads to increased absorption of iron and its accumulation in the liver, pancreas, heart, and endocrine glands. The process is a gradual one and remains asymptomatic until the fourth or fifth decade of life when affected patients present with cardiac failure, cirrhosis, and diabetes.

            (b) Secondary hemochromatosis occurs in association with or as the result of disorders such as anemias, which are treated by blood transfusion, or alcoholic cirrhosis, in which iron overload occurs.

        (2) Pathology. Primary hemochromatosis displays massive iron overload associated with micronodular cirrhosis, which becomes macronodular in later stages of the disease. In both primary and secondary hemochromatosis, iron deposits are seen within the hepatocytes and fibrous septa; however, secondary hemochromatosis differs from primary by the presence of iron in Kupffer's cells and a more severe cirrhotic process.

b. **Wilson's Disease.**
   (1) **Incidence.** This is an autosomal recessive disease, which occurs predominantly in geographical areas of high consanguinity and is characterized by deposition of copper in the liver. The primary defect is not known.
   (2) **Clinical Data.** The manifestations, rare before the age of 6 years, are more common in older children and adolescents and include weakness, lassitude, jaundice, angiomas, fever, and hypersplenism. **Kayser-Fleischer rings** are virtually diagnostic of this disease. Laboratory data include low serum ceruloplasmin (less than 20 mg/dl), increased hepatic copper concentration (250 µg/g in dry tissue), and increased urinary copper excretion.
   (3) **Pathology.** Grossly the liver appears shrunken and shows macronodular cirrhosis. Histologically there are macronodules separated by thin fibrous septa, with cholangiolar proliferation and inflammation. Mallory's bodies are seen. Distribution of the copper is variable throughout the parenchyma but is easily demonstrable by special stains.
   (4) **Treatment and Prognosis.** The prognosis is poor if the disease is not diagnosed early. Therapy with penicillamine generally succeeds in reversing many, if not all, of the clinical manifestations or in preventing their appearance in asymptomatic patients.

c. **Alpha$_1$-Antitrypsin Deficiency.**
   (1) **Etiology and Incidence.** Alpha$_1$-antitrypsin, an enzyme that is synthesized in the liver, inhibits trypsin and other proteases in the normal human serum. Thirty-four alleles have been identified in the protease inhibitor and have been designated as M, F, S, and Z, representing intermediate, fast, slow, and very slow mobility, respectively. The α_1-antitrypsin deficiency is associated with the Z variant. Homozygous individuals with ZZ phenotype have a serum concentration that is 20 percent of the normal levels of the enzyme. Although not firmly resolved, it has been suggested that the absence of sialic acid in hepatic antitrypsin is one of the basic defects caused by α_1-antitrypsin deficiency.
   (2) **Clinical Data.** Children with α_1-antitrypsin deficiency often present with jaundice, neonatal hepatitis, or cirrhosis. In adults, the association of panlobular pulmonary emphysema with α_1-antitrypsin deficiency is well-known.
   (3) **Pathology.** Histologically, the characteristic feature is the presence of round acidophilic bodies in the cytoplasm of the liver cells, which can be demonstrated clearly through periodic acid–Schiff (PAS) stain. Additional specific characteristics are lacking, and therefore care must be taken to rule out other disorders before diagnosis.
   (4) **Treatment.** Medical treatment for this progressive disease has been unsuccessful.

4. **Immunological Cirrhosis.**
   a. **Chronic Hepatitis.**
      (1) **Etiology and Incidence.** This term refers to an inflammatory condition of the liver in which no improvement is shown for at least 6 months. Less than one-half of the cases are associated with hepatitis B (i.e., the hepatitis associated with contaminated needles). The remaining cases are of unknown etiology. Men over 30 years of age are most often afflicted.
      (2) **Pathology.**
         (a) **Chronic Active Hepatitis.**
            (i) This form may be related to the hepatitis B virus, but other forms of the disease occur, such as that seen in young women, in which there are high levels of serum antibodies. This disease is sometimes referred to as lupoid hepatitis because of the presence of LE cells in the blood of the patients.
            (ii) The histopathologic feature is called **"piecemeal necrosis,"** and it consists of severe necrosis seen predominantly at the edge of the limiting plates, near the portal zones and areas of collapse and fibrosis. It is characteristically accompanied by lymphocytes and mononuclear cells that extend into the lobules. Occasionally the liver parenchyma is intersected by broad and narrow septa of fibrous tissue (bridging necrosis), with inflammatory cells seen in any part of the parenchyma.
            (iii) The prognosis of chronic active hepatitis is poor, and cirrhosis develops in the majority of the patients, who may die within 2 years of liver failure or hepatocellular carcinoma.
         (b) **Chronic Persistent Hepatitis.**
            (i) This is a relatively inactive form of hepatitis. In most cases a sequela of acute viral hepatitis is characterized by enlargement of the portal tracts

with infiltration of lymphocytes, other mononuclear cells, and plasma cells. Ductular proliferation is usually absent or mild, and the lobules may be normal.

(ii) Differentiation between chronic active and persistent hepatitis may be difficult sometimes, but the latter should not be diagnosed in the first 6 months after the onset of symptoms or signs (abdominal pain or abnormal liver function tests).

(iii) The course is usually benign, and in most cases the lesion remains static or resolves over a period of years.

b. Primary Biliary Cirrhosis.

(1) Incidence. This uncommon disease occurs in middle-aged women. The etiology is not known, but the abnormalities that accompany the disease suggest an immunological origin.

(2) Clinical Data. It has an insidious onset in which intense pruritus is the initial manifestation. Jaundice, hepatomegaly, xanthelasma, and portal hypertension appear later. Laboratory data include elevated levels of bilirubin, serum alkaline phosphatase, serum immunoglobulins, and copper. The most characteristic sign is the demonstration of serum M-antibody by the immunofluorescent technique.

(3) Pathology. Microscopic examination reveals inflamed and swollen portal tracts. The chronic inflammatory cells surround and are closely associated with the bile duct epithelium. Granulomas may be found disrupting the ducts and also in the portal tracts, where there is marked ductular proliferation. Eventually the inflammation resolves, but progressive fibrosis and cirrhosis occur.

(4) Treatment and Prognosis. The course of the disease is variable, with some patients dying within a few years of the onset of symptoms and others surviving for 10 or more years. There is no effective treatment.

IV. INFECTIONS

A. VIRAL INFECTIONS

1. Viral hepatitis is a diffuse inflammatory process of the liver that is accompanied by specific clinical abnormalities.

a. Etiology and Incidence. It is often caused by hepatitis viruses (A, B, or non-A, non-B). Hepatitis A and hepatitis B occur worldwide in a sporadic or epidemic fashion throughout the year.

(1) Hepatitis A, a naturally acquired infection transmitted by fecal-oral contamination, is more common in children and young adults of low socioeconomic status. The incubation period is short (15 to 40 days). The prevalence of infection in the general population is high, up to 70 percent of adults. There is no evidence of a carrier state. Immune response against the virus is strong, appears rapidly, and gives long-lasting protection.

(2) Hepatitis B occurs at any age and has a long incubation period (50 to 180 days). It is transmitted by blood or blood products (fibrinogen and antihemophilic globulin), or by personal contact. Newborns may be infected by antigen-positive mothers during delivery or in the first few weeks of life; intrauterine transmission has not been proven. An estimated 5 to 10 percent of infected patients become carriers.

(3) Viral antigens can be identified in liver tissue by immunofluorescence or electron microscopy (EM). The hepatic lesion is probably the result of an immunological host response aimed at eradicating affected liver cells.

b. Clinical Data. The prodromal phase of hepatitis A is from 7 to 10 days, while hepatitis B is characterized by a much longer prodromal phase and an insidious onset and progression of symptoms. Both types of hepatitis may be anicteric and difficult to diagnose clinically. The symptoms and signs of the two types are similar. The symptoms include malaise, anorexia, nausea, fever, and upper abdominal pain, followed by jaundice, dark urine, and light stools. Laboratory data include a normal leukocyte count with relative lymphocytosis and elevation of transaminase, serum bilirubin, and alkaline phosphatase. In hepatitis B, the antigen may be detected in the blood several weeks before the symptoms appear, but it disappears after the seventh week.

c. Pathology.

(1) Gross Appearance. The liver is enlarged with a smooth shiny surface and rounded edges. The capsule is tense, and the parenchyma has a characteristic reddish color. With submassive or massive necrosis, the liver is smaller than normal, has a wrinkled capsule, and may have yellow or green regenerating nodules.

(2) Histological Appearance. There is diffuse involvement of the liver parenchyma, characterized by a combination of degenerative, inflammatory, and regenerative changes. The hepatocytes are swollen, and their cytoplasms become eosinophilic and granular. Shrunken cells, very eosinophilic and necrotic without nuclei, appear in the sinusoids or tissue spaces and are known as **Councilman bodies**. The borders of the portal tracts remain sharp with ductular proliferation and marginal cholestasis, but the limiting plates are intact. The periportal inflammatory changes are seen in the predominance of mononuclear cells, lymphocytes, and Kupffer's cells. Neutrophils, eosinophils, and plasma cells are rare. Early regeneration is reflected by the presence of mitosis and the increased number of bi-, tri-, or multinucleated liver cells.

    (a) Confluent Bridging Hepatic Necrosis. In some severe cases of acute viral hepatitis there is extensive necrosis of the hepatocytes with central-to-portal bridging necrosis. The portal tracts are enlarged with marked ductular proliferation and bile duct ectasia, and the limiting plate may be distorted by inflammation and edema.

    (b) Massive Fulminant Hepatitis. In 1 percent of the patients with viral hepatitis, confluent necrosis is so extensive that it may affect multiple acini or a large part of the liver. In these cases, almost all of the hepatocytes disappear, leaving only the reticulin framework and a small periportal rim of surviving hepatocytes. The sinusoids may be filled with erythrocytes, and endophlebitis is present in patients who survive longer than 10 days (Fig. 10-3).

  d. Prognosis. The majority of patients with viral hepatitis recover with no sequelae, but some patients develop cirrhosis. This is more frequent with hepatitis B and non-A, non-B than with hepatitis A. Some patients with bridging hepatitis retain a scarred or substantially normal liver, while others die of hepatic coma or their disease evolves to chronic active hepatitis. Approximately 70 percent of patients with fulminant hepatitis with massive necrosis die of hemorrhage, hypoglycemia, impaired renal function, and liver failure within 2 to 4 weeks of the onset of the disease. Only a few patients survive without sequelae.

2. Reye's Syndrome.

  a. The **etiology** is not clear, but the syndrome usually follows a viral infection (varicella or influenza virus B). Additional factors, such as reaction to toxins or medications (aspirin), are necessary for the development of the disease.

  b. Clinical Data. It occurs predominantly in children who present with fever, convulsions, vomiting, coma, and alterations of muscular tone and reflexes. Laboratory data show marked elevation of serum ammonia and hypoglycemia.

  c. Pathology. Histologically microvesicular fatty infiltration of the liver is a diagnostic feature. The hepatocytes are packed with small fatty droplets easily demonstrated by lipid stains. There is no cholestasis or necrosis except in fatal cases.

  d. Treatment. There is no specific treatment except supportive efforts.

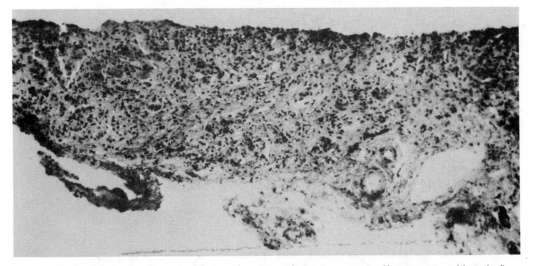

Figure 10-3. Liver biopsy showing acute fulminant hepatitis with massive necrosis of hepatocytes and foci of inflammatory cells (x 250).

3. Neonatal Hepatitis.
  a. Incidence. This presumed viral disease may be caused by a number of infectious agents such as cytomegalovirus, rubella, hepatitis B virus, and coxsackievirus.
  b. Pathology. Liver biopsy shows cholestasis, giant cell transformation, intralobular and portal inflammation, fibrosis, acidophilic bodies, and extramedullary hematopoiesis. The giant cells may have multiple nuclei and they contain bile pigment or hemosiderin in their cytoplasms. The number of giant cells decreases with age and are rare in patients over 1 year old.
  c. Prognosis. The majority of cases survive without serious complications.

B. PARASITIC INFECTIONS

1. Schistosomiasis is caused by *Schistosoma mansoni* in Central and South America, Africa, and the Middle East and by *Schistosoma japonicum* in Japan.
  a. Clinical Data. Lesions are caused by the host's immune response to the ova of the parasite. Patients may present with portal hypertension, splenomegaly, hematemesis, and ascites. Liver function tests are not greatly affected until the terminal stages of the disease.
  b. Pathology. The diagnosis is made by finding the eggs of the *Schistosoma*, which are characterized by their lateral spines. Large numbers of histiocytes, with formation of giant cells and granulomas, may surround the ova. Occasionally living adult *Schistosoma* may be seen within the veins. The liver parenchyma shows diffuse fibrosis, focal nodular regeneration, and inflammation. Portal vein branches are destroyed by endophlebitis, and the intrahepatic arterioles proliferate, forming a rich vascular network. The Kupffer's cells are hypertrophied and contain pigment. Scattered granulomas are present.
  c. Treatment and Prognosis. The treatment is directed toward prevention, with destruction of the intermediate hosts (snails of the *Australorbis Glabratus* species). Once liver damage is established, the lesions are irreversible.

2. Amebiasis. This infection of the liver, caused by *Entamoeba histolytica,* is relatively rare in this country.
  a. Clinical Data. The initial manifestations are related to the gastrointestinal tract, predominantly in the form of bloody diarrhea. Fever, jaundice, pain, and a tender mass in the right upper quadrant are indications of liver involvement. The right side of the diaphragm is raised, and direct extension of the infection to the pleural cavity occurs.
  b. Pathology. The right lobe of the liver is more frequently involved than the left lobe. Single or multiple abscesses develop and appear as reddish-brown necrotic cavities. Histologically, granulation tissue is present, containing acute and chronic inflammatory cells and degenerating hepatocytes. Amebae may be seen in the area of coagulative necrosis. They are round-to-oval bodies, 60 μm in size, with peripheral nuclei and the debris of red blood cells in their cytoplasms. Secondary infections may occur.
  c. Treatment consists of administration of amebicidal drugs and drainage of the abscesses.

3. Echinococcus cyst is rare in the United States but frequent in Argentina, Iceland, New Zealand, and Australia. The intermediary hosts are sheep, hogs, and cows. The infection is caused by the larvae of the dog tapeworm, *Echinococcus granulosus.*
  a. Pathology. The most common location of echinococcus cysts is the liver, but they can occur in other organs, such as the lungs and brain, and in soft tissues. Grossly, they appear as unilocular or multilocular cysts in the right lobe of the liver. Histologically the diagnosis is made by identifying fragments of germinal membranes or scoleces in the center of the cysts.
  b. Prognosis. Rupture of the cyst into the peritoneal cavity may result in a fatal anaphylactic reaction.

V. BENIGN NEOPLASMS

A. CYSTS. Intrahepatic nonparasitic cysts are rare and predominantly affect women (Fig. 10-4). They are usually multiple and vary from 0.5 to 1.0 cm in size. Larger cysts may be found in association with polycystic kidney disease.

B. BILE DUCT ADENOMAS present as multiple, whitish nodules scattered throughout the liver and are frequently misdiagnosed as carcinomas. Histologically they appear as a focal disorderly collection of bile ducts and ductules surrounded by fibrous stroma.

C. HEPATOCELLULAR ADENOMAS

1. Incidence. These are exceptionally rare neoplasms that occur in women between the ages of 17 and 60 years, with peak occurrence in the third and fourth decades of life. They are

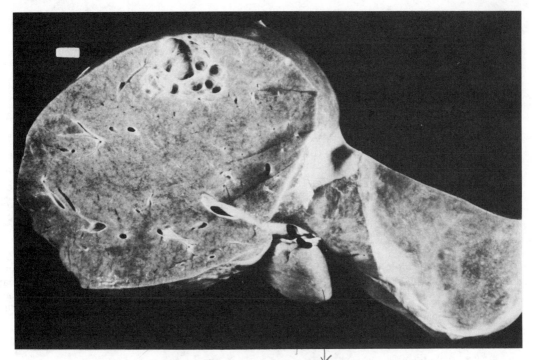

Figure 10-4. Benign cyst of the liver.

frequent autopsy findings. An association between oral contraceptives and adenomas has been established.

2. **Clinical Data.** Two-thirds of affected patients have a mass in the abdomen, but various gastrointestinal symptoms, such as nausea, anorexia, and pain, may be present. Other patients present with rupture of the tumor and hemoperitoneum. Hepatic function tests are usually normal, but a liver scan may show a filling defect.

3. **Pathology.** Grossly the tumors form a round-to-oval mass, well circumscribed, sometimes encapsulated, and lighter in color than the adjacent liver parenchyma. Histologically there may be pseudocapsules of fibrous tissue. The neoplastic cells are arranged in solid sheets and plates of hepatocytes 2 to 3 cells thick and separated by slit-like sinusoidal spaces. Definite trabecular patterns are missing. The neoplastic cells are larger than normal hepatocytes. Bile plugs may be present in canaliculae, but there are no bile ducts.

4. **Treatment and Prognosis.** If the lesion is not large, resection of the adenomas surrounded by a rim of liver parenchyma can be performed. There is no evidence to suggest that the lesion undergoes malignant transformation.

D. NODULAR HYPERPLASIA

1. **Incidence.** This unusual tumor can occur in both men and women, although it predominates in women in a 2:1 ratio. The ages of the patients range from 10 months to 75 years; the disease peaks in occurrence in the third to fifth decades of life. The etiology remains undetermined, but it has been associated with oral contraceptives.

2. **Clinical Data.** Affected patients are usually asymptomatic, but pain and hepatomegaly may be present. Rupture and hemoperitoneum are rare. Liver function tests are normal. Liver scans may show a defect.

3. **Pathology.** Grossly the right lobe of the liver is more often affected than the left. The lesion may be single or multiple and appears as a well-defined, unencapsulated mass, which on cut section has a typical stellate central scar, which divides the lesion into smaller areas. The nodules may be light brown, yellow, or white in color.

4. **Histologically**, the nodule is subdivided into smaller units by collagenous septa, which radiate outward from the central scar. Numerous bile ducts, blood vessels, and variable amounts of chronic inflammatory cells are present within the fibrous tissue. Large veins and

arteries are present at the periphery of the nodule. The hepatocytes in the nodule are richer in glycogen than are the normal liver cells. No bile retention is seen.

5. **Prognosis.** There is no evidence to suggest that nodular hyperplasia is premalignant; therefore, after the diagnosis is made by needle biopsy, the patients are followed carefully. There is no medical treatment.

VI. MALIGNANT NEOPLASMS

A. LIVER CELL CARCINOMAS (HEPATOMAS)

1. **Incidence.** Hepatocellular carcinomas are the leading cause of death in Africa and Southeast Asia and are rare in America and Europe. Young men are affected more often than women.

2. **Etiology.** Numerous synthetic chemicals, such as nitrosamines and Thorotrast, a colloidal solution containing thorium dioxide, used as a radiological contrast medium, have been shown to produce toxic damage in the liver, which leads to the development of carcinomas. Also, ingestion of aflatoxins (metabolites of the fungus, *Aspergillus flavus*), infections with hepatotrophic viruses (e.g., hepatitis B virus), and other elements can produce cirrhosis.

3. **Clinical Data.** Hepatomas do not produce characteristic symptoms or signs and therefore are difficult to diagnose. In patients affected by cirrhosis, the possibility of malignant transformation is considered when there is rapid and unexplained deterioration. The tumors may simulate liver abscesses or present as massive intraperitoneal hemorrhages. Laboratory data show elevated levels of serum alkaline phosphatase with normal or mildly elevated bilirubin. Alpha-fetoprotein can be detected in very high levels in the serum. Occasionally, systemic manifestations such as hypoglycemia, erythrocytosis, and hypercalcemia are present. Angiography and isotopic scanning delineate a mass in the liver.

4. **Pathology.**
   a. **Gross Appearance.** Hepatoma may present as single large masses, as multiple nodules, or as diffuse liver pathology. Most commonly, however, a large mass is identified surrounded by smaller satellite nodules. Portal vein thrombosis is found in a high proportion of cases.
   b. **Histological Appearance.** A variety of patterns, such as trabecular, pseudoglandular, scirrhous, or solid, can be recognized. In general, the tumor cells keep their liver appearance with different degrees of pleomorphism. Abundant mitoses and marked nuclear enlargement with multinucleation can be present. The tumors may contain clear cell areas, which rarely fill them entirely. Bile production, seen only in a minority of hepatomas, when present, is specific for these tumors.

5. **Treatment and Prognosis.** Liver cell carcinomas have a tendency to permeate quickly the intrahepatic veins and to spread to the lungs. Metastases to regional lymph nodes and the diaphragm often occur, but metastases to distant sites are rare. The prognosis is poor; most patients die within a few months of presentation. The only effective treatment is complete resection, but this is only possible in small, well-localized tumors.

B. CHOLANGIOCARCINOMAS (BILE DUCT CARCINOMAS)

1. **Incidence.** These tumors are less common than hepatomas. They are a disease of older individuals and affect both sexes equally.

2. **Etiology.** There is no association of cholangiocarcinomas with cirrhosis, but the increased incidence of cases in Japan is believed to be related to the infestation of patients with liver flukes (*Clonorchis sinensis*). The mechanism of action is not known.

3. **Clinical Data.** The patients may present with jaundice, pruritus, and weight loss.

4. **Pathology.** Bile duct carcinomas form scirrhous types of growth, which characteristically spread along neighboring bile ducts in a radiating fashion. The liver is bile stained, and secondary biliary cirrhosis may develop ultimately. Histologically, the tumors are adenocarcinomas with glandular formation as the most common pattern; however, papillary formation occasionally may be present. The tumors are frequently seen infiltrating the nerves.

5. **Treatment and Prognosis.** Intrahepatic spread is common, followed by lymphatic permeation to portal and peripancreatic lymph nodes. Peritoneal carcinomatosis with malignant ascites may occur. Although affected patients may survive for months or years, the ultimate prognosis is poor, with death occurring from liver failure.

C. **COMBINED LIVER CELL AND BILE DUCT CARCINOMAS.** Some primary malignant hepatic tumors demonstrate both a sinusoidal pattern of growth and bile production plus a glandular pattern with mucus secretion. The prognosis of patients with these tumors is very poor.

D. **HEPATOBLASTOMAS**

1. **Incidence.** These are rare but highly malignant tumors, which occur almost exclusively in children. They are twice as common in boys as in girls, with the majority of the cases presenting within the first 2 years of life.

2. **Clinical Data.** The usual presentation is abdominal enlargement, hepatomegaly, weight loss, fever, irritability, vomiting, and diarrhea. Jaundice is rare. Occasionally the tumors are associated with other congenital anomalies, such as renal malformations and cardiac defects. Some cases present with virilization as the result of ectopic sex hormone production.

3. **Pathology.** Grossly the tumors are solid, well-circumscribed, solitary masses, with areas of hemorrhage and necrosis. Microscopically two types of cells are seen. Epithelial cells resemble hepatocytes in varying degrees of maturity and are arranged in laminae that are two cells thick. Embryonal cells are small cells with small nuclei and scanty cytoplasm and may be arranged in ribbons, rosettes, or papillary formations. The mesenchymal stroma in these tumors may be undifferentiated and develop into immature bone or cartilage. A large number of cases demonstrate both epithelial and embryonal cells.

4. **Treatment and Prognosis.** These tumors are very aggressive and kill the patient by rupture of the tumor, leading to hemoperitoneum, through liver failure, or through metastasis to lymph nodes, lungs, and brain.

VII. VASCULAR NEOPLASMS

A. **HEMANGIOMAS**

1. Hemangiomas are the most common benign tumors of the liver. They occur at all ages and are usually incidental findings at surgery or autopsy. Rarely do they gain such size that they may rupture and lead to hemoperitoneum. Histologically they are identical to hemangiomas occurring elsewhere (see Chapter 5, "The Vascular System").

2. When hemangiomas occur in children (**"infantile hemangioendothelioma"**), they may be solitary or multiple; the latter frequently are associated with other vascular lesions. The mortality rate of these children is high, as the result of hepatic or congestive heart failure.

B. **PELIOSIS HEPATIS** is characterized by the presence of multiple blood-filled spaces not lined by endothelia. These hemorrhagic cysts communicate with sinusoids or central veins, and some may be filled with thrombi. Although not a true neoplasm, peliosis hepatis may be found in association with hepatic epithelial tumors. The etiology is not known, but some cases have been associated with the use of steroids.

C. **ANGIOSARCOMAS**

1. **Incidence and Etiology.** These rare tumors of the liver occur predominantly in adults. They are, however, the most common malignant mesenchymal tumors of the liver. Many cases have been reported in patients following the administration of Thorotrast. Also, workers exposed to vinyl chloride and arsenical insecticides may be afflicted with angiosarcomas.

2. **Clinical Data.** Patients present with hepatomegaly, jaundice, ascites, anemia, disseminated intravascular coagulation, or shock due to intraperitoneal hemorrhage.

3. **Pathology.** Grossly the tumors are usually multicentric, appearing as ill-defined, spongy, hemorrhagic nodules. The histologic characteristic is the presence of large, freely anastomosing blood channels lined by hyperchromatic and pleomorphic endothelial cells. Foci of extramedullary hematopoiesis are present.

4. **Prognosis.** The illness is brief and terminal. There is no effective treatment.

VIII. OTHER NEOPLASMS.
Tumors such as leiomyosarcomas, fibrosarcomas, teratomas, and lymphomas may occur in the liver, but they are very unusual there. When present, the tumors' histologies are similar to those of the same tumors occurring elsewhere.

IX. METASTASES.
The liver is frequently involved by metastases from tumors that arise in other organs such as the large bowel, breast, lung, pancreas, stomach, and skin. Practically all malignant neo-

plasms grow well in the liver parenchyma. Grossly they form multiple nodular masses that may elevate the capsule and cause central necrosis resulting in umbilication of the nodules (Fig. 10-5).

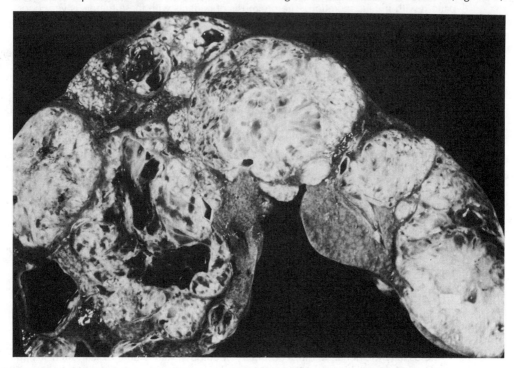

Figure 10-5. Metastatic carcinoma filling almost all of the liver parenchyma.

STUDY QUESTIONS

Directions: Each question below contains five suggested answers. Choose the **one best** response to each question.

1. Which of the following congenital defects of bilirubin metabolism is characterized by conjugated and unconjugated hyperbilirubinemia and causes a black coloration of the liver due to pigment accumulation in the hepatocytes?

(A) Rotor's syndrome
(B) Crigler-Najjar syndrome
(C) Dubin-Johnson syndrome
(D) Gilbert's syndrome
(E) Niemann-Pick disease

2. An adolescent who presents with lassitude, jaundice, fever, hypersplenism, and Kayser-Fleischer rings probably has which of the following disorders?

(A) Alpha₁-antitrypsin deficiency
(B) Wilson's disease
(C) Hepatitis B infection
(D) Gilbert's syndrome
(E) Idiopathic hemochromatosis

3. What is the clinical syndrome that is produced by obstruction of hepatic venous outflow?

(A) Reye's
(B) Crigler-Najjar
(C) Banti's
(D) Budd-Chiari
(E) Rotor's

4. What is the name that is given to the hyaline masses that are often seen in the cytoplasm of hepatocytes in patients with alcoholic hepatitis?

(A) Councilman bodies
(B) Negri bodies
(C) Mallory's bodies
(D) Zuckerkandl bodies
(E) Barr bodies

Directions: Each question below contains four suggested answers of which **one or more** is correct. Choose the answer

A   if **1, 2, and 3** are correct
B   if **1 and 3** are correct
C   if **2 and 4** are correct
D   if **4** is correct
E   if **1, 2, 3, and 4** are correct

5. Parasitic infections that occur internationally and affect the liver include

(1) schistosomiasis
(2) amebiasis
(3) echinococcus cyst
(4) filariasis

6. Liver cell carcinomas metastasize most often to which of the following sites?

(1) Lungs
(2) Portal lymph nodes
(3) Portal veins
(4) Central nervous system

7. Findings in liver biopsy of an infant with extrahepatic biliary atresia include

(1) periportal ductular fibrosis
(2) bile stasis
(3) bile duct proliferation
(4) peliosis hepatis

8. Conditions that have been commonly associated with the development of hepatoma include

(1) Laennec's cirrhosis
(2) aflatoxin ingestion
(3) hemochromatosis
(4) primary biliary cirrhosis

SUMMARY OF DIRECTIONS

A	B	C	D	E
1,2,3 only	1,3 only	2,4 only	4 only	All are correct

---

9. Conditions that can be associated with cirrhosis in <u>children</u> include

(1) galactosemia
(2) cystic fibrosis of the pancreas
(3) neonatal hepatitis
(4) α_1-antitrypsin deficiency

ANSWERS AND EXPLANATIONS

1. The answer is C. *(II H 3)* Dubin-Johnson syndrome is a chronic or intermittent form of jaundice with both conjugated and unconjugated bilirubin present in the plasma. Large amounts of yellow-brown to black pigment accumulate in the lysosomes of the hepatocytes. Rotor's syndrome is a benign, familial, chronic conjugated and unconjugated form of hyperbilirubinemia; it does not cause pigment deposition in the hepatocytes. Crigler-Najjar syndrome, types I and II, and Gilbert's syndrome are forms of chronic nonhemolytic unconjugated hyperbilirubinemia caused by a deficiency of hepatic bilirubin urinide diphosphoglucuronide transferase enzyme activity. Niemann-Pick disease (sphingomyelin lipidosis) can produce hyperbilirubinemia and obstructive jaundice in the neonatal period. The hepatocytes are pale yellow and vacuolated. Characteristic pale foam cells are scattered among the hepatocytes.

2. The answer is B. *(II B 4 b)* Wilson's disease is an autosomal-recessive condition that is characterized by deposition of copper in the liver. The clinical manifestations include lassitude, jaundice, spider angiomas, edema, ascites, splenomegaly, and the classical Kayser-Fleischer corneal rings. The nature of the primary abnormal gene product of Wilson's disease remains unknown. Laboratory findings include low levels of serum ceruloplasmin, increased hepatic copper concentration, and increased urinary copper excretion.

3. The answer is D. *(III B 2 b)* Budd-Chiari syndrome is the name given to the very rare condition that arises from obstruction of the hepatic veins. This obstruction can be produced by any one of many processes that impede blood flow from the liver. The result is acute severe congestion of the liver, with the sinusoids engorged by blood. The most important clinical manifestations of Budd-Chiari syndrome are abdominal pain, hepatomegaly, and ascites. Portal hypertension develops in all patients with this disorder.

4. The answer is C. *[III B 1 c (2)]* Hyaline bodies in the cytoplasm of the hepatocytes of patients with alcoholic hepatitis are termed Mallory's bodies. As observed under the light microscope, Mallory's bodies have a refractile eosinophilic appearance and are composed of a mass of cytoplasmic fibrils. The presence of Mallory's bodies is characteristic of alcohol-induced hepatic disease; however, they can be seen in other types of hepatic disease on occasion.

5. The answer is A (1, 2, 3). *(IV B)* Numerous parasitic diseases infect the liver, although many do not occur commonly in the United States. Schistosomiasis, amebiasis, and echinococcus cyst all can affect the liver. Filariasis, on the other hand, is caused by a parasite that enters through the skin, permeates the lymphatics, and localizes in regional lymph node groups, particularly in the lower extremities. The resulting lymphatic obstruction is termed elephantiasis.

6. The answer is A (1, 2, 3). *(VI A)* The metastatic patterns of hepatocellular carcinomas that arise in normal and in cirrhotic livers are somewhat different; however, in neither instance is metatasis to the central nervous system frequent. At autopsy, more metastases are found from hepatocellular carcinomas arising in normal livers than from those growing in cirrhotic livers. In either case, the prognosis for patients with these tumors is poor, with survival of only several months.

7. The answer is A (1, 2, 3). *(II F)* Extrahepatic biliary atresia accounts for about one-third of the cases of neonatal obstructive jaundice. This condition is not believed to result from failure of recanalization of the embryonic duct system but rather is an abnormality that develops during late pregnancy or soon after birth. Periportal ductular fibrosis, bile stasis, and bile duct proliferation are all seen in biopsies of affected infants. Peliosis hepatis is the presence of large, blood-filled cavities in the liver with accompanying areas of sinusoidal dilatation.

8. The answer is A (1, 2, 3). *(VI A)* Hepatocellular carcinoma (hepatoma) is a leading cause of death in parts of Africa and Southeast Asia yet is relatively uncommon in the United States. Exposure to a number of carcinogenic agents, including nitrosamines and thorium dioxide, ingestion of aflatoxins, hepatitis B viral infection, and chronic excessive alcohol ingestion have been related to development of hepatoma. Hepatocellular carcinoma is a very rare complication of primary biliary cirrhosis.

9. The answer is E (all). *(Chapter 10)* Congenital absence of galactose-1-phosphate uridyl transferase is a rare disorder that produces galactosemia; it is associated with cirrhosis in infants who survive more than a few months. Although a causal relationship of α_1-antitrypsin deficiency to cirrhosis has not been firmly proven, an association between the two clearly exists and was first recognized in children. The abnormal mucus secreted in cystic fibrosis of the pancreas can cause biliary tract obstruction, producing a true biliary obstructive cirrhosis. Neonatal hepatitis is a descriptive term for cases of prolonged obstructive jaundice with characteristic histologic changes but without a specific etiology. Approximately 15 to 25 percent of infants with neonatal hepatitis develop persistent liver disease or cirrhosis.

I. INTRODUCTION. The kidney has its origins in two mesodermal structures. The renal pelvis, renal calices, collecting tubules, and ureters are derived from the ureteric bud, an outgrowth of the mesonephric duct. The glomeruli, proximal and distal tubules, and Henle's loop are derived from the metanephric blastema.

Each adult kidney weighs between 120 and 150 g and is covered by a thin capsule known as Gerota's fascia, which peels off and contains different amounts of fatty tissue. A cut section shows a reddish-brown cortex approximately 1.5 cm in thickness and a lighter medulla. The latter contains the pyramids separated by fibrous tissue, ending in blunt tips or papillae that extend into the calices. The basic elements of the kidney are the glomeruli, tubules, interstitium, and blood supply.

This chapter will review disorders of the kidney and urinary tract system, which include the following.

A. CONGENITAL ANOMALIES

B. DISEASES OF THE GLOMERULI

C. TUBULAR DISORDERS

D. DISEASES OF THE INTERSTITIUM

E. HYPERTENSION

F. BENIGN RENAL NEOPLASMS

G. MALIGNANT RENAL NEOPLASMS

H. DISORDERS OF THE URINARY COLLECTING SYSTEM

II. CONGENITAL ANOMALIES

A. AGENESIS refers to absence of one or both kidneys. While bilateral agenesis is incompatible with life, unilateral agenesis is compatible with normal renal function. Agenesis may be due to congenital absence of the nephrogenic primordium or failure of the wolffian duct to contact the metanephric blastema.

B. HYPOPLASIA is the failure of the kidneys to develop to normal weight (150 g); each may vary in weight from 50 to 100 g. Hypoplasia is usually unilateral, and the affected kidney is a frequent site of infections.

C. HORSESHOE KIDNEY is produced by fusion of the renal blastema and most commonly involves the region of the lower pole, although it can occur in other regions of the kidney. The kidneys are connected by fibrous tissue or by an isthmus of renal parenchyma. It is not an uncommon finding at autopsy, and renal function is not impaired.

D. CYSTIC LESIONS

1. **Simple cysts** are common postmortem findings of little clinical significance. They result from inflammation and scarring, which create cystic dilatation of the proximal nephron. Rarely cysts may reach large sizes and are clinically palpable.

2. **Polycystic Kidneys.**
   a. **Incidence.** This condition is present in about 1 of 500 autopsies. The etiology is not completely understood, but the entity is believed to be due to some abnormalities in the formation of the fetal kidney.
   b. **Clinical Data.** The anomaly may lead to renal failure and death during infancy, or it may be asymptomatic until later decades, depending upon the type of abnormality. Occasionally, affected patients present with abdominal pain, hematuria, polyuria, hypertension, and renal failure.
   c. **Types.**
      (1) **Type I** is produced by dilatation and hyperplasia of the collecting tubules, which are lined by a single layer of low cuboidal cells. Varying numbers of normal glomeruli can be demonstrated under the renal capsule. The disease is bilateral, symmetrical, and usually fatal soon after birth. The occurrence in siblings suggests a heredofamilial trait believed to be the homozygous state of a recessive autosomal gene.
      (2) **Type II** is produced by inhibition of ureteral ampullary activity (i.e., failure of the ureteral ampullary region to branch). Histologically there are thick-walled cysts of variable sizes. Between the cysts there is an increased amount of fibroconnective tissue, which may contain blood vessels, nerves, and occasionally islands of cartilage. The disease may be bilateral, unilateral, or affect only a portion of one kidney. If the disease is bilateral, it is incompatible with life and therefore is only found in stillborns and infants.
      (3) **Type III** is characterized by an admixture of normal and abnormal nephrons. The disease is most frequently bilateral in adults, who present with impaired renal function during the fifth or sixth decade of life. Death occurs as a consequence of vascular or infectious complications. The disease appears to be inherited as an autosomal dominant gene of low penetrance.
         (a) **Gross Appearance.** The kidneys are enlarged, and normal parenchyma is replaced by multiple cystic cavities of different sizes (Fig. 11-1).
         (b) **Microscopic examination** shows the cysts filled with clear fluid and lined by cuboidal epithelia and scattered functioning nephrons. The cysts originate from the tubules, nephrons, or Bowman's capsule and are usually so large that they press upon any adjacent structure such as the renal pelvis.

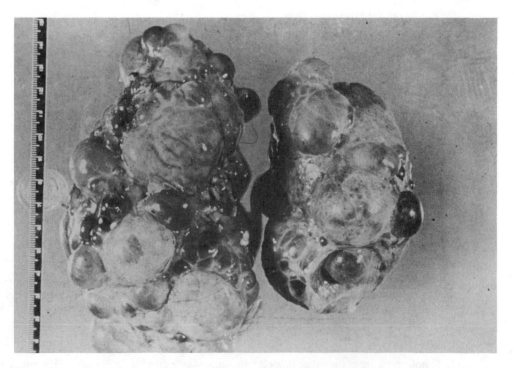

Figure 11-1. Adult polycystic kidney disease. The renal parenchyma is replaced by multiple cystic spaces.

III. DISEASES OF THE GLOMERULI

A. GENERAL CONSIDERATIONS

1. **Responses.**
   a. **Cellular Proliferation.** There is mesangial, endothelial, and epithelial proliferation.
   b. **Leukocytic infiltration** occurs in some inflammatory processes where the glomerulus is infiltrated by neutrophils and monocytes.
   c. **Thickening of the basement membrane** of the peripheral capillary loops is the result of deposition of abnormal amorphous dense material of immunocomplexes on the epithelial side of the membrane.
   d. **Sclerosis or hyalinization** occurs from the deposition of additional mesangial matrix.

2. **Mechanisms.** Most forms of glomerular injury are immunologically mediated by various mechanisms, such as complement leukocyte–independent injury and complement neutrophil–independent injury. In addition, the glomerulus may lose its normal structural organization. Two types of injury are recognized.
   a. **Immune complex nephritis** results from the deposition of antigen-antibody complexes on the glomerulus. These complexes may be formed in the circulation or in situ in the basement membrane.
   b. **Antiglomerular basement membrane** results from the fixation of antibodies directed against the glomerular basement membrane itself. This process may be the result of exogenous antigens, such as foreign protein and microbial antigens, or endogenous antigens derived from the patient's own tissues (DNA-antiDNA complexes seen in systemic lupus erythematosus).
   c. Following the deposition of immune complexes, injury is mediated by different mechanisms that include complement leukocyte–dependent injury and complement neutrophil–independent injury.

B. NEPHROTIC SYNDROME is the most common clinical syndrome associated with glomerular disease. The syndrome is characterized by marked proteinuria (more than 3 g/day), decreased levels of plasma proteins, an increase in serum lipids, and generalized edema.

1. **Lipoid Nephrosis.**
   a. **Incidence.** Lipoid nephrosis is the most common cause in children of nephrotic syndrome, comprising approximately 90 percent of all cases. In adults it accounts for 15 to 30 percent of all cases. There is no known immunologic mechanism involved.
   b. **Clinical Data.** Affected patients usually have selective proteinuria but otherwise demonstrate normal renal function.
   c. **Pathology.** The lack of specific lesions seen by light microscopy is called nil or minimal change disease. Electron microscopy (EM) studies show extensive foot process obliteration, and specialized histochemical studies reveal a reduction in negatively charged glycoproteins. There are no immune complex deposits.
   d. **Treatment.** The disease is highly responsive to steroid therapy, but a small proportion of patients progress to renal insufficiency. These patients may respond to combined steroid and cytotoxic agents.

2. **Membranous Glomerulonephropathy.**
   a. **Incidence.** It is the most common cause of nephrotic syndrome in adults and is very rare in children.
   b. **Etiology.** Most cases are idiopathic, but, in a small percentage, they are associated with known antigens such as infectious agents (e.g., malaria, schistosomiasis, and hepatitis BsAg), drugs such as gold therapy, or tumors such as colon carcinomas and lymphomas.
   c. **Clinical Data.** It is characterized by severe nonselective proteinuria, with both albumin and globulins excreted in the urine.
   d. **Pathology.** Thickening of the capillary wall is seen by light microscopy. EM studies show the presence of intramembranous and epimembranous dense deposits of immunoglobulin, which by immunofluorescence are proven to be immunoglobulin G (IgG) or immunoglobulin M (IgM), and the third component of complement (C_3) deposited in a granular pattern along the capillary wall.
   e. **Treatment and Prognosis.** Affected patients generally experience a long indolent course with occasional spontaneous remissions, but sometimes there is progression to renal insufficiency. Although no specific therapy has been proven successful, steroid therapy helps in preventing progression to renal insufficiency.

3. **Diabetes Mellitus.**
   a. **Incidence.** Diabetes mellitus is a systemic disease that involves the kidneys. "Diabetic

nephropathy" encompasses a variety of renal lesions such as nephrotic syndrome, arterionephrosclerosis, glomerulosclerosis, and pyelonephritis. The renal symptoms may appear from 10 to 20 years after the onset of the disease, and they usually accompany other microangiopathic manifestations such as retinopathy, coronary artery disease, and peripheral vascular insufficiency.

   b. Clinical Data. The predominant symptoms are proteinuria, glucosuria, and a progressive decrease in renal function. Dependent edema and hypertension may be late manifestations.

   c. Pathology. Histologically a variety of lesions involving the vessels, tubules, and interstitium can be found.

   (1) **Glomerulosclerosis** occurs several years after onset of diabetes mellitus and is characterized by two histologic forms. Combinations of nodular and diffuse glomerulosclerosis are common. Immunofluorescent studies show ultralinear IgG and IgM along the glomerular and tubular basement membranes.

   (a) In **nodular glomerulosclerosis** or **Kimmelstiel-Wilson lesions** there are nodules of acellular hyaline material in the glomerulus, surrounded by dilated capillary loops. There is an increase in the number of mesangial cells in the central masses and microaneurysmal dilatation of adjacent peripheral capillaries. The syndrome occurs 10 to 20 years after onset of the disease.

   (b) In **diffuse glomerulosclerosis** there is nonspecific capillary thickening with increased deposition of normal basement membrane—like material. The mesangial matrix is increased, and there are focal collections of lipid and calcium.

   (2) Advanced lesions are associated with glomerular atrophy, hyaline degeneration of the glomerulus, and narrowing of spiral papillary arteries, leading to anoxia of the inner renal medulla, papillary necrosis, and, eventually, renal failure. Diabetic patients are also susceptible to renal infections, specifically to pyelonephritis. The disease has a progressive course, and although glomerular abnormalities can be demonstrated soon after the onset of diabetes, clinical signs of renal dysfunction are indicative of poor prognosis. Treatment is directed at control of the diabetes.

4. Amyloidosis. Renal involvement, one of the most common and serious manifestations of amyloidosis, occurs with frequency in the secondary forms of the disease but also occurs in primary amyloidosis and in association with multiple myeloma.

   a. Clinical Data. Amyloidosis is found predominantly in adults who present with proteinuria, chronic renal failure, and nephrotic syndrome. Other symptoms may be related to organs other than the kidney, such as the heart, thyroid, or bowel if affected by amyloidosis.

   b. Pathology.
   (1) **Gross Appearance.** The kidneys are usually enlarged and have a waxy appearance, but cases in which the size of the kidney is normal or smaller than normal have been reported.

   (2) **Histological Appearance.** There is evidence of a pink, eosinophilic acellular material deposited in the mesangium and capillary walls, which causes irregular thickening and capillary narrowing with eventual obliteration of the glomerular capillaries. With progression of the disease, deposits of amyloid in the blood vessels, interstitium, and tubular basement membrane also appear, causing parenchymal atrophy and occasional papillary necrosis. This eosinophilic material stains positive with crystal violet and congo red and shows a characteristic green birefringence under polarized light with the latter stain. EM shows accumulation of fibrils, which are 75 Å to 80 Å in diameter. Immunofluorescence does not show a specific pattern.

   c. Treatment and Prognosis. There is no successful treatment for amyloidosis, but steroids and chemotherapeutic agents have been used in some cases. Prognosis is poor, with a 20 percent 5-year survival rate. In the secondary forms, treatment of the primary-associated disorder may result in clinical remission of the disease.

C. ACUTE NEPHRITIS is the second major clinical syndrome associated with glomerular disease. It is characterized by the presence of gross hematuria with red blood cell casts, oliguria, uremia, varying degrees of hypertension, and mild proteinuria. Edema is not a usual part of the syndrome, although puffiness of the eyes may occur in some cases.

1. Acute postinfectious glomerulonephritis occurs in both children and adults and usually follows a streptococcal infection with a nephritogenic strain, which may be sporadic or epidemic.

   a. Clinical Data. The initial sign is a pharyngeal or skin infection. Then, after a latent period of 1 to 2 weeks, hematuria, oliguria, and hypertension appear.

   b. Pathology. Microscopically there is endothelial and mesangial proliferation, with glomerular infiltration by polymorphonuclear leukocytes and mononuclear macrophages.

    c. Treatment and Prognosis. The syndrome is rapidly fatal due to pulmonary hemorrhages and uremia. Immunosuppressive agents and steroids are used but without definite beneficial effects.

5. **Wegener's granulomatosis** is a disease of unknown etiology, although it is believed to be of autoimmune origin. It predominantly affects men in their forties.

    a. Clinical Data. The presenting symptoms include sinusitis, nasal mucosal ulcerations, purulent otitis media, hemoptysis, and pleuritis. Renal involvement, found during the investigation of other disorders, includes proteinuria, hematuria, and erythrocyte casts.

    b. Pathology. The hallmark of generalized Wegener's disease, the classical renal lesion, is focal and segmental glomerulonephritis accompanied by necrotizing granulomatous vasculitis with giant cells present. The glomerulus may show differing amounts of inflammatory cells. EM shows subepithelial deposits of dense material arranged in a nodular fashion or encroaching on the basement membrane. Deposition of IgG and complement is detectable by immunofluorescence.

    c. Treatment and Prognosis. Cytotoxic immunosuppressive therapy is the treatment of choice; remissions lasting many years have occurred.

6. **Henoch-Schönlein purpura** is a disease associated with generalized skin rash, arthralgias, intestinal hemorrhages, and hematuria. The kidney may show focal or diffuse lesions, which are segmental or global. There are marked depositions of IgA in the complexes.

7. **Other systemic diseases** such as periarteritis nodosa, hypersensitivity, angiitis, and other forms of allergic vasculitis are associated with focal-segmental necrotizing glomerulonephritis.

IV. TUBULAR DISORDERS

  A. ACUTE TUBULAR NECROSIS (ATN) is the destruction of the tubular epithelial cells and presents clinically as acute renal failure.

1. **Etiology.** The **toxic form** results from ingestion or inhalation of toxic agents such as mercury, lead, gold, arsenic, ethylene glycol, pesticides, carbon tetrachloride, and methyl alcohol; the **ischemic form** occurs in cases of shock, specifically septic shock.

2. **Clinical Data.** Within the 24 hours following exposure to the etiological agents, there is oliguria, proteinuria, and elevation of blood urea nitrogen (BUN) and creatinine. There is a low specific gravity of the urine with loss of electrolytes.

3. **Pathology.**
    a. Gross Appearance. The kidneys are enlarged, swollen, and pale.
    b. Histology.
      (1) The **toxic form** affects principally the **proximal convoluted tubules.** The tubular cells may contain acidophilic inclusions in the cytoplasm or appear necrotic and desquamated toward the lumen of the tubule. Lipoid deposition within the cells or ballooning of the cytoplasm may occur, depending upon the toxicologic agent. The tubular basement membrane is intact, and the distal tubules are spared.
      (2) The **ischemic form** affects both the **distal tubules** and the Henle's loops, with necrosis of tubular cells and rupture of the tubular basement membrane.

4. **Prognosis** depends upon the etiological agent and the severity of the damage, but in one-half of affected patients renal failure is reversible with complete recovery.

  B. VACUOLAR NEPHROSIS

1. **Etiology.** The common cause is hypokalemia, brought about by electrolyte imbalance. Vacuolar nephrosis is also seen in patients who have been administered hypertonic solutions—mannitol or sucrose.

2. **Clinical Data.** It presents the same signs and symptoms as does ATN.

3. **Pathology.** The proximal convoluted tubule, Henle's loops, and collecting tubules may be affected. **Histologically**, the hallmark is the presence of large vacuoles in the cytoplasm, which fill the entire tubular cell.

4. **Prognosis.** Recovery occurs in almost all affected patients upon correction of the hypokalemia.

  C. FANCONI'S SYNDROME is a disease of hereditary origin that can affect children and adults and is characterized by urinary excretion of phosphates, amino acids, and glucose due to failure

Demonstrated by EM is a characteristic subepithelial hump. Immunofluorescent studi demonstrate a granular deposition of IgG, C_3, and mesangial fibrin.

c. **Treatment and Prognosis.** In 85 to 90 percent of affected children there is total recover A lower percentage of adults achieve total recovery; the majority enter a latent phase progress to chronic renal insufficiency.

2. **Rapidly progressive (crescentic) glomerulonephritis** represents a heterogeneous group glomerulonephritis with different etiological agents and pathogenetic mechanisms, only few cases of which are preceded by streptococcal infection.

a. **Clinical Data.** The symptoms are hematuria, oliguria, and hypertension.

b. **Pathology.** Extensive crescent formation is seen in the glomeruli, with deposition of strand of fibrin and necrosis of portions of the glomerular tufts. Immunofluorescent studies show granular pattern deposits of IgG, IgM, O_3, and fibrin in one-third of the cases, a linear pattern in one-third, and either no fluorescence or a nonspecific pattern in the remaining cases. The degree of crescent formation seems to correlate with the severity of the renal insufficiency.

c. **Prognosis** is poor as there is rapid progression of the disease.

3. **Systemic lupus erythematosus** is an autoimmune disease in which 50 to 80 percent of affected patients develop clinical evidence of renal involvement, but almost 100 percent show abnormalities if renal biopsy is performed. The onset of renal disease occurs in most patients within 2 years after the initial systemic symptoms. The majority of affected patients are women in the third decade of life.

a. **Clinical Data.** Most of the patients develop nephrotic syndrome with proteinuria (more than 2 g) and abnormal urine sediment. Hematuria, proteinuria, cylindruria, and renal failure also can occur.

b. **Pathology.** A wide spectrum of lesions can occur, but in 10 percent of the cases there is no recognizable change or only mild mesangial sclerosis.

   (1) **Focal glomerulonephritis**, in which there is a segmental glomerular proliferation and inflammatory reaction in the adjacent glomeruli, showing minor changes, occurs in 20 percent of systemic lupus erythematosus cases. There is no proven evidence that this localized process progresses to a more severe form.

   (2) **Diffuse Glomerulonephritis.** There is uniform involvement of all parts of the individual glomerulus. Areas of hypercellularity involving the capillary loops and associated foci of necrosis with fibrinoid degeneration and nuclear debris are present in the regions of intense inflammation. The hallmark of the lupus membranous glomerulopathy is the presence of **"wire loops,"** that is, eosinophilic thickening of capillary loops secondary to subendothelial deposits. These deposits are thought to represent aggregates of antigen-antibody complexes. Other associated changes are epithelial crescents, thrombi, and hematoxylin bodies. **Ultrastructurally** these immunocomplex deposits have a characteristic **"finger-print"** pattern with periodicity. They separate the basement membrane and the endothelial cytoplasm. There is secondary obliteration of epithelial cell foot processes. **Immunofluorescent studies** show granular deposits of IgG, C_3, IgM, IgA, C_1, and fibrin in the mesangium, as well as in the capillary loops.

c. **Treatment and Prognosis.** The symptoms usually disappear in cases of focal glomerulonephritis treated with steroids or chemotherapy. In contrast, diffuse glomerulonephritis is associated with an unrelenting progression to renal failure within 2 years of the onset of symptoms, despite the treatment. In general, the 10-year survival rate varies between 50 and 60 percent. The use of corticosteroids and cytotoxic drugs apparently results in an improved prognosis for patients with proliferative glomerulonephritis and systemic involvement.

4. **Goodpasture's syndrome** is a disease of unknown etiology, characterized by pulmonary hemorrhages and renal lesions. Immunological mechanisms have been postulated as causes of the syndrome.

a. **Clinical Data.** Hemoptysis, anemia, pulmonary infiltrates, and hematuria are seen. The syndrome affects predominantly young men in the second or third decade of life.

b. **Pathology.** On gross examination the kidneys are pale, soft, and enlarged. The cortical surfaces are smooth and covered with petechial hemorrhages. Histologically there is focal deposition of eosinophilic material or fibrinoid necrosis within the capillary tuft in the early stages of the disease. Eventually there is proliferative glomerulonephritis with prominent epithelial crescent formation and periglomerular fibrosis. Red blood cells and casts are seen in tubules, and giant cells may be present in the glomerulocapsular space. EM shows endothelial cell proliferation, deposition of basement membrane material, and fibrin beneath the capillary endothelium.

of tubular reabsorption. The clinical manifestations are those of skeletal disturbances (osteomalacia and a propensity to fractures), acidosis, and dehydration. The tubular cells are flattened, and there is an abnormal neck piece in the proximal convoluted tubule.

V. DISEASES OF THE INTERSTITIUM

A. ACUTE PYELONEPHRITIS is acute inflammation of the kidney and renal pelvis.

1. **Etiology.** The most common infecting agent is *Escherichia coli* (*E. coli*), but other agents include *Proteus, Pseudomonas,* and *Staphylococcus.* The most common pathway of infection is from the urinary bladder up to the kidneys. Frequent causes are the use of instruments in the urinary tract, obstruction, prostatism in older patients, vesicoureteral reflex, and diabetes mellitus. A predisposing factor is the female sex.

2. **Clinical Data.** Symptoms are fever, malaise, pain at the costovertebral angle, dysuria, and urgency. Urinalysis shows pyuria and bacteriuria.

3. **Pathology.**
   a. **Gross Appearance.** The affected kidney may be enlarged. Yellowish small microabscesses are present, scattered throughout the renal surface and rimmed by a hyperemic zone. The pelvic mucosa shows marked granularity and hyperemia.
   b. **Histological Appearance.** There is diffuse suppurative necrosis or abscess formation within the renal parenchyma. These abscesses contain neutrophils and cause tubular destruction. Occasionally the lesion may be very severe and produce necrosis of the renal papillae. "**Necrotizing papillitis**," occurring more frequently in diabetic patients, patients with sickle cell disease, or in those with a history of analgesic abuse, is characterized by yellow necrosis of the apical portion of the pyramids.

4. **Treatment and Prognosis.** Antibacterial therapy is the treatment of choice, but surgery may be necessary in unilateral severe cases of necrotizing papillitis. Cases of necrotizing papillitis have a far worse prognosis than do other cases of acute pyelonephritis. Cure is commonly achieved.

B. CHRONIC PYELONEPHRITIS

1. **Etiology.** There are two forms of this condition.
   a. **Obstructive chronic pyelonephritis** occurs in patients with chronic urinary obstructions caused by prostatic enlargement or renal calculi.
   b. **Nonobstructive chronic pyelonephritis** is produced probably by a derangement of the vesicoureteral function that causes reflex of urine and passage of bacteria from the bladder to the ureters.

2. **Clinical Data.** The patients present late in the course of the disease with renal failure and hypertension. Pyelograms are diagnostic and show the affected kidney asymmetrically contracted with deformity of the caliceal system.

3. **Pathology.**
   a. **Gross Appearance.** The affected kidney appears contracted and has an irregular granular surface. The parenchyma is atrophic and replaced by fat.
   b. **Histological Appearance.** There is chronic inflammation of the kidney and pelvis with papillary atrophy and fibrosis of the caliceal fornices. The tubules are dilated and show atrophic lining of the epithelium and pink material in the lumen, giving the kidney a thyroid-like appearance. The vessel walls show marked thickening (Fig. 11-2).

4. **Prognosis.** The disease follows a chronic course, and if there is bilateral involvement, the tubular damage is followed by glomerular involvement, azotemia, and death from uremia.

C. INTERSTITIAL NEPHRITIS

1. **Acute interstitial nephritis**, characterized by the presence of eosinophils in the inflammatory infiltrate, is often associated with allergic manifestations in other organs and may appear after the administration of a number of drugs. It causes rapidly progressive renal insufficiency, but it is reversible following discontinuation of the causative drug. If the process is not related to drugs, the rate of progression to renal insufficiency varies in relationship to the primary cause, but in general it is a slow indolent process.

2. **Chronic interstitial nephritis** is more common and may follow acute tubulointerstitial disease. Symptoms are related to distal tubular damage and are usually progressive and irreversible.

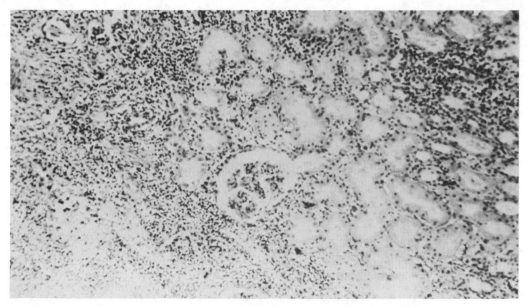

Figure 11-2. Chronic pyelonephritis showing diffuse infiltration by chronic inflammatory cells (x 125).

VI. HYPERTENSION. The renal vasculature may be the primary source of kidney disease as it contributes to a renal cause for hypertension as well as to the acceleration of other forms of vascular disease (e.g., thrombosis, embolization, and infarction).

The **etiology of hypertension**, unknown in the majority of affected patients, is known in approximately 10 percent.

The kidney influences blood pressure through several **mechanisms**: detoxification of pressor substances, secretion of vasodepressor prostaglandins, and secretion of renin from the juxtaglomerular apparatus, which is the result of obstruction of the renal artery (due to atherosclerosis, other diseases, or malformations of the intima and media). Renin acts on angiotensinogen to split it to angiotensin I, which is altered to become angiotensin II. This is a vasoactive substance, which causes arteriolar constriction and stimulates the production of aldosterone by the adrenal cortex. Blood pressure is increased also by an increase in intravascular volume.

A. BENIGN ESSENTIAL HYPERTENSION

1. **Clinical Data.** It is more common in men than in women and in black than in white patients. The blood pressure is persistently elevated, no higher than a diastolic of 110 to 120 mm Hg.

2. **Pathology.** Histologically there is deposition of amorphous hyaline material within the arteriolar wall, disrupting and replacing the elastic membrane and causing gradual narrowing of the lumen. Progression of the process causes atrophy and scarring of the tubules and glomerulus.

3. **Prognosis.** The course of the disease is prolonged, with a mean survival after onset of 20 years. In the black population, the disease starts at an earlier age and progresses more rapidly. Reduction of blood pressure by drug therapy increases longevity.

B. MALIGNANT HYPERTENSION

1. **Clinical Data.** This is a rare but severe form of hypertension in which the diastolic levels are higher than 110 to 120 mm Hg. It can appear de novo or as a complication of benign essential hypertension and is frequently associated with renal insufficiency and retinal hemorrhages.

2. **Pathology.** Light microscopy reveals a characteristic necrotizing arteriolitis. The arteriolar media becomes necrotic and is replaced by fibrin or fibrinoid material. The lumen of the vessel may be obliterated completely, leading to thrombosis and infarction of the parenchyma supplied by the vessel.

3. **Prognosis.** Progression of the disease leads to renal insufficiency and death.

VII. BENIGN RENAL NEOPLASMS

A. ANGIOMYOLIPOMAS are composed of a mixture of fat, blood vessels, and smooth muscle tissue. Their significance is that clinically and radiologically they are often misdiagnosed as carcinomas.

1. **Clinical Data.** They predominate in the fourth and fifth decades of life and are more common in women than in men in a ratio of 2:1. The most common symptom is flank pain, but hematuria and hypertension may be the initial manifestations.

2. **Pathology.**
   a. **Gross Appearance.** These tumors range from small (a few centimeters) to large. They affect the cortex and medulla equally, and there is no predilection for the right or left kidney. On a cut surface they exhibit a yellow-to-gray color, depending upon the amount of fat in them (Fig. 11-3).
   b. **Microscopic Appearance.** There is an admixture of mature adipose tissue with thick-walled vessels and varying amounts of smooth muscle tissue.

3. **Treatment** consists of complete resection of the lesion, even if a total nephrectomy is required.

B. MESOBLASTIC NEPHROMAS (benign nephroblastomas) are congenital hamartomas commonly confused with Wilms' tumors. Most mesoblastic nephromas are diagnosed in the early months of life.

1. **Pathology.**
   a. **Gross Appearance.** They are unilateral tumors of variable sizes. On a cut section they show the characteristic whitish firm surface resembling smooth muscle. Necrosis is usually absent, but cystic changes may be present. They lack clear encapsulation.
   b. **Microscopic Appearance.** The predominant features are interlacing bundles of mature connective tissue, which entrap the glomeruli and other renal elements. Foci of dysplastic cartilage and embryonic mesenchyma may be present.

2. **Treatment** is complete resection of the tumor and adequate margins of uninvolved tissue.

C. ADENOMAS are small (less than 2.5 cm) lesions present in the cortex or medulla of the kidney and are commonly found incidentally at autopsy.

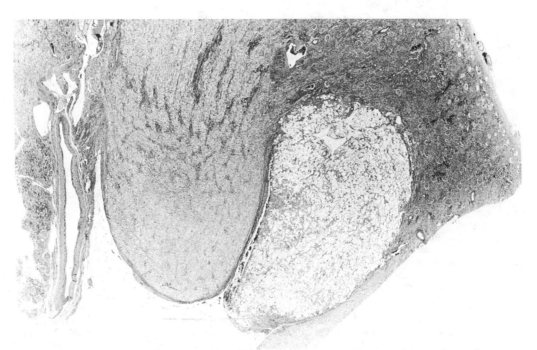

Figure 11-3. Cut section of an angiomyelolipoma. Notice the proliferation of mature fatty cells.

VIII. MALIGNANT RENAL NEOPLASMS

A. **WILMS' TUMORS** (nephroblastomas) are mixed neoplasms composed of metanephric blastemas and stromal and epithelial derivatives at variable stages of differentiation. They are the most common malignancy of renal origin in children.

1. **Etiology.** The origin of these tumors is not known with certainty, but several theories have been proposed.
   a. They originate from metanephric blastemas during fetal life.
   b. They originate from cells that retain their embryonic potential.
   c. They originate from cells that, under certain stimuli, will regain their embryonic potential.

2. **Clinical Data.** Wilms' tumors occur with equal frequency in both sexes. The tumors appear at any age, but the majority of cases are diagnosed before the age of 5 years, with the peak incidence in the second year of life. The most common presenting sign is an abdominal mass, which is seen in almost 90 percent of the cases. Other findings include hypertension, nausea, vomiting, hematuria, and occasionally leg edema. Arteriography reveals poorly vascularized tumors. Nephroblastomas may be part of several congenital malformations such as sporadic aniridia, microcephaly, mental retardation, and spina bifida. Another associated condition is hemihypertrophy of the body. Familial cases have been observed, including cases in monozygous twins.

3. **Pathology.** These tumors can be unilateral, bilateral, or show multifocal involvement of the same kidney.
   a. **Gross Appearance.** They are large, well delineated, and well encapsulated. On a cut section they are often grayish-white to tan in color, with areas of hemorrhage and occasional cystic changes. The junction between the tumor and the kidney is sharp, with a rim of normal kidney parenchyma often present. The renal pelvis is compressed, and local spread is frequent into the perirenal fat, the renal vein, and hilar nodes.
   b. **Histological Appearance.** These lesions are characterized by the formation of abortive or embryonic glomerular and tubular structures surrounded by an immature spindle cell stroma. The epithelial elements may be scanty or predominantly tubular. The stroma may show different elements, such as skeletal muscles, cartilage, and fat.

4. **Metastases.** The renal hilar and para-aortic lymph nodes are frequently the sites of metastatic spread. Also involved are the lungs, liver, adrenal gland, diaphragm, retroperitoneum, and bones. The presence of metastases is usually discovered within 2 years after diagnosis of the primary tumor.

5. The **prognosis** of these tumors depends upon several factors.
   a. Age of the patient—patients under 2 years of age have a good 5-year survival rate.
   b. Extent of the disease—capsular permeation, venous extension, and distant metastases are associated with a poor prognosis.
   c. Microscopic features—marked tubular and glomerular differentiation are associated with a good prognosis.

6. **Treatment** consists of surgical resection of the lesion and systemic chemotherapy, supplemented by radiation of the affected area.

B. **RENAL CELL CARCINOMAS** (hypernephromas) are adenocarcinomas that arise from the proximal convoluted tubule.

1. The **etiology** of these tumors remains obscure, but they have been produced in experiments with animals utilizing chemical, physical, and viral agents. The chemicals used include aromatic hydrocarbons, amines, amides, and some aliphatic compounds such as aflatoxins or metabolic products of the fungus *Aspergillus flavus*, which are found in a variety of foodstuffs.

2. **Clinical Data.** The majority of the cases occur in the adult population with the peak incidence around the sixth decade of life. Occasional cases have been recorded in children. Hypernephromas affect men more commonly than women in an approximate ratio of 2:1 and are usually not discovered until they are in an advanced stage. The characteristic triad of clinical symptoms is hematuria, pain, and a flank mass. Other symptoms include fever, fatigue, and anorexia.

3. **Laboratory Data.** Approximately 5 percent of affected patients have polycythemia with erythrocytosis. Other findings are leukocytosis, thrombocytosis, hypercalcemia, and an elevated erythrocyte sedimentation rate. Anemia is present in up to 25 percent of patients with these neoplasms. A selective arteriogram of the kidney demonstrates a mass with

increased vascular supply, irregular branching, and terminal blunting of vessels in the majority of the cases.

4. **Pathology.** These tumors affect both kidneys equally and have no predilection for a specific location within them.
   a. **Gross Appearance.** The tumor protrudes from the renal cortex as an irregular bosselated mass, which on a cut section shows a characteristic yellow-orange appearance. Hemorrhage and necrosis are common. At the periphery of the tumor the normal parenchyma is compressed, forming a pseudocapsule. Foci or myxoid degeneration and calcification can be present (Fig. 11-4).
   b. **Histological Appearance.** Several patterns can be recognized: papillary, tubular, granular, solid, or sarcomatoid. The majority of tumors, however, are composed of clear cells with distinct cytoplasmic membranes, abundant cytoplasm, and eccentric nuclei. The lesions are markedly vascularized with little stroma between the cells, but occasionally clusters of histiocytes and inflammatory cells are present (Fig. 11-5). These tumors frequently show areas of pleomorphism and giant cells, thus resembling different types of sarcomas.

5. **Metastases.** Hypernephromas metastasize mainly through the bloodstream but also through the lymphatic system. Approximately 95 percent of affected patients have evidence of metastatic spread at the time of death. The most common areas affected are the lungs, brain, bones, liver, adrenal glands, lymph nodes, and the opposite kidney.

6. **Prognosis.** Although spontaneous regressions of renal cell carcinomas have been reported, these tumors generally are associated with a poor prognosis, with a 20 percent 10-year survival rate. The unfavorable prognosis is not only due to the aggressive nature of the tumors but also to the fact that these lesions are silent until they reach a large size, frequently having metastasized at the time of presentation.

7. **Treatment.** Surgical resection of the lesion with removal of adjacent lymph nodes is the treatment of choice. Radiation and chemotherapy have not been very successful as regimens.

IX. **DISORDERS OF THE URINARY COLLECTING SYSTEM** (**Pelvis, Ureter, Bladder, and Urethra**). The entire urinary system is lined by transitional epithelia, and therefore inflammatory processes and tumors assume similar morphological patterns.

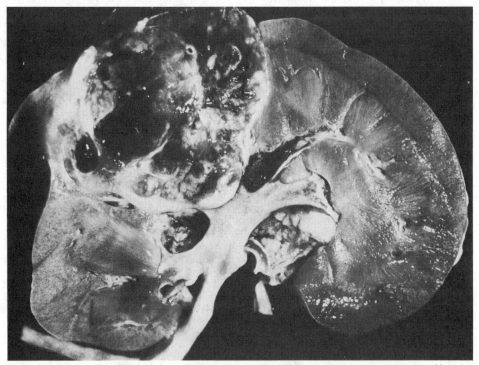

Figure 11-4. Renal cell carcinoma compressing the renal pelvis.

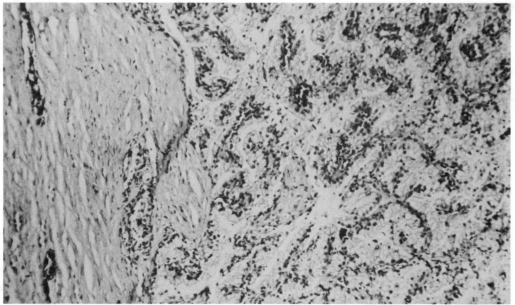

Figure 11-5. Renal cell carcinoma composed of cells with abundant clear cytoplasm (x 125).

A. CONGENITAL ANOMALIES

1. **Bladder diverticula** consist of pouch-like eversions of the bladder wall. They may be of congenital origin, due to a failure of development of the normal musculature, or acquired by means of obstruction in the urethra or bladder neck. They are more common in men than in women, and they are sites of urinary stasis infections and tumors.

2. **Persistent Urachus.** In fetal life the urachus connects the apex of the bladder with the allantois through the umbilical stalk. Normally the urachus atrophies and fibroses after birth, but occasionally it remains patent, creating fistulous tracts between the bladder and the umbilicus. It may also be the site of origin of epithelial malignancies.

3. **Exstrophy of the bladder** is the absence of the anterior musculature of the bladder due to a failure of downgrowth of the mesoderm over the anterior surface of the bladder. It is a site for severe infections. Exstrophy usually is associated with other developmental defects in the anterior abdominal wall.

4. **Double ureters** is an entity of little clinical significance. The two ureters may unite at some point before the junction to the urinary bladder or may pursue separate courses.

B. BENIGN CONDITIONS

1. **Inflammations.**
   a. **Clinical Data.** Affected patients complain of lower abdominal pain, increase in urinary frequency, and dysuria. Examination reveals mucosal edema, redness, and, occasionally, ulcerations. Cystitis is very common in women.
   b. **Pathology.** The transitional epithelium responds to inflammation by various forms of proliferation or by invagination of the epithelium within the lamina propria of the submucosa, forming nets that eventually lose their continuity with the surface. These changes are referred to as **cystitis** (occurring in the urinary bladder), **ureteritis** (occurring in the ureter), or **pyelitis** (occurring in the renal pelvis). Occasionally, a condition occurs such as glandular metaplasia, which resembles the epithelium of the large intestine. This change is associated with infections, irritants, or calculi, and there is no evidence that it implies a premalignant condition.
   c. **Treatment** is correction of the condition that causes the inflammation (such as obstruction, calculi, and prostatic enlargement) by means of specific antibiotics or surgery.

2. **Hydronephrosis** is the dilation of the renal pelvis due to a partial block of urinary outflow. The obstruction can occur at any level in the urinary tract, and the most common causes are nodular hyperplasia of the prostate, calculi, or malignant tumors such as cervical or bladder carcinomas.

a. **Clinical Data.** The dilation may remain silent for long periods of time. When present, the symptoms are usually related to the cause of the hydronephrosis.

b. **Pathology.**

   (1) **Gross Appearance.** The kidneys may show some degree of enlargement. A cut section shows renal calices blunted and the cortex narrowed. The pelvis is dilated massively and is filled with urine (Fig. 11-6).

   (2) **Histological Appearance.** The tubules may be atrophic, but the glomeruli become hyalinized only in the late stage of the disease. Chronic inflammatory cells may be present in the interstitium.

c. **Treatment** is directed toward the cause of the hydronephrosis. In some unilateral cases produced by calculi nephrectomy is performed.

3. **Malacoplakia** are rare lesions produced by *E. coli* and are characterized by multiple yellowish thickenings of the mucosa and submucosa. Clinically they may appear as cancer. Histologically multiple histiocytes with granular cytoplasms accumulate beneath the surface epithelium. Round, concentric, intracytoplasmic inclusions are present in some of these histiocytes. These are known as Michaelis-Gutmann bodies, and they stain positive for calcium.

4. **Endometriosis** is the presence of ectopic endometrial tissue beneath the intact mucosa. These lesions undergo cyclic changes during the menstrual cycle. Clinically, they may mimic carcinomas.

5. **Caruncles** are small, red, painful masses present in the external urethral meatus of the affected women. Histologically they are composed of vascularized stromas covered by squamous or transitional epithelium. The lesions may recur if not completely excised.

C. MALIGNANT TUMORS

1. **Transitional cell carcinomas** of the urothelium have similar features wherever they are located along the urinary collecting system. They are characterized by their multifocality and tendency to recur.

   a. **Incidence.** Malignant tumors of the urinary collecting system account for more than 10,000 deaths per year in this country.

   b. **Etiology.** These tumors, especially those that occur in the bladder, have been linked to environmental factors, such as industrial carcinogens (e.g., aniline dyes), metabolites of tryptophan, cigarette smoking, mechanical irritations such as calculi and diverticuli, or parasites. Longer time of exposure means a greater chance to develop these tumors.

   c. **Clinical Data.** They produce painless hematuria. On examination they may appear as papillary lesions or plaque-like ulcers. The region of the trigone in the bladder is the most common location.

   d. **Pathology.** Histologically the transitional cell epithelium is thickened with an increase in the number of layers of cells with varying degrees of nuclear atypia and pleomorphism (Fig. 11-7). There are four histologic grades that are significant for prognosis.

   (1) **Grade I** is composed of a central core of fibrovascular tissue covered by uniform transitional cells. Pleomorphism and mitoses are rare, and necrosis is absent. The epithelium is 7 to 10 cells thick (Fig. 11-8).

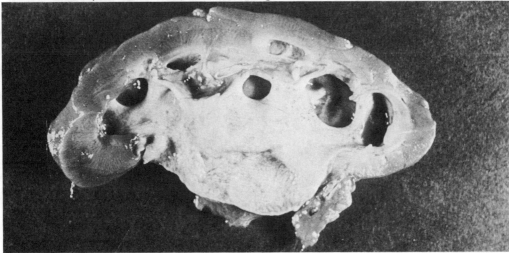

Figure 11-6. Hydronephrosis. Notice the massive pelvic dilatation.

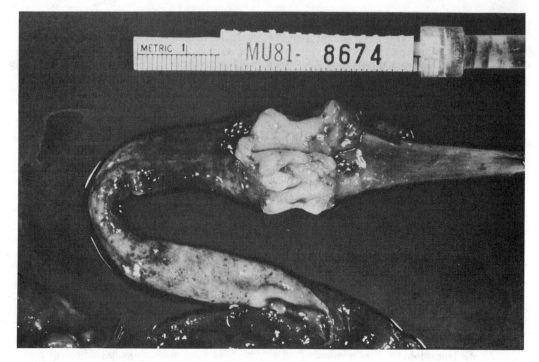

Figure 11-7. Transitional cell carcinoma of the ureter.

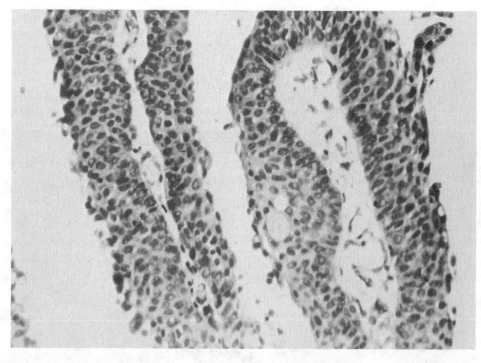

Figure 11-8. Papillary transitional cell carcinoma. Notice the stalk of fibroconnective tissue and the proliferation of cells (x 200).

        (2) Grade II. The papillary configuration persists, but there is more crowding of cells, with enlargement and hyperchromatism of nuclei. Mitoses are present in variable numbers.

        (3) Grade III tumors have a sessile, cauliflower-like appearance. Necrosis and ulceration are frequent. The cell masses form groups. Necrosis, atypia, and mitoses are abundant.

        (4) Grade IV. Most of these lesions are necrotic masses, and they show marked pleomorphism, atypia, and areas of squamous differentiation.

    e. Prognosis depends on the histologic grade and the stage of the disease. The more undifferentiated the tumor, the worse is the prognosis. There are six stages of the disease.

        (1) Stage O   carcinoma in situ (limited to the mucosa)

        (2) Stage A   invasion of the submucosa

        (3) Stage B$_1$ invasion of superficial muscle

        (4) Stage B$_2$ invasion deep into the muscle

        (5) Stage C   invasion of perivesical tissue and the lymphatic system

        (6) Stage D   distant metastases

    f. The **treatment** is resection of the lesion (local or total cystectomy) followed by radiation. The overall 5-year survival rate is approximately 30 percent.

2. Squamous cell carcinoma is rare, representing 5 percent of all bladder tumors. These tumors occur in individuals in geographical areas such as Egypt, where close association between parasitic infections, such as schistosomiasis, and carcinomas are known to occur. Grossly they are ulcerated and necrotic masses. Histologically they are poorly differentiated, but areas of keratinization may be present. These tumors imply a poor prognosis.

3. Adenocarcinomas may arise from urachal remnants, from cystitis cystica, cystitis glandularis, or from metaplasia of transitional epithelium. Histologically the glands produce abundant mucin and are frequently well differentiated.

4. Sarcomas or mesenchymal tumors of the bladder are rare. Of these, sarcoma botryoides is the most common. The histological appearance is identical to that of sarcoma botryoides in the vagina.

STUDY QUESTIONS

Directions: Each question below contains five suggested answers. Choose the **one best** response to each question.

1. Lipoid nephrosis of the kidneys characteristically produces changes that may be observed by electron microscope (EM) in which of the following renal glomerular elements?

(A) Endothelial cells
(B) Epithelial cells
(C) Mesangium
(D) Blood vessels
(E) Basement membrane

2. Necrotizing papillitis (renal papillary necrosis) of the kidneys is seen most often in which of the following conditions?

(A) Lupus erythematosus
(B) Diabetes mellitus
(C) Goodpasture's syndrome
(D) Renal transplantation
(E) Heavy-metal poisoning

3. A computed tomography (CT) scan of the kidney of a 55-year-old patient shows a large, partially necrotic mass replacing the upper pole of the right kidney. Statistically, this lesion is most likely

(A) tuberculosis
(B) transitional cell carcinoma
(C) renal cell carcinoma
(D) endometriosis
(E) adrenal cortical adenoma

4. A 55-year-old man was admitted to the hospital with impaired renal function. He underwent ultrasound examination, which showed bilateral large multicystic masses in the normal location of the kidneys. Shortly thereafter, the patient died of sepsis that was presumed to originate from a renal infection. What is the most likely diagnosis?

(A) Polycystic kidneys—type I
(B) Multiple simple renal cysts
(C) Polycystic kidneys—type II
(D) Lobar nephronia
(E) Polycystic kidneys—type III

Directions: Each question below contains four suggested answers of which **one or more** is correct. Choose the answer

A   if **1, 2, and 3** are correct
B   if **1 and 3** are correct
C   if **2 and 4** are correct
D   if **4** is correct
E   if **1, 2, 3, and 4** are correct

5. True statements concerning Goodpasture's syndrome include

(1) pulmonary hemorrhage leads to hemoptysis
(2) eosinophilic material is deposited in the renal glomeruli
(3) death occurs because of uremia and pulmonary hemorrhage
(4) electron microscopy (EM) of affected kidneys shows characteristic fibrin deposits beneath the endothelium

6. Immunofluorescent-stained kidney specimens from a patient with poststreptococcal glomerulonephritis show increased deposits of which of the following serum components?

(1) Immunoglobulin G (IgG)
(2) Fibrin
(3) Complement component C₃
(4) Immunoglobulin M (IgM)

7. Which of the following conditions may lead to hydronephrosis?

(1) Prostatic hypertrophy
(2) Pelvic tumor
(3) Renal calculi
(4) Renal vein thrombosis

8. True statements concerning diffuse glomerulosclerosis include which of the following?

(1) It is associated with protein loss into the urine
(2) It is a frequent cause of hypertension
(3) It is seen frequently in patients with chronic diabetes
(4) It may occur secondary to necrotizing papillitis

9. Mercury poisoning causes which of the following conditions in the kidneys?

(1) Papillary necrosis
(2) Amyloid deposition
(3) Oncocytoma
(4) Acute tubular necrosis

ANSWERS AND EXPLANATIONS

1. The answer is B. *(III B 1)* Lipoid nephrosis is sometimes termed minimal change glomerulonephritis because of the paucity of histologic findings. Accumulation of lipids in the renal tubular epithelial cells and loss of the foot processes of the glomerular epithelial cells are seen in electron micrographs. This entity is the most common cause of nephrotic syndrome in children, particularly in those under 15 years of age.

2. The answer is B. *(V A 3 b)* Necrotizing papillitis is a form of acute pyelonephritis, which is seen in diabetics and in patients with chronic severe urinary tract obstruction. The distal portion of the renal papilla becomes ischemic and undergoes necrosis. Sloughing of the necrotic tissue may then occur.

3. The answer is C. *(VIII B)* Renal cell carcinomas show no predilection for a specific location within a kidney and arise from both kidneys with nearly equal incidence. However, a large, partially necrotic mass replacing the upper pole of the right kidney in a 55-year-old patient is a classical sign of the lesion. These tumors are irregular masses that typically protrude from and distort the renal cortical surface. Renal cell carcinomas often show hemorrhage and necrosis. The sixth decade of life is the age of peak incidence.

4. The answer is E. *[II D 2 c (3)]* Polycystic kidneys are an unusual congenital abnormality resulting from failure in normal development of the fetal kidneys. These conditions may lead to early renal failure with death in infancy or may not cause symptoms until later in life—depending upon the type. Type I is bilateral and fatal soon after birth; type II, if bilateral, is also incompatible with life. Therefore, the patient in question must have had type III polycystic kidneys. Patients with type III have impaired renal function by the fifth or sixth decade of life and often die as a consequence of cardiovascular or infectious complications.

5. The answer is E (all). *(III C 4)* Goodpasture's syndrome is characterized by glomerulonephritis and proliferative pulmonary hemorrhages. Electron microscopic (EM) examination of the renal biopsy shows linear deposition of immunoglobulin G (IgG) and complement along the glomerular basement membrane. Deposits of fibrin can be demonstrated between the capillary endothelium and the glomerular basement membrane.

6. The answer is A (1, 2, 3). *(III C 1 b)* Poststreptococcal glomerulonephritis is a form of immune complex nephritis that can develop as a result of immune reaction to an infection. Kidney biopsies from patients with this condition show endothelial and mesangial cell proliferation, granular deposits of fibrin, immunoglobulin G (IgG), C_3, and sometimes other components of the complement system. Immunoglobulin M (IgM) is not deposited in detectable amounts in this disease.

7. The answer is A (1, 2, 3). *(IX B 2)* Hydronephrosis is the term given to dilatation of the renal pelvis due to complete or incomplete obstruction of the urine flow from the pelvis. Although there are many causes, including prostatic hypertrophy, pelvic tumors, and the presence of renal calculi, renal vein thrombosis is not a known cause of hydronephrosis.

8. The answer is A (1, 2, 3). *(III B 3)* Both diffuse and nodular forms of glomerulosclerosis occur in diabetic patients. Both forms cause sufficient basement membrane damage to produce nephrotic syndrome with its characteristic protein loss in the urine. While necrotizing papillitis may also occur in the diabetic patient, it is not associated with diffuse glomerulosclerosis.

9. The answer is D (4). *(IV A)* Acute tubular necrosis is the destruction of the tubular epithelial cells, which causes acute renal failure. The toxic agents that can produce acute tubular necrosis include mercury, lead, gold, arsenic, ethylene glycol, numerous pesticides, carbon tetrachloride, and methyl alcohol. Because mercury is excreted through the urine, the proximal convoluted tubular cells are damaged, causing disruption of intracellular organelles, breaks in the plasma membrane, and the appearance of curious eosinophilic droplets within the cytoplasm.

12
The Male Reproductive System

I. INTRODUCTION. The male reproductive system consists of the testes, epididymis, the prostate gland, and the penis and scrotum. The lesions involving the system can be divided into three main groups, which include **congenital anomalies**, **inflammations**, and both benign and malignant **neoplasms**.

II. TESTES

A. NORMAL DEVELOPMENT

1. **Embryology.** The testicular germ cells originate from the endoderm of the yolk sac and migrate toward the gonadal or genital ridge by active movement of individual cells.

2. **Anatomy.** Normal adult testes are surrounded by a thick, dense fibrous capsule called the tunica albuginea. At the hilus of the testis, there is a condensation of fibrous tissue that extends into the testicular stroma and divides it into several compartments. Each compartment contains seminiferous tubules and clumps of interstitial cells localized in the surrounding connective tissue.

B. CONGENITAL ANOMALIES

1. Both testes may be absent (**anorchia**), or only one may be missing (**monorchia**).

2. In **cryptorchidism** (the absence of usually one testis, occasionally both testes, from the scrotal sac), the testes may be retained in the abdominal cavity, inguinal region, or somewhere within the inguinal canal. The cause of cryptorchidism often is not evident.
   a. If the condition is not discovered and corrected until after puberty, the testes are smaller than normal in size (atrophy), and, in the majority of cases, there is no evidence of normal spermatogenesis.
   b. Undescended testes have a higher likelihood of developing malignant neoplasms than normal testes.

C. INFERTILITY PROBLEMS

1. **Hypospermatogenesis** is a condition involving a decreased number of cells of the spermatogenic series; the normal number is 2 million. The cells that are present appear histologically normal. Clinically, there is oligospermia.

2. **Maturation arrest** consists of a failure of normal spermatogenesis at some stage and is manifested by either oligo- or azoospermia.

3. **Klinefelter's syndrome** is one of the most common causes of hypogonadism in males.
   a. The condition is characterized by testicular hypoplasia, azoospermia, gynecomastia, eunuchoid build, and elevated urinary gonadotropin levels and may be associated with mental retardation.
   b. Chromosome studies usually reveal 47 chromosomes with an XXY karyotype.

4. **Atrophy** is characterized by small testes (less than 10 g) with no histologic evidence of sper-

matogenesis. **Acquired atrophy** occurs in old age, in conditions such as hypothyroidism and cachexia, and in patients receiving estrogen therapy for prostatic carcinoma.

5. Torsion and Infarction. Free mobility of the testes predisposes to twisting of the spermatic cord with compression and occlusion of the blood vessels.

    a. The decrease in blood flow leads to hemorrhagic infarction of the testis and epididymis. If there is only partial or temporary torsion of the cord, there is hyperemia and edema but not necrosis.

    b. Predisposing factors include anomalies in the insertion of the vas deferens, a wide tunica vaginalis, absence of the scrotal ligaments, or an atrophic testis.

D. INFLAMMATIONS

1. Acute orchitis refers to an acute inflammation of the testicular parenchyma due to an infectious process, which usually reaches the testis and epididymis by ascending through the vas deferens or via lymphatics.

    a. The most **common sources** of acute orchitis are acute urethritis, acute cystitis, and prostatitis. Rarely, the condition occurs as a complication of mumps, affecting patients (postpubescent more commonly than prepubescent) approximately 1 week after the onset of parotitis.

    b. The most common organisms that produce orchitis are *Escherichia coli (E. coli)*, staphylococci, and streptococci.

    c. Common **clinical manifestations** are fever, pain, tenderness, and swelling of the testis.

    d. Histologically, a diffuse infiltrate of neutrophils, lymphocytes, and plasma cells involves both the interstitium and the tubules.

    e. Sterility may result as a consequence of extensive fibrosis, scarring, and damage to the tubules.

2. Granulomatous orchitis has an obscure etiology and is characterized by unilateral testicular enlargement occurring predominantly in middle-aged men. Trauma and autoimmune disorders have been postulated as causes of the lesion.

    a. Histologically, the hallmark is the presence of epithelioid granulomas with abundant plasma cells, lymphocytes, and neutrophils surrounding ruptured tubules and nests of spermatozoa.

    b. The condition should be differentiated from tuberculous orchitis, in which necrotizing granulomas containing acid-fast bacilli can be demonstrated.

E. MALIGNANT TUMORS.
Approximately 95 percent of malignant testicular neoplasms are of germ cell origin, and more than 40 percent of **germ cell tumors** exhibit more than one histologic type. These tumors are one of the most common forms of cancer in males between the ages of 15 and 34 years, although they account for only approximately 1 percent of all male cancer deaths.

1. The **etiology** of these tumors is not known. However, patients with undescended testes are known to have up to 14 times as high a chance of developing these tumors as normal individuals, and other predisposing factors are known to include infection and trauma. A hereditary or genetic influence on the pathogenesis of these tumors is suggested by the increased occurrence of testicular tumors in siblings and other family members of affected patients.

2. Classification. Germ cell tumors can be classified into five types: seminoma, teratoma, embryonal cell carcinoma, infantile embryonal cell carcinoma (yolk sac tumor), and choriocarcinoma.

3. Seminoma is the most common of the testicular tumors and the most common tumor to occur in the undescended testis. It comprises approximately 70 percent of primary germ cell tumors of the testis.

    a. Clinical Data. Seminoma occurs predominantly during the fourth and fifth decades of life and only rarely in children. Enlargement of the testis with or without pain is the most common symptom.

    b. Gross Pathology (Fig. 12-1).

        (1) The involved testis maintains its normal contour and configuration, although it is enlarged in size. The tunica albuginea is intact, and frequently the epididymis and spermatic cord are spared.

        (2) A cut surface shows a bulging, white-gray, homogeneous mass of firm consistency. Hemorrhage and necrosis are not present.

    c. Histology (Fig. 12-2).

        (1) Seminomas are composed of sheets of uniform, polyhedral cells with large hyperchromatic nuclei and abundant, clear cytoplasm, rich in glycogen.

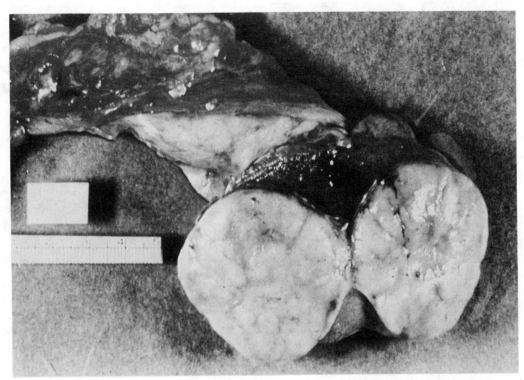

Figure 12-1. Cross section of a testis involved by a seminoma showing an encapsulated homogeneous tumor and compressed normal testicular parenchyma.

      (2) Strands of fibroconnective tissue and lymphocytes are common, interspersed with the tumor cells. Occasionally, multinucleated giant cells are present.

      (3) Approximately 10 percent of seminomas show marked anaplasia and increased mitotic activity (**anaplastic seminoma**). These tumors, in the opinion of certain authors, behave more aggressively than ordinary seminomas.

   d. Prognosis.

      (1) The tumors have a good prognosis with a 90 percent to 98 percent 5-year survival rate.

      (2) Metastases to regional lymph nodes and viscera are rare but can occur.

   e. Treatment. Orchiectomy followed by radiotherapy is the treatment of choice.

   f. Spermatocytic seminoma accounts for no more than 10 percent of seminomas and occurs in older patients.

      (1) Histologically, it is characterized by three types of cells: medium-sized cells with round nuclei and abundant eosinophilic cytoplasm, which constitute the main population; large mononuclear or multinucleated cells; and small cells resembling spermatocytes.

      (2) Patients with these tumors have an excellent prognosis.

4. Teratoma is characterized by the presence of elements from the three germinal layers (ectoderm, endoderm, and mesoderm). It comprises about 30 percent of the testicular tumors.

   a. Clinical Data. Teratomas can occur at any age but are most common in the first, second, and third decades of life. The symptomatology is identical to that of other testicular tumors.

   b. Gross Pathology.

      (1) The testis is enlarged, the tunica is distorted, and occasionally the lesion can extend beyond the capsule.

      (2) Cut section of the tumor reveals a lobulated, soft-to-firm, **partly cystic** mass encompassed by a rim of compressed normal testicular tissue.

      (3) Areas of calcification, hemorrhage, and necrosis are present.

   c. Histology.

      (1) A variety of heterogeneous tissues are present, including bone, cartilage, neural elements, and gastric, respiratory, and squamous epithelium.

      (2) Immature elements may be present, and sarcomatous transformation may occur.

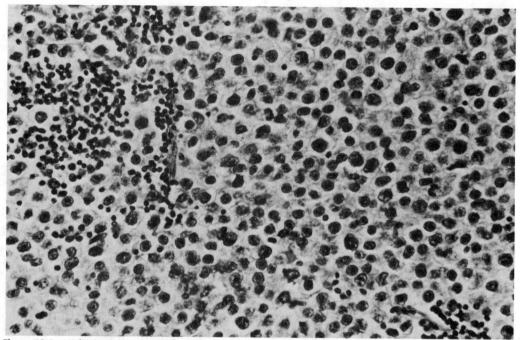

Figure 12-2. High-power view of a seminoma showing sheets of uniform cells with clear cytoplasm and prominent nuclei. Occasional lymphocytes are present.

      (3) Metastasis via lymphatics or blood vessels can occur even when no histologic evidence of malignant transformation can be demonstrated. Metastases can be composed of one or several histologic patterns, which may be poorly or well differentiated.

      (4) Elements from other germ cell tumors, such as seminoma or embryonal cell carcinoma, may be present.

    d. Prognosis. The 2-year mortality rate for teratoma is approximately 30 percent.

    e. Treatment. Orchiectomy, followed by chemo- and radiotherapy, is the treatment of choice.

  5. Embryonal cell carcinomas comprise between 15 percent and 20 percent of testicular germ cell tumors and occur predominantly during the second and third decades of life.

    a. Clinical Data. Gradual swelling of the testis, with or without pain, is the most common clinical complaint, and about one-third of affected patients have evidence of metastatic spread at the time of diagnosis.

    b. Gross Pathology.

      (1) These tumors are usually small with no evidence of encapsulation and produce asymmetrical distortion of the testis.

      (2) Cut section reveals nodules with extensive areas of hemorrhage and necrosis.

      (3) Infiltration of the tunica albuginea, spermatic cord, and epididymis is common.

    c. Histology.

      (1) The tumors are composed of pleomorphic epithelial cells that vary in size and shape. They have large nuclei, prominent nucleoli, and abundant eosinophilic cytoplasm.

      (2) The cells can be arranged in a variety of patterns such as glandular, papillary, tubular, or solid sheets of cells.

      (3) Mitosis, hemorrhage, and necrosis are common.

    d. Prognosis.

      (1) These tumors are far more aggressive than seminomas, and metastatic spread to lymph nodes and viscera (e.g., lungs or liver) is not uncommon.

      (2) The 5-year mortality rate is about 65 percent.

    e. Treatment. Orchiectomy should be performed in all cases, usually followed by radiotherapy. Because these tumors are less radiosensitive than seminomas, chemotherapy may be the treatment of choice after orchiectomy in some cases.

  6. The **infantile embryonal cell carcinoma** (yolk sac tumor) is so named because it resembles the endodermal sinus and amniotic cavity of a yolk sac.

a. Clinical Data.
(1) It occurs predominantly in children.
(2) Serum levels of α-fetoproteins are elevated in affected patients.
b. Histology. The hallmark of this tumor is the presence of organoid structures that simulate embryoid (Schiller-Duval) bodies.
c. Prognosis. This is a highly aggressive neoplasm with a 5-year mortality rate of 50 percent.

7. **Choriocarcinoma** is the most malignant of the testicular tumors, comprising about 1 percent of the germ cell neoplasms.
   a. Clinical Data.
   (1) It occurs predominantly in males 15 to 25 years of age.
   (2) Enlargement of the testis is common; however, sometimes the presenting symptoms are those produced by metastatic spread of the tumor. Some patients may have gynecomastia.
   (3) Serum and urine levels of chorionic gonadotropins are elevated.
   b. Gross Pathology.
   (1) This tumor can either be very small and difficult to identify or involve the entire testis, producing distortion and nodularity.
   (2) On cut section, extensive hemorrhage and necrosis are present, with small foci of white-gray, well-preserved tissue interspersed among hemorrhagic areas.
   c. Histology.
   (1) In order to make the diagnosis of choriocarcinoma, two types of cells must be present—the **syncytiotrophoblast** and the **cytotrophoblast**. Syncytiotrophoblasts are large multinucleated cells with abundant eosinophilic cytoplasm and occasionally vacuolated cytoplasm. Cytotrophoblasts are cuboidal cells with dark nuclei and clear cytoplasm, arranged in sheets or cords.
   (2) In some instances, these cells are arranged around stalks of fibroconnective tissue, resembling the normal architecture of the mature placenta.
   (3) Extensive hemorrhage always is present, and foci of other germ cell tumors may be found.
   d. Prognosis. The poor prognosis associated with these neoplasms is often ascribed to their tendency to invade blood vessels and disseminate to viscera (lungs, liver, and brain).
   e. Treatment. These tumors are sensitive to chemotherapy, which usually is given after orchiectomy is performed.

F. TUMORS OF SPECIALIZED GONADAL STROMA. The testicular stroma has the capacity to differentiate into a variety of patterns and to elaborate androgens, estrogens, or both.

1. The **interstitial (Leydig) cell tumor** originates from the interstitial cells of the testis and accounts for approximately 1 percent of all testicular neoplasms.
   a. Clinical Data.
   (1) Most cases occur between the fourth and sixth decades of life, but cases have been reported at all ages.
   (2) The symptoms are due to the ability of the tumor to produce hormones.
      (a) If the tumor occurs before puberty, the clinical manifestations are those of precocious puberty due to androgen production.
      (b) In adults, gynecomastia and feminization resulting from excess estrogen are the main symptoms, present in up to 35 percent of patients.
   b. Gross Pathology. Most interstitial cell tumors are made up of several 1- to 2-cm nodules with a characteristic yellow-brown color.
   c. Histology.
   (1) This neoplasm consists of sheets of a fairly uniform population of cells with round nuclei and abundant eosinophilic cytoplasm.
   (2) A cigar-shaped structure (Reinke's crystal) is present in the cytoplasm as are lipid vacuoles and brown pigment.
   d. Prognosis. The tumor usually behaves in a benign fashion, but malignancies can develop in up to 10 percent of cases. Malignancy is determined by the presence of invasive or metastatic spread.

2. **Metastatic tumors to the testis** are rare; malignant lymphoma and leukemia are the most common tumors to involve the testis secondarily.

III. EPIDIDYMIS

A. INFLAMMATORY LESIONS

1. **Tuberculosis** (Tuberculous Epididymitis).

      a. This condition can result from hematogenous spread from the diseased kidneys or lungs. The inflammation usually begins in the interstitial tissue and then spreads to the testis.

      b. The hallmark of the condition is the presence of caseating granulomas in which acid-fast bacilli can be demonstrated either by culture of the tissue or by special stains.

  2. Spermatocytic granuloma is a granulomatous reaction to a lipid fraction released by the sperm.

      a. The lesion is probably the result of damage to the tubular epithelium and basement membrane by inflammation or trauma.

      b. Histologically there is a prominent histiocytic reaction intermixed with numerous spermatozoa.

B. TUMORS

  1. Tumors of the epididymis are rare and usually are of mesenchymal origin. They can occur at any age but predominantly affect males in the third, fourth, and fifth decades of life. They manifest clinically as asymptomatic nodules that usually are discovered as incidental findings on routine physical examinations.

  2. Adenomatoid tumor is a benign neoplastic growth of mesothelial origin.

      a. Grossly the tumor is a small, white, solitary, well-demarcated nodule.

      b. Histologically it is composed of acidophilic cells arranged in solid cords. The cells are low columnar and cuboidal with a vacuolated cytoplasm. Variable amounts of stroma and smooth muscle fibers are present.

IV. THE PROSTATE

A. NORMAL DEVELOPMENT

  1. Embryology. The prostate gland is formed by evagination from the posterior urethra and is, therefore, considered to be of endodermal origin. Normal development is dependent upon endocrine stimulation.

  2. Anatomy. The prostate is divided into five lobes: anterior, middle, posterior, and two lateral. These lobes are purely anatomical without functional significance.

  3. Histology.

      a. There are three major types of glands in the prostate: the periurethral glands, which are the smallest; the submucosal glands; and the external glands, which comprise the largest portion of the prostate.

      b. The glands are composed of two layers of cells: flat cuboidal cells that are found in the basal layer and tall columnar cells oriented towards the lumen of the gland. The glands are surrounded by an eosinophilic basement membrane.

B. CONGENITAL ABNORMALITIES of the prostate usually are associated with malformations of the urogenital system. The prostate may be small or absent, or abnormal communications may develop between the prostate and the ureter, the urethra, or both. Such communications may form cavities called diverticula, which resemble cysts in the prostate.

C. INFLAMMATIONS

  1. Acute Prostatitis.

      a. This is a common condition usually resulting from local extension of an inflammatory process in the urethra or bladder. It may follow a local operative maneuver such as urethral catheterization. The inflammatory process may involve the entire organ, or localized abscesses may be formed.

      b. Etiology. Gonococcus was for a long time the most common cause, but recently other organisms such as *E. coli*, staphylococcus, and streptococcus have become the most common causes.

      c. Clinical Data. Fever and lower abdominal pain are common symptoms.

      d. Histology. Both stroma and glands are infiltrated by polymorphonuclear cells.

  2. Chronic Prostatitis.

      a. Clinical Data. This condition is clinically more significant than acute prostatitis because it is frequently recurrent and probably is the most common cause of relapsing urinary tract infections in men.

         (1) It predominately affects older men and can cause low back pain, dysuria, frequency, urgency, and prostatic enlargement and tenderness, but it often may be totally asymptomatic.

(2) Both a bacterial and a nonbacterial form of the condition exist. The forms may have similar clinical manifestations, but only the bacterial form predisposes to urinary tract infections. In most cases, bacterial prostatitis occurs insidiously and is not a sequela of acute prostatitis, although the causative organisms are the same as for the acute condition. Nonbacterial prostatitis, in some cases, is thought to have a viral origin.

    b. Histology.

        (1) Chronic prostatitis causes an inflammatory reaction characterized by the aggregation of numerous lymphocytes, plasma cells, and macrophages as well as neutrophils within the glandular acini and fibrotic stroma. Corpora amylacea, large laminated calcifications, commonly are contained within the glands.

        (2) The nonspecific aggregations of lymphocytes that occur as part of the normal aging process should not be diagnosed as chronic prostatitis in the absence of other inflammatory cells.

  3. Granulomatous prostatitis occurs in two forms.

    a. In the first, nonspecific granulomas occur secondary to either acute or chronic prostatitis and are believed to be caused by retained prostatic secretions. Histologically, in addition to inflammatory cells, there are well-circumscribed granulomas of epithelial giant cells with few eosinophils.

    b. The second form represents tuberculosis of the prostate, usually following tuberculosis of the genitourinary tract.

  4. Malacoplakia is a rare inflammatory reaction caused by *E. coli*. It can affect the prostate and urinary tract. The lesion is predominantly composed of histiocytes and small calcified bodies (Michaelis-Gutmann bodies).

D. BENIGN NODULAR HYPERPLASIA (benign prostatic hypertrophy) is an enlargement of the prostate that usually affects men over 40 years of age. The cause is not known, but it is believed to be due to certain hormonal changes such as decreased androgen and increased estrogen production.

  1. Clinical Data.

    a. The condition occurs in more than 95 percent of men over 70 years of age but produces symptoms in only a small percentage of affected patients.

    b. When symptoms do occur, they are secondary effects related to compression of the urethra or to retention of urine in the bladder. These two problems in turn may be further complicated by distention and hypertrophy of the bladder, hydroureter, hydronephrosis, prostatitis, cystitis, renal infections, calculi, and infarctions.

    c. Hyperplasia **does not predispose to prostatic cancer** according to most experts.

  2. Gross Pathology.

    a. The enlarged prostate is firm and rubbery and weighs over 50 g. (A normal prostate weighs 20 g to 30 g.)

    b. The middle lobe appears to be most commonly affected, in contrast to carcinoma of the prostate, which often involves the posterior lobe.

    c. Cut surface may disclose numerous closely packed nodules exuding small amounts of milky fluids. Cystic changes may be present.

    d. In nodules that are primarily glandular, the tissue has a yellow-pink color, a soft consistency, and is fairly discretely demarcated. In those nodules that are primarily fibromuscular, the tissue is pale gray, tough, fibrous, and less clearly demarcated.

  3. Histology. The appearance of the nodules varies greatly, depending on whether the nodules are composed of only glandular structures, equal amounts of glandular and stromal elements, or predominantly smooth muscle and connective tissue.

E. MALIGNANT TUMORS

  1. Carcinoma of the prostate is a malignant tumor of the glandular epithelium. Although it is the third most common cause of cancer death in men over 50 years of age, it is also commonly an incidental finding at the time of autopsy.

    a. Etiology. The cause of prostatic cancer is not known.

        (1) However, a clear association has been established with advancing age (greater than 50 years) and with certain racial backgrounds (a high prevalence in blacks and a low prevalence in Orientals).

        (2) Some studies suggest the possibility of an endocrine (or hormonal) relationship; other factors such as viral infection and environmental influences (e.g., cadmium exposure) also have been contemplated as causes.

    b. Clinical Data.

        (1) Carcinoma of the prostate may arise in any lobe, but it most commonly originates in the posterior lobe near the outer margins.

        (2) The clinical diagnosis of prostatic carcinoma usually is based on the finding of an indurated area in the gland on rectal examination.

(3) Small (occult) cancers are asymptomatic, and urinary symptoms appear only after the tumors have spread. Pain is a late symptom, reflecting involvement of capsular perineural spaces.

c. Laboratory Data. By using sensitive immunoassay techniques to test for an elevated level of serum acid phosphatase, specifically of prostatic origin, prostatic carcinoma in many cases can be detected before it has extended beyond the capsule.

d. Bone scans and x-rays may reveal multiple osteoblastic metastatic lesions in the pelvis, ribs, skull, and spine when the disease has spread.

e. Morphology.

(1) **Grossly** prostatic carcinomas characteristically appear as nodular, ill-defined areas of a stony hard consistency with a color varying from gray-white to yellow.

(2) **Microscopically** the majority are adenocarcinomas, consisting of glandular structures.

(a) Two types of cells may be seen: clear cells with abundant foamy cytoplasm or dark spindle cells with condensed cytoplasm. The cells have prominent nucleoli, and different degrees of anaplasia can be present (Fig. 12-3).

(b) The normal lobular architecture is destroyed because the malignant acini grow irregularly.

(c) Perineural invasion is a common finding.

f. Prognosis. Those tumors that are well differentiated histologically and have not metastasized are associated with a good 5- to 15-year survival rate. Eventually, however, there is a relapse and spread of the disease, with the most frequent sites of metastases being regional lymph nodes, bones, lungs, liver, and brain.

g. Modalities of treatment include antiandrogenic therapy (orchiectomy and estrogen therapy), radiotherapy, and chemotherapy.

2. **Sarcomas** are uncommon tumors of the prostate and usually have a rapid growth, a high malignant potential, and are predominantly of two types.

   a. Rhabdomyosarcomas most commonly affect children.

   b. Leiomyosarcomas most commonly affect adults.

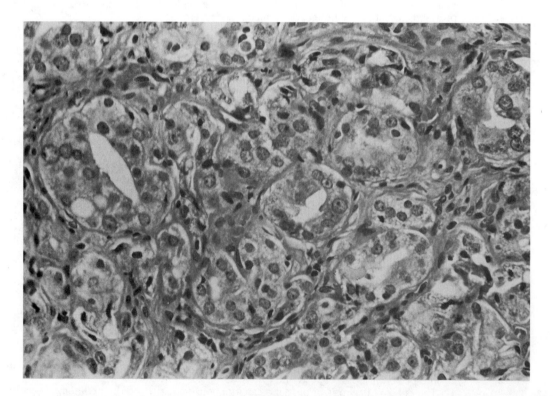

Figure 12-3. High-power view of an adenocarcinoma of the prostate showing glandular formation.

V. PENIS AND SCROTUM

A. NORMAL ANATOMY

1. Body. The penis is composed of two lateral corpora cavernosa and one medial corpus spongiosum containing the urethra. These elements are covered by pigmented skin that folds at the distal extremity to form the prepuce.

2. The **glans** is formed by the distal molding of the three corpora.

B. CONGENITAL ABNORMALITIES

1. Hypospadias. This condition is a developmental arrest in which the urethral meatus is present on the under (ventral) surface of the penis. When the urethral opening is on the upper (dorsal) surface, it is referred to as **epispadias**.

2. Phimosis is constriction of the orifice of the prepuce so that the prepuce cannot be retracted. This process often is associated with **balanitis,** a chronic inflammation.

3. Bifid scrotum is the presence of two separate scrotal sacs.

C. INFLAMMATIONS

1. The variety of specific infections that may involve the glans and prepuce include herpes, syphilis, chancroid, granuloma inguinale, and lymphopathia venereum.

2. Dermatologic conditions of the scrotum may occur, such as scabies, pediculosis, eczema, and prurigo.

D. TUMORS

1. Benign condyloma acuminatum is a papillary excrescence in the coronal sulcus and inner surface of the prepuce.
   a. Histologically, a complicated papillary structure characterized by pronounced acanthosis and hyperplasia of the prickle cell layer is present. The basement membrane of the lesion is always intact.
   b. The condition is caused by a virus.

2. Malignant Tumors.
   a. Erythroplasia of Queyrat is a squamous cell carcinoma in situ (Bowen's disease) in which the malignant cells are well confined by the basement membrane. No evidence of invasion is present.
   b. Squamous Cell Carcinoma.
      (1) Etiology. As with most cancers, the etiology is not known, but chronic inflammation and accumulations of smegma have been postulated as predisposing factors.
      (2) Clinical Data.
         (a) This tumor represents about 1 percent to 2 percent of all cancers of the male genital tract and occurs predominantly in men between the ages of 40 and 70 years.
         (b) It is most common in uncircumcised males and appears as an ulcerated, painful lesion that bleeds easily.
      (3) Gross Pathology. The lesion appears as an elevated ulcerated papule of variable dimensions.
      (4) Histology. The tumor is identical to the squamous cell cancer that occurs in the skin, tending to be well differentiated and keratinized.
      (5) Prognosis.
         (a) The lesion has a 50 percent 5-year survival rate.
         (b) It grows slowly, although it frequently metastasizes to regional lymph nodes.
      (6) Treatment consists of amputation.

STUDY QUESTIONS

Directions: Each question below contains five suggested answers. Choose the **one best** response to each question.

1. A grossly apparent, well-circumscribed white nodule in the epididymis of a patient undergoing testicular surgery is most likely to be which of the following lesions?

(A) Tuberculous granuloma
(B) Adenomatoid tumor
(C) Spermatocytic granuloma
(D) Congenital malformation
(E) Focal infarct

2. Leydig cell tumors of the testis have a unique histologic finding, which is termed

(A) Michaelis-Gutmann body
(B) Schiller-Duval body
(C) psammoma body
(D) Reinke's crystal
(E) oxalate crystal

3. Which of the following tumor markers has been associated with the yolk sac tumor of the testis?

(A) Carcinoembryonic antigen (CEA)
(B) Acid phosphatase
(C) Beta-human chorionic gonadotropin (HCG)
(D) Alpha-fetoprotein
(E) Alpha$_1$-antitrypsin

Directions: Each question below contains four suggested answers of which **one or more** is correct. Choose the answer

A   if **1, 2, and 3** are correct
B   if **1 and 3** are correct
C   if **2 and 4** are correct
D   if **4** is correct
E   if **1, 2, 3, and 4** are correct

4. Characteristics of cryptorchidism include

(1) failure of one or both testes to migrate into the scrotum
(2) gynecomastia
(3) higher than normal likelihood of developing testicular tumors
(4) complete agenesis of one or both testes

5. Klinefelter's syndrome includes which of the following conditions?

(1) Hypogonadism
(2) Infertility
(3) Gynecomastia
(4) Forty-six chromosomes with an XY karyotype

6. Free mobility of the testis may allow testicular torsion. True statements concerning this condition include

(1) it can be the result of an abnormally wide tunica vaginalis
(2) it results in twisting of the spermatic cord
(3) it can result in infarction of the testis
(4) it can result in a temporary phenomenon with only edema without necrosis

7. True statements concerning testicular seminoma include

(1) it is the most common form of testicular malignancy
(2) it usually does not involve the epididymis
(3) it is most common in middle-aged men
(4) it is the most common tumor found in the cryptorchoid testis

8. Which of the following conditions may be responsible for the symptoms produced by prostatic hypertrophy?

(1) Urethral compression
(2) Urine retention in the bladder
(3) Recurrent cystitis
(4) Infiltration of the bladder wall

9. The prostatic lobes most often affected by benign nodular hyperplasia include the

(1) anterior
(2) posterior
(3) lateral
(4) middle

ANSWERS AND EXPLANATIONS

1. The answer is B. (*III A, B*) The adenomatoid tumor, which is a benign neoplasm of the epididymis, is thought to originate from mesothelial cells. It is a small, white, solitary tumor. Multiple confluent tubercles with caseous necrosis are present in tuberculous epididymitis. Spermatocytic granuloma is presumed to be the result of inflammatory reactions toward a component of semen or spermatocytes. Infarction of the epididymis would not leave a well-circumscribed nodule but, more typically, a fibrous scar.

2. The answer is D. (*II F 1*) The interstitial or Leydig cell tumor originates from the interstitial cells of the testis. Symptoms resulting from this tumor usually relate to the ability of the tumor to produce hormones. Histologically, Leydig cell tumors consist of uniform sheets of cells with eosinophilic cytoplasm. A cigar-shaped inclusion—Reinke's crystal—is present in the cytoplasm along with lipid vacuoles and brown pigment.

3. The answer is D. (*II E 6*) The infantile embryonal cell carcinoma is often termed a yolk sac tumor because of its resemblance to the endodermal sinus and amniotic cavity of a yolk sac. It is predominantly a testicular tumor of children and is identified by the presence of elevated serum levels of α-fetoprotein.

4. The answer is B (1, 3). (*II B 2*) Individuals with cryptorchidism typically have one or both testes located outside of the scrotum. The testis or testes that fail to migrate may be located anywhere along the path of descent from the embryonic urogenital ridge to the inguinal canal. If the cryptorchidism is not corrected prior to puberty, there is usually progressive atrophy of the undescended testis. A male with uncorrected cryptorchidism is more likely to develop neoplasia than is a male with a scrotal testis. Agenesis of one or both testes is distinct from cryptorchidism. No gynecomastia results from the disorder.

5. The answer is A (1, 2, 3). (*II C 3*) Klinefelter's syndrome is characterized by testicular hypoplasia, azoospermia, gynecomastia, eunuchoid habitus, and sometimes mental retardation. Individuals with this syndrome have 47 chromosomes with an XXY karyotype.

6. The answer is E (all). (*II C 5*) Testicular torsion can result in twisting of the spermatic cord, in infarction of the testis, and in a temporary condition with edema but no necrosis. It can be the result of an abnormally wide tunica vaginalis. If the twisting of the spermatic cord is severe with prolonged compression of the blood vessels supplying the testis, infarction and necrosis will occur. The clinical differentiation between torsion and infection is critical since rapid treatment of torsion can save the ischemic testis.

7. The answer is E (all). (*II E 3*) Testicular seminomas account for nearly 70 percent of all testicular tumors. The greatest incidence in the affected male population occurs during the fourth and fifth decades of life. They are the most common neoplasms of the cryptorchoid testis as well. Fortunately, patients with testicular seminomas have a 90 to 98 percent 5-year survival rate.

8. The answer is A (1, 2, 3). (*IV D 1*) Nodular benign hypertrophy, although a very common condition in older men, produces symptoms in only a small percentage of affected patients. These symptoms are usually the result of urethral compression, causing difficulty in micturition and retention of urine within the bladder. Urine retention predisposes to secondary problems such as cystitis, renal infections, and distention of the bladder, ureters, and even the renal pelvis.

9. The answer is D (4). (*IV A, D*) Benign nodular hyperplasia occurs most commonly in the middle lobe of the prostate gland. In contrast to this, adenocarcinoma of the prostate most often involves the posterior lobe.

I. INTRODUCTION. The pathology of the female reproductive system can be considered according to the following schema.

A. Lesions associated with decreased fertility

B. Lesions associated with fertility, pregnancy, and contraception

C. Infectious diseases

D. Inflammatory lesions and neoplastic lesions and their precursors

1. Diseases of the uterus

2. Tumors of the ovaries

3. Tumors of the fallopian tubes

4. Vulvar disorders

5. Disorders of the vagina

II. LESIONS ASSOCIATED WITH DECREASED FERTILITY

A. GONADAL AGENESIS AND DYSGENESIS. Abnormalities in the formation of the ovaries include complete or partial failure of development and the abnormal presence of both ovarian and testicular structures in the same individual. Phenotypic females may be genotypically abnormal (i.e., instead of an XX karyotype, they may have an XO, XY, or a mosaic karyotype).

1. Turner's Syndrome (usually an XO genotype). Individuals with this condition have infantile external genitalia, short stature, webbed neck, and various skeletal abnormalities. Typically, the uterus is small. The gonads are represented by fibrous tissue or ovarian stroma without germ cells (streak gonads).

2. XY Dysgenetic Syndromes.
   a. Pure Gonadal Dysgenesis. Patients with this very rare syndrome have a normal female habitus with primary amenorrhea. The gonads may be streak or ovotestes. A uterus is present.
   b. Testicular Feminization. Certain individuals with a feminine appearance have bilateral, undescended, very immature testes lying in an intra-abdominal or inguinal location. Thirty percent of patients with dysgenetic gonads develop gonadal **neoplasms**, one-third of which are malignant.

B. ENDOMETRIOSIS is defined as benign but displaced endometrial tissue (glands and stroma) occurring outside of the uterine fundic mucosa. The condition can occur anywhere in the pelvis or, less often, in extrapelvic sites (Fig. 13-1). **Adenomyosis** is endometriosis in the wall of the uterus.

1. Clinical Data. Pelvic endometriosis is most common in women who delay childbearing. The major symptom is pain. Abnormal uterine bleeding also is common and results from the ectopic endometrial tissue responding to the hormonal variations of the menstrual cycle. Infertility may develop because the uterine tubes are involved in almost all cases, and the

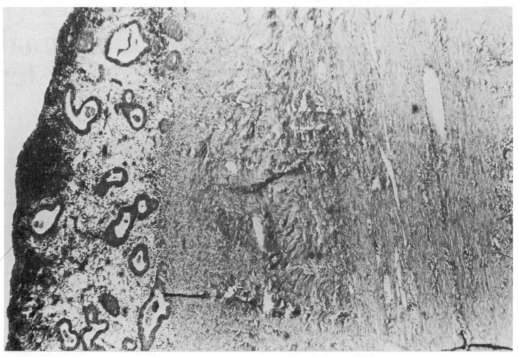

endometrial glands

Figure 13-1. Low-power view of endometriosis. Glands and stroma of endometrial type are present *(left)* in the ovary.

response of the endometrial tissue to cyclic changes can lead to fibrosis and distortion or narrowing of the tubes.

  2. Pathogenesis.
    a. Sampson's theory postulates that endometriosis is caused by **reflux menstruation** through the fallopian tubes and beyond into the ovaries and pelvis, with implantation of endometrial tissue.
    b. Novak's theory suggests that any part of the müllerian system may undergo change to endometrial tissue via a **metaplasia** of the specialized surface epithelium (mesothelium). Most modern investigators favor this theory.
    c. Others have postulated that lymphatic or blood-borne **emboli** are responsible. This theory offers the best explanation for endometriosis in rare sites such as the retroperitoneal lymph nodes and the lungs.

  3. Pathology.
    a. Grossly, endometriosis appears as tiny-to-large blue cysts, often on peritoneal surfaces. In the ovary, large **"chocolate" cysts** can occur as a result of repeated hemorrhage.
    b. Microscopically, endometrial glands and stroma are found, frequently surrounded by hemorrhage, hemosiderin, and fibrosis.

  4. Location. Endometriosis most often affects the uterine tubes, ovaries, cervix, and vagina. Extragenital sites include the urinary bladder, intestines, appendix, laparotomy scars, and hernia sacs.

  5. Complications. The response of the ectopic endometrium to cyclic hormonal changes can lead to smooth muscle hypertrophy and fibrosis in some affected organs such as the intestine, which in turn may lead to **obstruction**. In scars and hernia sacs, monthly **swelling** and pain can result, and in the bladder, endometriosis can cause **hematuria**.

C. PELVIC INFLAMMATORY DISEASE (PID) is an inflammatory (predominantly infectious) condition of the fallopian tubes (salpingitis) and paratubal tissues, which can lead to fibrosis, scarring, and obstruction of the tubes.

  1. Etiology and Pathogenesis.
    a. The infection usually results from *Neisseria gonorrhoeae* and is venereally transmitted.

b. Coliform organisms, especially *Escherichia coli (E. coli)*, also may be responsible. Recently, coliform organisms producing salpingitis have been found with increasing frequency in women wearing **intrauterine devices** (IUDs).

c. Tubal tuberculosis is a rare cause of chronic salpingitis in the Western Hemisphere.

2. Clinical Data. Fever, pain, and other signs of infection are common. Although therapy may allow subsidence of the infection, once damage to the tubal epithelium has occurred, it is irreversible, and chronic salpingitis ensues.

3. Pathology.

a. The **acutely** inflamed fallopian tube is red and swollen; microscopically, the capillaries are congested and there is pus in the lumen, wall, and serosa. As the infection continues, the tubal plicae adhere to each other. The infection extends outside the tube, producing paratubal and tubo-ovarian abscesses. Both tube and ovary become incorporated into an inflammatory mass, plastered together by fibrinopurulent exudate.

b. In **chronic** salpingitis, the adherent plicae fuse, and fibrosis occurs. Adhesions may obliterate the lumen of the tube, leading to pyosalpinx or hydrosalpinx. The adhesions and stenosis produced are major causes of **sterility** and **tubal pregnancy**.

D. OVARIAN CAUSES OF STERILITY

1. **Stein-Leventhal (polycystic ovary) syndrome** is characterized by infertility, hirsutism, obesity, and secondary amenorrhea in young women who have enlarged cystic ovaries.

a. The **etiology** is unknown. The common finding is a persistent failure to ovulate. Biochemically, 17-ketosteroid production usually is normal, follicle-stimulating hormone is normal, and androgens are found in excessive quantity in cyst fluid and urine.

b. **Pathology.** The ovaries are large (4 cm to 6 cm) and have a pale gray color, produced by a thick fibrous capsule. Beneath the capsule are seen many small cystic spaces containing clear, watery fluid.

c. **Histologically**, normal structures are seen, but the pattern is abnormal. The capsule is composed of dense fibrous tissue and is markedly thicker than is usual. The cysts are graafian follicles, developing or atretic. The theca layer is overly luteinized, although the granulosa layer is not. Ova are present generally in normal numbers. The stroma, especially in the medulla, is prominent.

d. Some patients with this syndrome develop endometrial hyperplasia and, rarely, carcinoma.

2. Hyperthecosis and stromal hyperplasia tend to be more masculinizing than the Stein-Leventhal syndrome and may cause true virilism. Onset of these conditions may not occur until middle or older age, in contrast to Stein-Leventhal syndrome, which affects young women.

a. Etiology. The cause and biochemical changes involved are unknown.

b. Pathology. The ovaries are large and solid, lacking cysts. Large, luteinized theca cells are distributed in groups throughout hyperplastic ovarian stroma.

III. LESIONS ASSOCIATED WITH FERTILITY, PREGNANCY, AND CONTRACEPTION

A. THE MENSTRUAL CYCLE. The various hormonal changes that occur during the ovarian cycle lead to characteristic histologic alterations in the endometrium, affecting glands and stroma. Evaluation of the stage of the menstrual cycle, and thus estimation of ovulation, can be ascertained by endometrial biopsy.

B. PREGNANCY

1. Spontaneous abortion may result because of trauma, blighted ova, viral infections, and fetal death or, most commonly, unknown reasons.

2. At or near term, problems of intrauterine pregnancy are often mechanical and chiefly involve fetal position, cephalopelvic disproportion, or abnormal placental implantation sites.

3. Abnormalities of the Placenta.

a. Placenta previa refers to the condition in which the placenta develops in the lower uterine segment and partially or completely covers the internal os, necessitating delivery of the placenta before the fetus. **Painless vaginal bleeding** is the most common symptom of the condition. Because the abnormality compromises the infant at partum and predisposes to maternal hemorrhage, its presence generally requires that delivery be made by cesarean section.

b. Placenta accreta, a rare condition, is implantation of the placenta in the myometrial surface: chorionic villi may penetrate the uterine muscle (**placenta increta**) or penetrate

the entire myometrial wall and extend into the uterine serosa **(placenta percreta)**.
   (1) Such placentas occur in uteri that previously have been scarred by infection or trauma, and they implant in areas of denuded endometrium, which lack normal decidua.
   (2) **Clinical Data.** These lesions are associated with excessive hemorrhage both intra- and postpartum because the placentas cannot separate normally from the uterus.
c. **Placental abruption (abruptio placentae)** is separation of the placenta from the uterine wall *before* delivery of the infant.
   (1) The separation, which may run for only a few millimeters or be complete, impedes normal postpartum vascular constriction, and bleeding results (retroplacental hemorrhage).
   (2) **Clinical Data.** While mild abruption may be asymptomatic, severe abruption produces uterine rigidity, severe abdominal pain, shock, and occasional disseminated intravascular coagulation in the mother, as well as severe fetal distress or fetal death. Abruption is associated with preexisting maternal hypertension in 25 percent to 50 percent of cases; it is the most common **recognizable** cause of fetal death.
d. Preexisting maternal **vascular disease** is often reflected in the extremely vascular placenta. Maternal hypertension, diabetes, lupus erythematosus, and renal disease may all cause vascular abnormalities. Such lesions may be accompanied by degenerative changes, hyalinization of villi, and infarcts.
e. **Chorioangioma** is a true hemangioma of the placenta. Found in only 1 percent of pregnancies, it is still the most common benign tumor of the placenta. It is rarely very large (usually under 5 cm) and has no clinical manifestations unless it becomes big enough to compromise the placenta by replacement.
f. **Multiple-Gestation Placentas.** With monozygotic twins, there may be a single placenta or two individual ones. When there is only one placenta, gross and histologic examination of the placental membranes at the separation zone will disclose, with a high degree of accuracy, whether the pregnancy is mono- or diamniotic and mono- or dichorionic.

4. **Ectopic pregnancy** (i.e., pregnancy outside the uterus) may occur in the ovary or pelvic peritoneum, but it affects the fallopian tubes in over 95 percent of cases (Fig. 13-2). The incidence of ectopic pregnancy is increased in women who have a history of pelvic inflammatory disease. Tubal pregnancies comprise about 2 percent of all pregnancies, but if a patient has 1 such pregnancy, her chance of having another is 1 in 10.
   a. **Pathology.** As a tubal pregnancy progresses, the wall of the tube is distended and weakened by infiltration of chorionic villi. With progressive enlargement, tubal rupture and

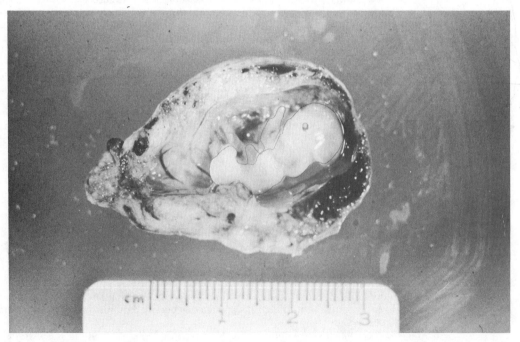

Figure 13-2. Cross section of a tubal (ectopic) pregnancy with the fetus in place.

hemorrhage become inevitable. Most tubal pregnancies progress for 6 weeks to 12 weeks and then abort.
   b. Ectopic pregnancy is life-threatening to the mother and must be surgically treated.
5. Preeclampsia and Eclampsia (Toxemia of Pregnancy). In the last trimester of pregnancy, about 6 percent to 7 percent of women develop hypertension, edema, albuminuria, and salt retention, a syndrome known as preeclampsia; eclampsia is the more severe form of the syndrome, in which the above symptoms are accompanied by convulsions. Eclampsia is a frequent cause of maternal and fetal mortality.
   a. Cause. The etiology is unknown. The condition tends to occur in young primigravid women. The pathologic findings are similar to those in the generalized Shwartzman reaction, suggesting the possibility that degenerative products of necrotic decidua or the trophoblast may be an inciting factor.
   b. Pathology. Maternal autopsies have shown hemorrhage, necrosis, and fibrin deposition in the liver, kidneys, and brain. The placenta shows aging changes, necrosis, trophoblastic degeneration, and large infarcts.

6. Disorders of the Trophoblast.
   a. Hydatidiform mole results from the missed abortion of a pathologic ovum. The condition occurs when the death of an embryo at 3 weeks to 5 weeks gestation is followed by hydropic changes in the vascular villi; because the trophoblast survives the embryo, the villi accumulate fluid and swell.
      (1) Incidence. In the United States hydatidiform moles occur in 1 in 2000 pregnancies; in the Orient, in 1 in 125 to 250 pregnancies. Poor nutrition, consanguinity, and either very young or very old maternal age seem to increase the incidence.
      (2) Pathology. The uterus often enlarges more rapidly than normal, and human chorionic gonadotropin (HCG) serum levels are elevated. When the mole aborts, a large mass of edematous tissue with grape-like bulbs of hydropic villi is found.
      (3) Histologically, the hydropic villi are sparsely cellular and avascular; they are covered by a syncytiotrophoblast. Occasionally, highly proliferative trophoblastic lesions are seen.
      (4) Course. In 80 percent of affected patients, the condition has a benign course after uterine evacuation. The remainder of patients eventually manifest evidence of an **aggressive malignant lesion** (invading the myometrium or extrauterine tissues).
   b. Choriocarcinoma of gestational origin is a rare neoplasm composed of malignant trophoblast. Of these lesions, 50 percent are **preceded by molar pregnancy**, 25 percent by abortion, 22 percent by normal pregnancy, and 3 percent by ectopic pregnancy.
      (1) Pathology. Choriocarcinoma is composed of soft (necrotic?) hemorrhagic nodules, microscopically showing admixtures of syncytio- and cytotrophoblastic cells and vascular invasion. The tumor produces HCG, the measurement of which is used clinically to follow response to therapy and determine prognosis.
      (2) Course. Actinomycin D or methotrexate can cure patients with a low-risk tumor, and combination chemotherapy with the two drugs plus cyclophosphamide often is effective for patients with widespread metastases; overall, chemotherapy produces a 75 percent to 80 percent cure rate. Hysterectomy is not needed and, in fact, normal pregnancies with viable offspring are not unusual in women cured of choriocarcinoma.

C. DISORDERS ASSOCIATED WITH ORAL CONTRACEPTIVES AND INTRAUTERINE DEVICES

1. Oral Contraceptives.
   a. Most endocervical changes produced by oral contraceptives are recapitulations of the microglandular hyperplasia seen in pregnancy.
   b. In the endometrium, oral contraceptives can produce atypia in glandular epithelium and hyperplasia. Recently, adenocarcinoma of the endometrium (usually a disease of postmenopausal women) has been found with abnormally high frequency in young women who take sequential oral contraceptives.

2. Intrauterine Devices. In the endometrium, squamous metaplasia and chronic endometritis are found in about 1 in 5 women using IUDs. The incidence of tubo-ovarian infections (and possibly of ectopic pregnancies) appears to be increased in women using IUDs.

IV. INFECTIOUS DISEASES

A. VIRAL DISEASES

1. Herpes genitalis is caused by herpes simplex type 2 virus, which is venereally transmitted.

    a. In over 90 percent of cases, the infection is subclinical. If symptomatic, **painful focal vesicles** or blisters are found on the cervix, vagina, and vulva. Associated dysuria, fever, and malaise may occur.

    b. **Pathologically**, the gross lesions are 1-mm vesicles surrounded by an erythematous base; focal ulceration may be present. Histologically and on Pap smears, the hallmark is the finding of **multinucleated giant epithelial cells with homogeneous intranuclear inclusions**.

    c. The herpetic lesion usually resolves spontaneously in 1 to 3 weeks. Recurrences are common. The possibility of a relationship between herpesvirus infection and **cervical cancer** is discussed in V B 6 a (5) (a). Active herpetic infection occurring in pregnant women usually necessitates cesarean section to avoid systemic, **possibly fatal, disease in the newborn infant**.

  2. **Condyloma Acuminatum [Papillomavirus Infection]** (Fig. 13-3).

    a. This viral infection is extremely common in sexually active women; it is an incidental finding in 2 percent to 10 percent of Pap smears. The infection is usually asymptomatic.

    b. **Grossly**, 2 percent to 4 percent of affected women have verrucuous (warty) papillary tumors on the cervix, vagina, or vulva. However, according to recent evidence, most papillomavirus infections cause **flat lesions**, which especially involve the cervix.

    c. **Histologically**, the affected epithelium is thickened, with superficial cells showing large crinkled nuclei surrounded by clear cytoplasm (balloon cells: koilocytosis). Studies have shown that 20 percent to 30 percent of affected women have a coexistent dysplastic lesion of the cervix. A possible etiologic association with cervical cancer is discussed in V B 6 a (5) (b).

B. **SYPHILIS**, caused by the spirochete *Treponema pallidum*, is transmitted either by venereal contact or transplacentally by an infected mother to her unborn child (congenital syphilis).

  1. **Clinical Data.** Three stages of the disease are recognized.

    a. The **primary stage** is characterized by the development of a chancre (a **painless hard-based ulcer**) at the point of inoculation (usually in the genital area), but this stage often is asymptomatic.

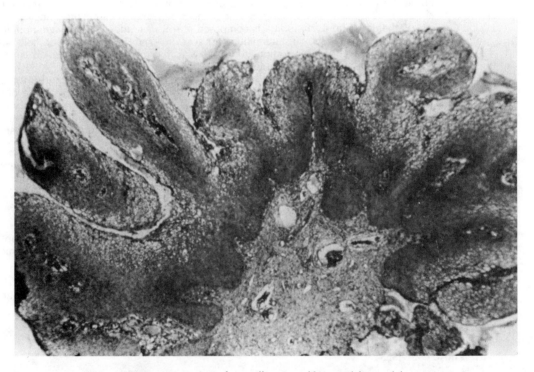

Figure 13-3. Low-power view of a papillary (wart-like) condyloma of the cervix.

b. In the **secondary stage,** usually 1 month to 4 months later, a diffuse skin rash (which may develop into **condylomata lata** in moist areas) is associated with generalized (especially inguinal) lymphadenopathy and often is accompanied by fever and malaise.

c. Tertiary syphilis affects the cardiovascular and central nervous systems often after latent periods of 1 to 30 years. Other areas, especially the liver, bones, and joints may be affected by gummas.

2. Pathologically, the lesions in the three stages are different.

   a. A chancre is a grossly shallow ulcer. Microscopically, the epithelium is ulcerated and the ulcer base shows an intense, predominantly plasmacytic infiltrate, accompanied by an obliterative endarteritis. Spirochetes are numerous.

   b. Skin biopsies of the rash of secondary syphilis show a subepidermal mononuclear cell (plasma cell) infiltrate, chiefly perivascular. Spirochetes may be found. The lymph nodes demonstrate an extensive capsular fibrosis and plasmacytic perivasculitis.

   c. The cardiac and nervous system lesions are described in the appropriate chapters.

3. The diagnosis of syphilis is either made by dark-field examination of material from the primary chancre (when present) or by serologic tests.

C. GONORRHEA is the most common venereal disease in the United States. It is caused by the diplococcus *Neisseria gonorrhoeae*. This organism has surface pili that preferentially attach to endocervical and fallopian tube epithelium, allowing access of the organism into host cells.

1. Clinical Data. The most common symptoms in infected women include vaginal discharge and dysuria, but up to 50 percent of infected women are asymptomatic. Some patients may present with constitutional symptoms including fever, abdominal pain, and vomiting, which are indicative of acute salpingitis with pelvic peritonitis (PID). Gonorrheal infection is responsible for about 50 percent to 65 percent of cases of PID.

2. Pathologically, the initial involvement may affect Bartholin's glands or the endocervix and often is followed by ascending infection that reaches the fallopian tubes. The tubal epithelium is exquisitely sensitive to the gonococcus, and acute salpingitis with purulent exudate (pyosalpinx) results. Extension into the ovaries and pelvic peritoneum may ensue, with formation of adhesions and decreased fertility (see II C 3).

3. The **diagnosis** of gonorrhea necessitates identification of the organism either by gram-stained direct smears of infected material or by appropriate bacteriologic cultures.

D. CHANCROID

1. Caused by *Hemophilus ducreyi (H. ducreyi)*, this venereal disease is endemic in tropical countries, although it is of minor significance in the United States.

2. Clinical Data. One or frequently multiple **painful, soft ulcers** are noted at the site of inoculation (incubation period: 3 to 5 days). Early, rapid enlargement of regional lymph nodes may occur.

3. Pathologically, the chancroid ulcer shows superficial necrosis, with underlying granulation tissue and fibrosis. Acute, tender, suppurative lymphadenitis is found, often unilaterally, in draining nodes.

4. Specific **diagnosis** requires isolation of *H. ducreyi* from an ulcer or bubo. The disease is usually self-limited, eventually resulting in scarring of affected nodes and ulcer sites.

E. CHLAMYDIAL INFECTIONS. The *Chlamydia* genus consists of small microorganisms that are considered to be bacteria despite the fact that they undergo obligate intracellular development in the cytoplasm of infected cells. *Chlamydia trachomatis (C. trachomatis)* causes lymphogranuloma venereum (LGV), and some subtypes produce nonspecific urethritis and cervicitis.

1. Lymphogranuloma Venereum.

   a. LGV is much less common in the United States than the other diseases that were described previously.

   b. Clinical Data. It is characterized by transient genital or anal ulcers (which often are overlooked by the affected patient), followed 2 to 6 weeks later by regional lymphadenitis. The lymph node involvement is associated with abscesses and fistula formation, often involving the rectal, vaginal, and inguinal areas; at later stages, these lesions heal by scarring and can produce **strictures**.

   c. The **diagnosis** usually is made by serologic testing (microimmunofluorescent antibody test or LGV complement fixation).

2. Other Chlamydial Infections.
  a. Clinical Data. Other genital chlamydial infections (e.g., cervicitis and salpingitis) are usually asymptomatic in women and are brought to clinical attention by a concomitant symptomatic venereal disease. The greatest importance in recognizing these types of chlamydial infection lies in the possible transmission to neonates at parturition, resulting in **neonatal conjunctivitis and pneumonia**.
  b. The **diagnosis** can be made by finding characteristic intracytoplasmic inclusion bodies in cervicovaginal cytologic smears.

F. GRANULOMA INGUINALE

1. Caused by the organism *Donovania (Calymmatobacterium) granulomatis*, this presumably venereally transmitted disease is most common in tropical areas and is rare in the United States.

2. Clinical Data. At the site of inoculation, an initial papule gives rise to a large serpiginous ulcer. Many satellite lesions may occur and become infected secondarily. Regional lymphadenopathy may ensue.

3. Pathologically, there is acute and chronic inflammation with vacuolated macrophages containing the causative organisms (Donovan bodies), which are demonstrable by Giemsa stain.

4. Diagnosis requires identification of Donovan bodies in smears, scrapings, or biopsies of active lesions.

G. CANDIDIASIS (moniliasis) is the most common type of vulvovaginitis. The causative fungus *Candida albicans* normally is a commensal organism but can become pathogenic under certain conditions (e.g., pregnancy, diabetes, cancer, immunosuppression, and ingestion of oral contraceptive pills and systemic antibiotics).

1. Clinical Data. Affected patients present with intense vulvar pruritus.

2. The vulva and vagina may be reddened, and characteristic white patches may be present. Vaginal secretions usually have a white, curdled appearance.

3. The diagnosis is made on clinical grounds, although cytologic smears can confirm it by demonstrating the causative fungus.

H. TRICHOMONIASIS is an infection of the vagina in women of reproductive age.

1. The major **clinical** symptom is a copious, malodorous, green-yellow or gray vaginal discharge, sometimes accompanied by pruritus. The prevalence of asymptomatic infection is high, especially in men.

2. The **diagnosis** often can be made by clinical examination and can be confirmed by cytologic smears or wet-mount preparations. Atypia in cervicovaginal epithelium may be noted in cytologic preparations.

V. DISEASES OF THE UTERUS

A. MYOMETRIUM

1. Leiomyomas (fibroids) are extremely common benign tumors found in 30 percent to 60 percent of women at autopsy (Fig. 13-4).
  a. Usually they are **multiple** tumors. They arise from uterine muscle and may be found in subserosal, intramural, or submucosal locations.
  b. Usually asymptomatic, they may undergo degenerative changes leading to pain; if submucosal, they may cause bleeding.
  c. During pregnancy or in women using oral contraceptives, leiomyomas, which are hormone-dependent, may increase in size. Rarely, they may produce mechanical problems at the time of delivery.
  d. Fibroids can interfere with conception.

2. Leiomyosarcomas comprise only 0.5 percent to 1 percent of mesenchymal uterine tumors but are the most common sarcoma of the uterus.
  a. It is doubtful if leiomyomas undergo malignant change, and most leiomyosarcomas arise de novo.
  b. Prognosis depends upon the extent of the lesion, the size, and mitotic activity. With well-differentiated leiomyosarcomas, there is a 40 percent to 50 percent 5-year survival rate following surgery and chemotherapy. Premenopausal women fare better than older patients.

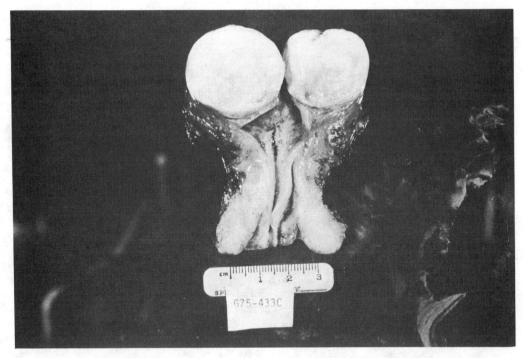

Figure 13-4. Leiomyoma of the uterus showing a circumscribed homogeneous mass in the wall of the uterus.

B. CERVIX

1. **Acute cervicitis** may be associated with ulceration, especially following trauma at parturition or following specific bacterial infections. The endocervical glands may proliferate in response to inflammation; the lumina of the glands may become occluded, resulting in cystic dilation of the glands, which produces **nabothian cysts**.

2. **Chronic cervicitis** with **squamous metaplasia** is found almost universally in postmenopausal women. The severity of inflammation varies considerably.

3. **Cervical erosion** is the extension of endocervical mucosa beyond the external os onto the exocervix where it overgrows destroyed squamous epithelium. This process is probably not inflammatory but is either congenital or a response to a factor such as vaginal pH. In a reparative attempt, the squamous epithelium of the exocervix grows back over the eroding endocervical mucosa in a process called **epidermidization**. Also, squamous cells may originate from reserve cells of the endocervix, giving rise to **squamous metaplasia**. These competing processes may alter the position of the squamocolumnar junction in the so-called transformation zone.

4. Pregnancy or the use of oral contraceptives may stimulate **glandular hyperplasia**, leading to what has been called the pill tumor. This florid pattern of hyperplasia must be differentiated from adenocarcinoma.

5. **Endocervical polyp** is really an overgrown fold of endocervical mucosa. It may have a papillary pattern and contain cystic glands. It is extremely vascular (bleeds easily), is never malignant, and is common in postmenopausal women.

6. **Cancer of the Cervix.**
   a. **Cervical Intraepithelial Neoplasia.**
      (1) **Dysplasia** usually refers to a combination of nuclear atypia, focal hypercellularity of the epithelium, and loss of cellular polarity involving only part of the epithelial thickness (thus preserving some evidence of normal cellular maturation toward the surface).
      (2) **Carcinoma in situ** (preinvasive cancer) implies a high mitotic rate, marked cellularity, and loss of polarity and maturation throughout the full thickness of the cervical epithelium (Fig. 13-5).

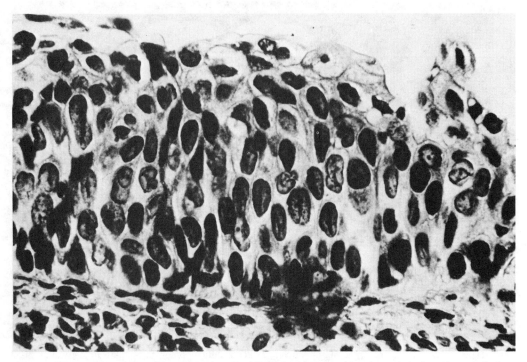

Figure 13-5. Carcinoma in situ of the cervix showing full-thickness mucosal involvement by neoplastic cells (low power).

(3) Because these two premalignant changes produce no gross visible effects, diagnosis depends on biopsy or exfoliative cytology [Papanicolaou's (Pap) test]. Biopsy may be directed by use of Lugol's solution, which fails to stain dysplastic areas, or by colposcopy, which identifies abnormal areas by changes in vascular pattern. (Cytology has the advantage in that it is atraumatic and easy to repeat.)

(4) **Etiology.** The single cell theory is the most widely accepted etiologic theory concerning cervical squamous carcinoma and the premalignant states of dysplasia and carcinoma in situ. Studies of glucose-6-phosphate dehydrogenase isoenzymes suggest that in 95 percent of cases dysplasia and carcinoma in situ originate in one cell. Thus, cancer of the cervix is believed to begin in a single cell at the squamocolumnar junction as mild dysplasia, to pass through a carcinoma in situ stage, and then to involve the transformation zone and the endocervix. The entire stage of cervical intraepithelial neoplasia has a mean duration of 12 to 15 years from mild dysplasia to carcinoma in situ.

(5) **Epidemiology.**
   (a) Women who have had a **herpesvirus type 2 infection** have a higher incidence of cervical cancer than controls; women who have cervical cancer have a higher incidence of antibodies to herpesvirus than controls.
      (i) In vitro experiments have shown the oncogenic potential of herpesvirus type 2. Recently, hybridization studies demonstrated part of the herpesvirus genome incorporated within the genetic makeup of cervical cancer cells.
      (ii) Proof of causation requires further evidence, however, and it should be noted that individuals may be affected by a high incidence of two diseases without a causal relationship existing.
   (b) Recent studies indicate an association between cervical intraepithelial neoplasia and **condyloma** (papillomavirus) infection of the cervix and vagina. Careful studies are needed for adequate interpretation of this relationship.
   (c) A positive **epidemiologic relationship** exists between cancer of the cervix and the following factors.
      (i) Early age at first coitus
      (ii) Multiple sexual partners
      (iii) Low socioeconomic status

- **(iv)** Multiparity, which suggests birth trauma may play a role
- **(v)** Poor hygiene: smegma may be a factor as the incidence of cervical intraepithelial neoplasia is low in Jews and Moslems who practice circumcision.
  - **(6)** The **prognosis** for cervical intraepithelial neoplasia is 100 percent cure with treatment.
- **b. Squamous Cell Carcinoma.**
  - **(1)** Ninety-five percent of cervical cancer is squamous cell carcinoma.
  - **(2)** The stage after carcinoma in situ is microinvasive cancer (an invasion of less than 3 mm in depth), followed by invasive cancer, which appears as a granular, papillary, or ulcerated lesion, which bleeds easily, near the external os. When invasion begins, the cells penetrate into the stroma, keratinize, and may reach the lymphatics and disseminate to parametrial, iliac, and hypogastric nodes, later to sacral and obturator nodes, and finally to lumbar and inguinal nodes. The average age (40 to 50 years old) at diagnosis of invasive cancer is 8 to 10 years older than that at diagnosis of carcinoma in situ.
  - **(3)** The **incidence** of invasive cervical cancer has been halved in the past 40 years as a result of routine cytologic screening that allows identification of dysplasia, the presumed precursor of the lesion. Invasive cervical cancer now occurs in about 2 percent of women in the United States. Previously, carcinoma of the cervix was 20 times more common than endometrial cancer; now the incidence is roughly equal.
  - **(4)** **Treatment** consists of hysterectomy for the microinvasive stage and radiotherapy for the frankly invasive stage. The **prognosis** is related to the clinical stage, with lymphatic spread being the most important consideration. For stage I lesions with negative nodes, the 5-year survival rate is almost 90 percent; for stage IV lesions, it is closer to 10 percent.
- **c. Adenocarcinoma** of endocervical glands represents about 5 percent of cervical cancers.
  - **(1)** Its behavior and degree of malignancy are roughly comparable to those of cervical squamous carcinoma because its lymphatic spread is similar.
  - **(2)** **Clinical Data.** Patients with endocervical adenocarcinoma more closely resemble those with endometrial carcinoma than do those with squamous cervical cancer. They tend to be postmenopausal, nulliparous (or have few children), obese, hypertensive, and diabetic.
  - **(3)** The **prognosis** depends upon the degree of differentiation and the extent of the lesion.

C. ENDOMETRIUM

1. **Acute endometritis** usually is caused by a bacterial infection of the endometrium that is associated with septic abortion. Occasionally, specific viruses (cytomegalovirus) or fungi *(Aspergillus)* may be responsible.

2. **Chronic endometritis** is defined by the presence of plasma cells in inflamed endometrial stroma, which may be seen in postabortal states, postpartum (especially if retained placental fragments are present), in the presence of an IUD, and following instrumentation of the endometrial cavity. Over 50 percent to 60 percent of cases have no known cause, which may reflect an immunologic response, possibly to sperm. Affected patients have abnormal uterine bleeding, which often is painful.

3. **Polyps** of the endometrium occur at or near menopause and may cause bleeding.
   - **a.** They are composed of endometrial glands and stroma and represent a portion of basalis endometrium that is unresponsive to the hormonal cycle.
   - **b.** They may become necrotic at their tips, ulcerate, and bleed. (Rarely, they contain carcinoma.)

4. **Hyperplasia** of the endometrium (excessive endometrial proliferation) is found in patients with relative or absolute hyperestrogenism (as is found in obesity, functioning ovarian tumors, exogenous estrogen intake, and Stein-Leventhal syndrome).
   - **a. Cystic** hyperplasia is characterized by the presence of ectatic glands that are lined by plump, benign endometrial cells. It is associated with a 1 percent to 2 percent risk of progression to endometrial adenocarcinoma.
   - **b. Adenomatous** hyperplasia is characterized by the presence of an increased number of glands with budding and subgland formation. An increase in the gland-to-stroma ratio is found. There is a 10 percent risk of cancer.
   - **c. Atypical adenomatous** hyperplasia is characterized by the presence of cytologic atypia in the individual glandular cells. There is a 20 percent to 25 percent risk of cancer.

5. **Metaplasia.** Changes in endometrial glandular tissue include squamous, tubal, papillary, and eosinophilic varieties. The changes occur near or after menopause, often in women

taking exogenous hormones, and may be associated with various degrees of hyperplasia. They have been misinterpreted as adenocarcinoma of the endometrium, from which they differ in their lack of cytologic atypia.

6. **Adenocarcinoma.**
   a. The **incidence** of adenocarcinoma of the endometrium has increased over the past 20 years and is now roughly equal to that of cervical cancer (12 to 15 cases per 100,000). The highest incidence occurs at the age of endometrial atrophy (i.e., postmenopausally) in middle-class, often obese, women.
   b. **Etiology.** Unopposed **estrogen** action during prolonged anovulatory cycles (premenopausal) appears to lead to hyperplasia of the endometrium, which is a possible precursor of endometrial cancer. The etiologic role of estrogen is supported by an increased incidence of endometrial cancer in women who have functioning ovarian tumors, Stein-Leventhal syndrome, delayed menopause, or who have received prolonged exogenous estrogen therapy.
   c. **Histologically**, adenocarcinoma of the endometrium can be well or poorly differentiated (Fig. 13-6). About 25 percent of these tumors show benign squamous metaplasia (**adenoacanthoma**); 25 percent have malignant squamous elements (**adenosquamous cancer**). In 70 percent of cases, the cancer is confined to the uterine corpus at the time of diagnosis; in 3 percent, it spreads outside the pelvis.
   d. **Prognostic features** include anatomic extent, histologic differentiation, depth of myometrial invasion, size of the uterine cavity (there is decreased survival with increasing size), age of the patient, and presence of metastases. The average 5-year survival rate is 63 percent.
   e. **Treatment** consists of surgery, usually combined with radiotherapy.

7. **Carcinosarcoma and mixed müllerian tumors** are lesions that show a variety of histologic patterns, often combining sarcomatous and carcinomatous patterns. They usually occur in postmenopausal women. The 5-year survival rate is 15 percent.

8. **Stromal Tumors.**
   a. A **stromal nodule** is a circumscribed nodule resembling a leiomyoma; it is usually an incidental finding.
   b. **Endolymphatic stromal myosis** is a low-grade malignant tumor of endometrial stromal cells with a peculiar propensity to invade the myometrial wall and vascular spaces.

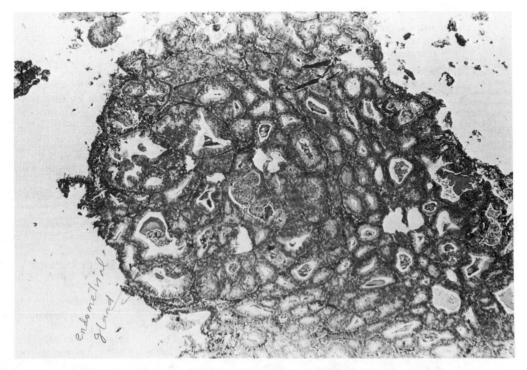

Figure 13-6. Well-differentiated adenocarcinoma of the endometrium (low power).

Although the 5-year survival rate is fairly high, recurrences and death usually occur within 10 to 15 years of onset.

c. **Stromal sarcomas** resemble leiomyosarcomas clinically and in terms of prognosis. These fully malignant tumors have a 5-year survival rate of less than 50 percent.

VI. TUMORS OF THE OVARIES.
Neoplastic lesions of the ovaries are the most diverse group of tumors affecting any organ in the human body. Although malignant ovarian tumors occur less frequently than malignant tumors of the cervix or endometrium, they are the fourth most common cause of **cancer death** in American women (ranking after cancer of the breast, colon, and lung).

A. EPITHELIAL TUMORS

1. **Incidence.** Epithelial tumors are by far the most common tumors of the ovaries, comprising approximately 60 percent of ovarian neoplasms.

2. **Clinical Data.** Epithelial tumors usually come to attention as large abdominal masses, often discovered as incidental findings during routine pelvic examination. Presentation is non-specific; affected patients may complain of abdominal discomfort, distention, constipation, urinary frequency, or abnormal bleeding.

3. **Classification.** Each epithelial tumor is classified according to its epithelial cell type [e.g., serous, mucinous, and so forth] (Table 13-1). Most tumors are then further categorized as benign, borderline, or malignant.

   a. **Serous tumors** are characterized by the presence of ciliated epithelial cells that resemble the epithelium of the fallopian tube. These tumors arise from the surface epithelium of the ovary.

   (1) **Incidence.** These neoplasms account for approximately 20 percent to 50 percent of ovarian tumors.

   (2) **Clinical Data.** They may occur at any age but predominate between the ages of 30 and 60 years. Bilateral neoplasms can be seen in as high as 50 percent to 60 percent of cases.

   (a) **Benign serous cystadenomas** comprise 20 percent of all serous tumors and are usually unilateral.

   (i) **Grossly**, these tumors are uni- or multilocular, thin-walled cysts filled with yellow, clear fluid. They can be very large but rarely attain huge dimensions. The surface of the ovary is smooth and lacks papillae.

   (ii) **Microscopically**, the cysts are lined by a single layer of ciliated cuboidal epithelium. There is no mitosis, pleomorphism, or necrosis. Occasionally the cyst lining is not identified.

Table 13-1. Classification of Ovarian Tumors

Epithelial (60 percent)

Serous tumors
Mucinous tumors
Brenner tumors
Endometrioid carcinomas
Clear cell carcinomas
Mixed mesodermal tumors

Germ Cell (15 percent to 20 percent)

Teratomas
   Benign dermoid cysts (mature cystic teratomas)
   Immature teratomas
Dysgerminomas
Endodermal sinus tumors
Mixed germ cell tumors

Gonadal Stromal (5 percent to 10 percent)

Thecomas and fibrothecomas
Granulosa cell tumors
Sertoli cell tumors
Lipid cell tumors

Metastatic (5 percent to 10 percent)

      (iii) Treatment and Prognosis. Oophorectomy is usually curative.

   (b) Borderline serous tumors (carcinomas of low malignant potential) constitute 9 percent to 15 percent of all serous tumors. The tumors are bilateral in 25 percent of cases.

      (i) Grossly, these lesions are recognizable by the presence of firm papillary excrescences, which may involve the serosal surface of one or both ovaries, as well as being present within the cavity of a cyst. Yellow, clear fluid fills the cystic spaces.

      (ii) Microscopically, the epithelium reveals complicated papillae lined by stratified epithelium, generally not exceeding two or three layers of cells, with variable degrees of cellular atypia. A cribriform pattern may be present, but **true stromal invasion is absent**. Calcified psammoma bodies are found in one-fourth of all cases.

      (iii) Prognosis. These tumors often spread beyond the ovary, especially in the form of peritoneal implants (present in up to 40 percent of cases); the implants may regress, remain stationary, or progress and become invasive. True metastases to viscera or lymph nodes do not, however, occur. The stage (degree of spread) appears to be the single most important prognostic factor. The 10-year survival rate is approximately 90 percent, but recurrences may develop after this time period.

      (iv) Treatment typically consists of bilateral salpingo-oophorectomy, hysterectomy, and omentectomy with as much removal of the tumor as possible, but may be more conservative if the patient is young and wants to preserve fertility and if there is no biopsy-proven involvement of the opposite ovary.

   (c) Serous cystadenocarcinomas represent at least 65 percent of serous tumors and are the most common of all malignant ovarian tumors, constituting approximately 40 percent of this group. As many as two-thirds of the cases are bilateral.

      (i) Grossly, these carcinomas range from being predominantly cystic and papillary to being entirely solid masses with areas of hemorrhage and necrosis. The ovarian surfaces usually are covered with diffuse papillary excrescences.

      (ii) Microscopically, serous carcinomas are characterized by obvious invasive growth, the formation of papillary structures lined by pluristratified epithelium, and abundant calcified psammoma bodies. These poorly differentiated carcinomas may grow in solid sheets of cells with marked cellular pleomorphism, atypia, and abnormal mitoses.

      (iii) Prognosis. The overall 5-year survival rate for these tumors is 20 percent to 30 percent, with most deaths occurring within the first few years after diagnosis. The prognosis depends upon the stage of the tumor at the time of initial treatment. **Stage I** tumors involve one or both ovaries. **Stage II** tumors involve one or both ovaries with pelvic extension. **Stage III** tumors involve one or both ovaries with intraperitoneal metastases outside the pelvis, positive retroperitoneal nodes, or both. **Stage IV** tumors involve one or both ovaries with distant metastases (e.g., lung or parenchymal liver metastases). Peritoneal and omental implants occur rapidly, and only 20 percent of patients have stage I lesions at the time of diagnosis.

      (iv) Treatment consists of bilateral salpingo-oophorectomy and hysterectomy followed by radiation or chemotherapy, according to the stage of the disease.

  b. Mucinous tumors are characterized by the presence of tall columnar epithelial cells with abundant intracytoplasmic mucin. The cells resemble the epithelium that lines the endocervix and the intestine. These tumors are believed to originate from metaplasia of the coelomic epithelium of the ovary.

   (1) Incidence. Mucinous tumors account for 15 percent to 20 percent of all ovarian tumors.

   (2) Clinical Data. They occur most frequently in the third through the sixth decades of life.

    (a) Benign mucinous cystadenomas are bilateral in less than 5 percent of cases.

      (i) Grossly, these neoplasms tend to form very **large masses** (15 cm to 30 cm), which may either have a single locule or be polycystic on cut section. The cysts are filled with mucoid, gelatinous material. Papillae are rare, and the surface is always smooth.

      (ii) Microscopically, the cysts usually are lined by a single layer of well-differentiated epithelium. The cells have one nucleus towards the base, and the cytoplasm is filled with mucin. Atypia and mitoses are absent.

      (iii) Prognosis. These tumors almost always follow a benign clinical course.

      (iv) Treatment consists of oophorectomy.

  (b) Borderline mucinous cystadenocarcinomas are bilateral in up to 20 percent of cases.

      (i) Grossly, they appear as multiloculated cysts with common intracystic papillary projections. Solid zones are seen in some cases and may contain foci of hemorrhage and necrosis. The ovarian surface is involved in less than 10 percent of cases.

      (ii) Microscopically, the tumors are characterized by an overgrowth or papillary projection lined by mucinous epithelium (no more than three layers thick) with moderate atypia and stratification of the nucleus. No invasion of adjacent stroma is noted.

      (iii) The **prognosis** is similar to that for the serous counterparts of these tumors.

      (iv) Treatment usually consists of bilateral salpingo-oophorectomy and hysterectomy, but a more conservative approach may be taken in young women to preserve fertility.

  (c) Mucinous cystadenocarcinomas represent about 10 percent of mucinous tumors and constitute approximately 15 percent of malignant epithelial tumors.

      (i) Grossly, the tumors exhibit large solid areas with differing amounts of hemorrhage and necrosis. Intracystic papillae frequently are present.

      (ii) Microscopically, the tumors are characterized by numerous irregular, glandular structures lined by multilayered atypical epithelium with numerous mitoses. The stroma is infiltrated by cords and malignant glandular epithelium. Some authors believe that the diagnosis of mucinous carcinoma can be reached in the absence of frank invasion if the atypical lining epithelium is more than four cell layers thick.

      (iii) The **prognosis** depends upon the stage of the lesion; the overall 5-year survival rate is less than 60 percent.

  (d) Pseudomyxoma peritonei is a condition that accompanies 3 percent to 5 percent of cases of ovarian mucinous neoplasms. It consists of gelatinous masses scattered throughout the peritoneal cavity, which result from the implantation of cells that secrete abundant mucus.

      (i) These cells are thought to originate either from the epithelium of benign or low-grade malignant mucinous ovarian tumors or from mucoceles of the appendix, conditions that commonly coexist. They are believed to reach the peritoneum by means of spillage or rupture of these tumors at the time of surgery or because of spontaneous rupture of the tumors.

      (ii) Although histologically benign, pseudomyxoma can compromise vital structures by local spread and cause death. **Treatment** consists of surgical excision (often repetitive because of recurrences). The 5-year survival rate is approximately 45 percent.

c. Brenner tumors are epithelial tumors that are characterized by the presence of a transitional type of epithelium embedded in dense fibrous connective tissue. These tumors may rarely secrete hormones. Brenner tumors are associated with mucinous cystadenomas and cystic teratomas in 5 percent to 10 percent of cases.

  (1) Incidence. Brenner tumors are rare, constituting approximately 1.7 percent of all ovarian neoplasms. The age of affected patients ranges from 6 years to 81 years, with a mean age at diagnosis of 50 years. Approximately 7 percent of cases are bilateral.

  (2) Clinical Data. Most tumors are incidental findings, but some patients may present with an abdominal mass or complain of irregular menstrual bleeding.

    (a) Benign Brenner Tumors.

      (i) Grossly, these tumors are solid and firm with a gray-white, whorled cut surface. They vary in size from microscopic (about 50 percent of cases) up to 10 cm. They are encapsulated, and there are no papillary excrescences.

      (ii) Histologically, they are comprised of solid to partly cystic epithelial nests of polygonal cells, with oval nuclei and distinct nucleoli that have a longitudinal groove (coffee-bean appearance), embedded in a dense proliferative stroma. These nests resemble the transitional type of epithelium of the urinary bladder and may undergo mucinous metaplasia.

      (iii) Treatment and Prognosis. The majority of Brenner tumors fall in the benign category and can be treated by resection or oophorectomy; the prognosis is excellent.

    (b) Proliferative Brenner Tumors.

      (i) Grossly, these lesions form large tumor masses characterized by large cystic spaces into which polypoid growths project through the lumina.

    (ii) **Microscopically**, there is an exuberant proliferation of papillae lined by eight to twenty layers of transitional epithelium with only mild focal atypia. Occasionally normal mitoses are present, but there is no evidence of stromal invasion. Areas of typical benign Brenner tumors may be found adjacent to the tumor. Proliferative Brenner tumors resemble grade I transitional cell tumors of the urinary bladder.

    (iii) **Prognosis.** The malignant potential of these tumors has yet to be determined.

    (iv) **Treatment** varies from unilateral salpingo-oophorectomy to total hysterectomy, with bilateral salpingo-oophorectomy in postmenopausal patients.

  (c) **Malignant Brenner Tumors.**

    (i) **Diagnosis** is based on frank evidence of malignancy, abnormal mitosis, pleomorphism, and necrosis, the presence of a benign Brenner tumor, and demonstrable stromal invasion.

    (ii) **Histologically**, the transitional-cell type of the epithelium is markedly atypical, and areas of hemorrhage and necrosis are identifiable. There can be foci of squamous metaplasia and frank squamous carcinoma.

    (iii) **Treatment and Prognosis.** In most instances, the tumors are treated by total hysterectomy and bilateral salpingo-oophorectomy. The 5-year survival rate is approximately 50 percent.

  d. **Endometrioid carcinomas** of the ovaries are histologically identical to endometrial adenocarcinomas or adenoacanthomas. They may arise in association with preexisting ovarian endometriosis.

   (1) **Incidence.** Endometrioid carcinomas account for 10 percent to 25 percent of primary ovarian adenocarcinomas.

   (2) **Clinical Data.** The mean age of affected patients is 53 years, and at the time of surgery, 30 percent to 50 percent of patients have bilateral tumors.

   (3) **Grossly**, the tumors appear as multilocular cystic structures, partly filled with soft papillary tumor tissue.

   (4) **Microscopically**, the tumors are composed of glands that are arranged in a cribriform pattern, similar to endometrial cancer, although this pattern may not be easy to identify in poorly differentiated tumors. In some cases, benign endometriosis may be present in areas adjacent to the tumor. In about 50 percent of cases, the glandular component contains benign squamous elements, warranting the diagnosis of **adenoacanthoma**. When the squamous component shows malignant changes, the diagnosis of **adenosquamous carcinoma** is made.

   (5) **Prognosis.** Endometrioid carcinoma has a 5-year survival rate of approximately 50 percent. The prognosis depends on the stage and histology of the tumors; adenosquamous carcinoma, for example, has a lower 5-year survival rate than pure adenocarcinoma.

   (6) **Treatment.** Total hysterectomy with bilateral salpingo-oophorectomy constitutes the major modality of treatment, followed by supplementary radiation or chemotherapy.

  e. **Clear cell carcinoma** develops from the surface epithelium of the ovary and is found in association with endometriosis in 25 percent of cases.

   (1) **Incidence.** Clear cell carcinomas constitute 5 percent to 11 percent of primary ovarian tumors.

   (2) **Clinical Data.** The average age of affected patients is 50 to 55 years. The tumors are bilateral in about 5 percent of cases.

   (3) **Grossly**, the appearance of these tumors is not specific; they may be entirely cystic or have a combination of solid and cystic areas.

   (4) **Histologically**, the cells are columnar or cuboidal with abundant clear cytoplasm and large hyperchromatic nuclei, which may fill the cytoplasm and bulge into tubular lumina, imparting a hobnail appearance to the cells. The cells may be arranged in three different patterns: solid, tubular, or papillary.

   (5) **Prognosis.** The 5-year survival rate when all stages are included is 50 percent to 55 percent.

   (6) **Treatment** consists of total hysterectomy with bilateral salpingo-oophorectomy, followed by radiation and chemotherapy.

  f. **Mixed mesodermal tumors** are composed of both malignant epithelial and mesenchymal components.

   (1) **Incidence.** These neoplasms are rare and occur predominantly in postmenopausal women; the median age is from 53 to 65 years.

   (2) **Grossly**, mixed mesodermal tumors tend to be large, with a median diameter of 15 cm. Some are solid, but most are multiloculated cystic neoplasms with solid areas

and extensive foci of hemorrhage and necrosis. Approximately 50 percent to 70 percent of these tumors extend beyond the ovary.

(3) **Microscopically**, there are two types.

    (a) **Mixed mesodermal tumors with homologous elements (carcinosarcomas)** are composed of an epithelial malignancy (carcinoma) and a sarcoma made up of spindle-shaped cells with nuclear pleomorphism and mitotic activity. The sarcomatous element resembles the stroma of the endometrium.

    (b) **Mixed mesodermal tumors with heterologous elements** contain malignant elements such as striated muscle, cartilage, bone, and fat in addition to the malignant epithelial components.

(4) The **prognosis** is very poor; the median survival time is 6 to 12 months from diagnosis.

(5) **Treatment** consists of total hysterectomy with bilateral salpingo-oophorectomy, followed by radiation or chemotherapy.

B. GERM CELL TUMORS arise from germ cells, which embryonically originate in the yolk sac and which are present in the ovaries at birth.

  1. Incidence. These tumors account for 15 percent to 20 percent of ovarian neoplasms.

  2. Clinical Data. They occur primarily in children and young women. The presentation is nonspecific and similar to that of the epithelial tumors.

  3. Classification. Ovarian germ cell tumors can be divided into five major types (see Table 13-1).

    a. Benign dermoid cyst (benign cystic teratoma) is the **most common** type of ovarian neoplasm. It usually occurs during the reproductive years and is discovered incidentally.

      (1) **Grossly**, benign dermoid cysts are usually unilateral and are of varying sizes. The cut surface reveals a cavity that is filled with fatty material and hair and surrounded by a capsule of variable thickness. The fatty material is similar to normal sebum. Other elements such as bone, teeth, cartilage, and fetus-like structures may be present (Fig. 13-7).

      (2) **Microscopically**, the tumor is characterized by the presence of elements from the three germ layers: ectoderm, endoderm, and mesoderm. These elements are all histologically benign and mature. The most frequent elements found are keratinized skin, bronchial and gastrointestinal epithelium, mature glial elements, apocrine glands, and thyroid and salivary glands. (When thyroid elements compose more

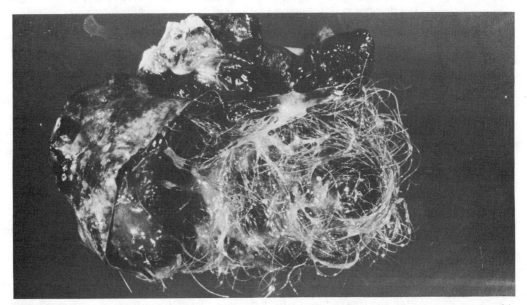

Figure 13-7. Gross photograph of a benign cystic teratoma (dermoid cyst) of the ovary. Note the cystic nature of the lesion and hair.

than 80 percent of a tumor, the lesion is called **struma ovarii**.) The outer portions of dermoid cysts frequently are composed of compressed ovarian stroma, which may appear hyalinized or which may show inflammation with a foreign body giant cell reaction, induced by spillage of the contents of the tumor into the adjacent stroma.

(3) **Prognosis and Treatment.** Dermoids are benign tumors, which can be cured by oophorectomy.

b. **Immature teratomas** constitute about 1 percent of teratomas and usually occur in young females; the median age of onset is 18 years. The tumors are composed entirely or in part of partially differentiated structures that resemble tissues of a developing embryo.

(1) **Grossly**, these tumors are usually unilateral, have a median size of 18 cm, and generally are more solid than benign teratomas. The external surface is smooth. The cut surface is soft, gray-to-pink, and contains areas of hemorrhage and necrosis. Hair, calcifications, and cartilage are present in 40 percent of the tumors.

(2) **Histologically**, immature teratomas are characterized by elements that are derived from the three germ layers. Immature neural tissue is especially common and is the critical element to diagnose immature teratomas. It may form tubular structures, rosettes, or solid nests of immature cells. Other elements, such as immature cartilage, may be present. Additionally, histologically mature epithelium may be present, including that of the skin, sweat glands, hair, respiratory and gastrointestinal tracts, muscle, and bone.

(3) The **prognosis** is related to the grade and stage of the tumor but in general is poor.

(4) **Treatment** consists of surgical removal followed by chemotherapy.

c. **Malignant dysgerminoma** constitutes 50 percent of the germ cell tumors and 2 percent of all ovarian neoplasms. It occurs predominantly in children and women under 30 years of age.

(1) **Grossly**, dysgerminomas are solid, fleshy tumors, well encapsulated, and with a homogeneous white-to-tan cut surface. Hemorrhage and necrosis usually are absent.

(2) **Histology.** The tumor is composed of large polygonal cells with abundant clear cytoplasm and vesicular nuclei that contain one or more nucleoli. Dysgerminoma is similar to seminoma of the testis and often is infiltrated by lymphocytes and multinucleated giant cells.

(3) The **prognosis** depends upon the stage of the disease; the 5-year survival rate is 90 percent when the tumor is confined to one ovary and approximately 40 percent when the tumor has progressed to an advanced stage.

(4) **Treatment.** Unilateral oophorectomy is performed in most young women, but a total hysterectomy with bilateral salpingo-oophorectomy is necessary when the disease is disseminated, regardless of a patient's age. The tumor is highly radiosensitive.

d. **Endodermal sinus tumor** (yolk sac tumor) is rare, accounting for approximately 20 percent of malignant germ cell tumors. It is characterized by the rapid growth of an abdominal mass, and one-half of the affected patients have symptoms for 1 week or less before seeking medical attention. The tumor seldom affects patients over 40 years of age.

(1) **Grossly**, it is a large tumor (median size, 15 cm) with a smooth surface. Cut surface shows a solid mass with extensive hemorrhage and necrosis.

(2) **Microscopically**, the germ cells may be arranged in several patterns: **reticular**, composed of a loose network of spaces and channels lined by cuboidal cells with scanty cytoplasm; **festoon**, characterized by glomeruloid structures composed of a central papillary core surrounded by germ cells (Schiller-Duval bodies); **alveolo-glandular**; **polyvesicular vitelline**; and **solid**. Hyaline eosinophilic droplets, which contain α-fetoprotein and stain strongly with periodic acid-Schiff (PAS) reagent, are common in these tumors.

(3) The **prognosis** is poor, with a low 5-year survival rate.

(4) **Treatment** consists of oophorectomy followed by chemotherapy.

e. **Malignant Mixed Germ Cell Tumors.**

(1) Tumors of other cell types, such as **embryonal carcinoma** and **choriocarcinoma**, may occur in the ovary but are rare.

(2) Germ cell tumors that contain two or more malignant components represent 8 percent of all germ cell tumors. The most common is dysgerminoma combined with endodermal sinus tumor and immature teratoma.

(3) The **prognosis** depends mainly on two elements.

(a) The size of the tumor—those larger than 10 cm have a worse prognosis than smaller ones.

(b) The cell types involved—if more than one-third of a mixed germ cell tumor is composed of endodermal sinus tumor, choriocarcinoma, or immature teratoma, the prognosis is poorer than when less malignant elements predominate.

C. **GONADAL STROMAL TUMORS** (stromal tumors of the sex cord) are comprised of a variety of cells that give rise to neoplasms, such as theca, granulosa, Sertoli, hilus, or Leydig cells and fibroblasts of stromal origin, singly or in combinations of one or more types. They arise from the stromal cells of the ovary.

1. **Incidence.** As a group, these lesions account for approximately 5 percent to 10 percent of ovarian tumors. They can occur at any age.

2. **Clinical Data.** These tumors have the potential to produce hormones (steroids), and affected patients may present with specific clinical manifestations due to the hormones.

3. **Classification.** Gonadal stromal tumors can be divided into four major types (see Table 13-1).

   a. **Thecoma and fibrothecoma** are composed exclusively of theca cells and fibroblasts of ovarian stromal origin. They can elaborate **estrogen**, producing precocious puberty in premenarchal girls and irregular bleeding in adults.

      (1) **Grossly**, the neoplasms range in size from small, unpalpable tumors to large, firm, solid masses. On cut section, there is a characteristic yellowish color, which is more prominent in pure thecomas.

      (2) **Microscopically**, there are two types of cells: a spindle-like cell with a round-to-oval nucleus and scant cytoplasm and a round luteinized cell with abundant cytoplasm and a central nucleus. Mitosis almost always is absent. Fat stains usually are positive.

      (3) **Prognosis and Treatment.** Thecomas almost always are unilateral and **almost never are malignant**. Resection of the tumors (oophorectomy) is usually curative.

   b. **Granulosa Cell Tumors.**

      (1) **Clinical Data.** Although these tumors affect a wide age range of females, from newborn infants to postmenopausal women, most occur after menopause. Granulosa cell tumors can produce a variety of steroid hormones, resulting in either feminizing or virilizing effects. The majority, however, cause signs and symptoms that are related to excessive **estrogenic** hormones.

      (2) **Grossly**, the tumors are commonly unilateral, well encapsulated, and of varying sizes. Cross section shows a solid neoplasm with areas of hemorrhage and necrosis.

      (3) **Microscopically**, the hallmark of these tumors is the presence of a small, round or spindle-shaped cell, with small amounts of cytoplasm. The nucleus has a longitudinal groove and occasionally a small nucleolus. The cells may grow in several patterns: microfollicular (resembling Call-Exner bodies), macrofollicular, trabecular, and diffuse. A combination of patterns is common. Endometrial hyperplasia accompanies granulosa cell tumors in approximately 50 percent of cases, and endometrial adenocarcinoma accompanies the tumors in approximately 15 percent of cases.

      (4) **Prognosis.** All granulosa cell tumors are thought to be potentially aggressive, but, in general, the tumors have a good prognosis, despite a tendency to recur after long intervals. Factors that worsen the prognosis include advanced tumor stage, patient age of over 40 years, solidity and large size of tumors, bilateral occurrence, mitoses, and atypia.

      (5) **Treatment** consists of hysterectomy and bilateral salpingo-oophorectomy (except when preservation of the reproductive function is a major concern).

   c. **Sertoli Cell Tumors.**

      (1) **Clinical Data.** Patients with this type of tumor may have symptoms either of **virilization or of excess estrogen** production.

      (2) **Grossly**, Sertoli cell tumors are unilateral, well-circumscribed, solitary masses. The cut surface shows a characteristic yellow-tan color. The tumors are usually large.

      (3) **Histologically**, they resemble Sertoli tumors of the testis. The cells grow following three different patterns: simple tubular, complex tubular, and folliculoma lipidique; the patterns are frequently admixed.

      (4) **Prognosis.** Most of these tumors are benign.

      (5) **Treatment** consists of oophorectomy.

   d. **Lipid cell tumors** include hilus cell and Leydig cell tumors.

      (1) **Incidence.** They account for less than 0.1 percent of all ovarian neoplasms.

      (2) **Clinical Data.** They predominantly affect adults. In 75 percent to 90 percent of cases, they have **androgenic** activity and produce virilization; patients present with hirsutism, amenorrhea, deepening of the voice, and clitoral enlargement. Estrogenic activity occurs in 20 percent of cases. Approximately 5 percent to 10 percent of patients have associated Cushing's syndrome.

      (3) **Grossly**, lipid cell tumors are unilateral, lobulated, soft, yellow or brown masses of varying sizes, with areas of hemorrhage and necrosis.

(4) **Histologically**, the tumors are composed of cuboidal or polyhedral cells with round nuclei and eosinophilic granular cytoplasm, which may contain crystals of Reinke. Areas of fibrosis and hyalinization may be present.

(5) **Prognosis.** The tumors are generally benign, but about 10 percent to 15 percent are aggressive and may cause death.

(6) **Treatment** consists of unilateral oophorectomy in most cases; for the rare malignant tumor, more radical surgery is required.

D. METASTATIC TUMORS of the ovary account for 5 percent to 10 percent of ovarian neoplasms and can represent a significant diagnostic problem. They are usually bilateral. The most common sites of origin include the stomach (Krukenberg's tumor), gastrointestinal tract (colon), breast, and genital tract.

VII. TUMORS OF THE FALLOPIAN TUBES

A. BENIGN TUMORS of the fallopian tubes are uncommon and are frequently confused with inflammatory processes such as chronic salpingitis or pyosalpinx.

1. **Inclusion cysts** are benign mesothelial inclusions formed by invaginations of the tubal serosa. The cystic cavities are lined by columnar or cuboidal cells and are filled with yellow, clear fluid. They are usually incidental findings of no clinical significance.

2. **Adenomatoid tumors** are benign mesothelial growths identical to those occurring in the testes (see Chapter 12, "The Male Reproductive System"). Their only significance resides in their possible confusion with carcinomas.

3. **Leiomyomas** are tumors of smooth muscle that arise from the tubal muscularis. They are rare and histologically are identical to leiomyomas of the uterus (V A 1).

B. MALIGNANT TUMORS

1. **Carcinomas** of the fallopian tubes are rare neoplasms, accounting for approximately 0.5 percent of all gynecologic malignancies.

   a. **Clinical Data.** The highest incidence occurs in the fifth and sixth decades of life. The classic symptomatology consists of a clear or serosanguineous vaginal discharge, pelvic pain, and an adnexal mass. The diagnosis of tubal carcinoma is rarely made prior to surgery.

   b. **Grossly**, the tube is swollen due to the neoplastic intraluminal growth. The serosal surface is congested, and, on cut section, the lumen is dilated and filled with a papillary or solid tumor, which may infiltrate through the muscularis in advanced cases. The fimbriated end is frequently obliterated.

   c. **Microscopically**, there is a complex papillary and solid pattern with occasional small glandular formations. The cells pile up and show different degrees of nuclear pleomorphism. Mitosis and necrosis are present. Areas of abrupt transition from normal to neoplastic epithelium may be found as well as areas of atypical proliferation. The tumor may invade the muscularis and the serosa.

   d. **Prognosis.** Primary tubal carcinoma must be differentiated carefully from metastases from other primary sites (such as the ovary) because the histology is very similar. The prognosis of tubal carcinoma depends upon the stage of the disease; the overall 5-year survival rate is thought to be approximately 19 percent.

   e. **Treatment** consists of total hysterectomy and bilateral salpingo-oophorectomy, followed by radiation therapy.

2. **Sarcomas** of the fallopian tubes are very rare. They may be pure or mixed with carcinomatous elements. The clinical manifestations are identical to those produced by carcinomas, but sarcomas are associated with an even more dismal prognosis.

VIII. VULVAR DISORDERS

A. BENIGN DISORDERS

1. **Bartholin's cysts** are cystic dilatations of Bartholin's glands caused by obstruction of the duct and followed by progressive accumulation of secretions. The cysts are filled with mucoid, clear fluid, and the wall is lined by transitional-type epithelium. Such cysts may be recurrent and occasionally become infected. **Abscess** of Bartholin's gland is an acute process, commonly caused by *Neisseria gonorrhoeae* and *Staphylococcus*. It is associated with severe acute inflammation and a purulent exudate. The acute process may subside and give rise to a chronic form.

2. **Mucinous cysts** usually are located deep in the lamina propria, and there is no evidence of communication with the surface. The cysts usually are lined by tall columnar cells, similar to those of the endocervical glands, but occasionally undergo squamous metaplasia. They probably arise from elements of the urogenital sinus, representing, therefore, examples of dysontogenetic formation.

3. The **papillary hidradenoma**, which is rare before puberty, occurs predominantly in white women.
   a. **Clinical Data.** Hidradenomas typically appear as small, firm, well-encapsulated nodules in the labia majora, but they may evert to the surface and have a cauliflower-like appearance. They are usually asymptomatic, but if they ulcerate, they may cause bleeding and soreness.
   b. **Histologically**, these lesions resemble intraductal papillomas of the breast. They are composed of long stalks of connective tissue lined by one or two layers of cuboidal-to-columnar cells. Although they may exhibit apocrine metaplasia and some atypia, they are not malignant.
   c. **Treatment** consists of surgical excision, which is curative.

4. **Vulvar dystrophies** are epithelial disorders that often appear clinically as white, pruritic lesions in the vulva. Any of these lesions may show variable degrees of atypia, but less than 10 percent are thought to progress to invasive or in situ cancers. There are three main types.
   a. **Hyperplastic dystrophy** may occur at any age but predominantly affects patients from 30 to 60 years of age.
      (1) **Clinical Data.** The lesions may appear as both white and red patches, and the affected skin surface appears raised and scaly.
      (2) **Histologically**, elongation, widening, and confluence of the rete ridges of the epidermis are present with marked hyperkeratosis and parakeratosis. The dermis is edematous and contains moderate amounts of chronic inflammatory cells. Normal mitosis may be present in the basal layer.
      (3) **Prognosis and Treatment**. Hyperplastic dystrophy is considered to be a benign disorder that responds to conservative topical management. Local excision is recommended in small lesions.
   b. **Lichen sclerosus** is most common in postmenopausal women but can occur at any age.
      (1) **Clinical Data.** This dystrophy can produce gross changes in the vulvar architecture, with flattening of the labia minora and edema of the preputial folds. The affected area is white because of avascularity of the superficial layers and may be pruriginous, which leads to scratching and irritation of the area.
      (2) The **histologic** hallmark of lichen sclerosus is sclerosis or homogenization of the upper dermis, which appears markedly edematous and exhibits destruction of the collagen bundles. The epidermis is thin, with marked keratosis and parakeratosis and loss of rete ridges. Subepidermal bullae may be found. The capillaries are thin, and there may be extravasation of blood in the dermis.
      (3) **Treatment and Prognosis.** The lesion is not considered premalignant and responds to topical treatment. Surgery is not recommended because of a high incidence of recurrences.
   c. **Mixed Dystrophies.** Both forms of vulvar dystrophy can affect different areas of the vulva in the same patient.

B. MALIGNANT TUMORS

1. **Carcinoma In Situ** (Bowen's Disease).
   a. **Incidence.** The mean age at onset of this disease is 41 years, although the lesion may occur at any age. It is more common in black than white females and has a significant association with infectious processes such as condyloma acuminatum.
   b. **Clinical Data.** Squamous cell carcinoma in situ causes asymptomatic, multicentric, raised, patchy, white plaques that retain toluidine blue dye.
   c. **Histologically**, the lesion is identical to Bowen's disease of the skin (see Chapter 20).
   d. **Prognosis and Treatment**. In 30 percent to 40 percent of cases, patients with Bowen's disease of the vulva have dysplasias or carcinomas in other areas of the genital tract. Local resection is recommended for small lesions; superficial vulvectomy is recommended for widespread disease. Topical chemotherapy has been used with variable success. The lesion usually recurs if it is not completely excised.

2. **Squamous Cell Carcinoma.**
   a. **Incidence.** This lesion accounts for approximately 4 percent of all genital cancers and more than 90 percent of all vulvar malignancies. It predominantly affects women between 60 and 90 years of age.

    b. Clinical Data. Squamous cell carcinoma appears as either an endophytic or exophytic lesion, usually ulcerated. Pruritus and bleeding may occur. The mass extends progressively to involve the entire vulva and sometimes the vagina and cervix. It is associated with other primary malignancies in 10 percent or more of cases.

    c. Histologically, the lesion is identical to squamous cell carcinoma of the skin and mucous membranes.

    d. Prognosis and Treatment. In general, the 5-year survival rate is approximately 70 percent, but the rate drops if inguinal lymph node involvement is present. Total vulvectomy combined with **bilateral** groin node dissection (even when the tumor is unilateral) is the treatment of choice.

3. Paget's disease of the vulva is a rare tumor that essentially is identical to Paget's disease of other areas such as the skin or nipple.

    a. If the lesion invades the dermis, there is a high incidence of lymph node metastases.

    b. Approximately 14 percent of cases are associated with adenocarcinoma of Bartholin's glands and other sites.

    c. Treatment and prognosis of the disease depend upon the presence or absence of associated carcinomas. Vulvectomy is recommended, and, if an associated invasive cancer is found, regional lymphadenectomy should be performed. Positive lymph nodes worsen the prognosis and reduce the survival rate.

4. Other malignancies such as **melanomas** and **basal cell carcinomas** can occur in the vulva. The histology of these lesions is identical to that of the respective tumors occurring in the skin or salivary glands. Sarcomas such as leiomyosarcoma, malignant neural tumors, rhabdomyosarcoma, and angiosarcoma also have been reported.

5. Metastatic Tumors. The vulva is infrequently involved by metastatic spread of carcinoma from the cervix and endometrium, and even more infrequently it is involved by metastases from other sites such as the kidneys and urethra.

IX. DISORDERS OF THE VAGINA

A. ADENOSIS is the presence of ectopic mucinous endocervical glands in the vagina. It has been linked to prenatal exposure to diethylstilbestrol (DES) and predominately affects girls and young women. Its true incidence is not known because the condition is probably asymptomatic and not recognized in many patients.

    1. The epithelium usually is tall and columnar but may undergo squamous metaplasia. Areas of adenosis do not stain with iodine because the cells do not produce glycogen but mucin.

    2. Adenosis has been associated with vaginal deformities, such as ridges, hoods, and collars, and with malignant processes such as **clear cell adenocarcinoma**.

B. BENIGN TUMORS

    1. Gartner's duct cysts are commonly located in the anterolateral wall of the vagina and originate from vestigial remnants of the wolffian duct. The cysts are lined by low-cuboidal epithelium and are usually small.

    2. Fibroepithelial polyps are polypoid, rubbery lesions covered by vaginal mucosa that protrude from the introitus as multiple finger-like projections, which, in children, may be confused with sarcoma botryoides.

        a. Histologically, the stroma is made of fibrous connective tissue with dilated capillaries and occasional large atypical cells.

        b. Treatment. Surgical resection is curative.

    3. Other benign tumors include leiomyomas, neurofibromas, rhabdomyomas, and granular cell myoblastomas.

C. MALIGNANT TUMORS. Primary malignant tumors of the vagina are very rare and probably account for less than 1 percent of all gynecologic neoplasms.

    1. Epithelial Tumors. The vagina can undergo the same dysplastic and neoplastic changes that have been described already for the cervix and vulva—dysplasia, carcinoma in situ, and invasive squamous cell carcinoma. The latter affects older patients and has been associated with chronic irritative processes such as the use of pessaries. The most common location is the upper portion of the posterior wall. The 5-year survival rate is approximately 80 percent to 90 percent.

    2. Clear cell adenocarcinoma is associated with vaginal adenosis and occurs in approximately

0.14 to 1.4 females in 1000 who have been exposed to DES in utero. The tumor predominantly affects young women.

   a. **Histologically**, several patterns, such as solid, tubular (with hobnails), and papillary, can be recognized.

   b. These tumors have a survival rate of 50 percent, similar to that of clear cell adenocarcinoma of the cervix.

3. **Sarcoma botryoides** is a very rare tumor that occurs predominantly in infants and children, with a peak incidence at 1 to 2 years of age.

   a. **Clinical Data.** Affected children present with polypoid, confluent masses, which resemble bunches of grapes and protrude through the vaginal introitus.

   b. **Histologically**, the lesion originates in the mesenchyma of the lamina propria. A distinct subepithelial zone, known as the grenz zone, is always present. The cells are round or spindle-like with dark nuclei and scanty cytoplasm. Occasional mitotic figures can be identified. Striated muscle cells may be present.

   c. **Treatment and Prognosis.** The 5-year survival rate has been reported to be 10 percent to 35 percent, although recently it has been improving when patients are treated with pelvic exenteration, regional lymphadenectomy, and vaginectomy, followed by radiation and chemotherapy.

4. The vagina also can be the primary site for other tumors such as **melanoma** and **leiomyosarcoma**.

STUDY QUESTIONS

Directions: Each question below contains five suggested answers. Choose the **one best** response to each question.

1. Condylomatous cervicitis will most likely be found in which of the following patients?

(A) An 18-year-old woman with multiple sex partners

(B) A 38-year-old woman with ovarian carcinoma

(C) A 20-year-old virgin

(D) A 28-year-old mother of two with chlamydial infection

(E) A 35-year-old multigravida woman with herpetic vulvitis

2. The most common benign germ cell tumor of the ovaries in premenopausal women is

(A) Brenner tumor

(B) hilus cell tumor

(C) benign dermoid cyst

(D) mucinous cystadenoma

(E) dysgerminoma

Directions: Each question below contains four suggested answers of which **one or more** is correct. Choose the answer

A if **1, 2, and 3** are correct
B if **1 and 3** are correct
C if **2 and 4** are correct
D if **4** is correct
E if **1, 2, 3, and 4** are correct

3. The endometrial biopsy obtained from a 30-year-old woman shows a proliferative phase endometrium with chronic endometritis. This represents

(1) a premalignant endometrial lesion

(2) an inadequate luteal phase

(3) a hyperestrogenic state

(4) an intrauterine device (IUD) present in the uterus

4. Endometrial hyperplasia, which appears as an exuberant overgrowth of endometrial tissue, typically is

(1) common in patients with granulosa cell tumors

(2) considered to be a precancerous condition

(3) seen in postmenopausal women with bleeding

(4) treated with radium implants

5. Invasive squamous cell carcinoma of the vulva can arise de novo or in cases of previous cervical cancer. In patients with prior histories of cervical cancer, this invasive vulvar cancer

(1) is frequently multifocal

(2) often extends into the vagina

(3) is treated by surgical vulvectomy

(4) is referred to as Bowen's disease

6. A 70-year-old woman presents clinically with a pruritic excoriated lesion on her vulvar skin, which has been present for several months. A biopsy shows the lesion to be Paget's disease invading the dermis. Complications may include

(1) inguinal lymph node metastases

(2) infiltrating ductal breast carcinoma

(3) adenocarcinoma of Bartholin's glands

(4) elevated levels of serum calcium and alkaline phosphate

7. Characteristics of serous cystadenocarcinomas of the ovary with so-called borderline malignant potential include

(1) grossly evident papillary excrescences on the ovary

(2) complicated papillae lined by stratified epithelium less than three cell layers thick

(3) nuclear atypia

(4) stromal invasion of the ovary

8. True statements concerning choriocarcinoma include

(1) it can arise from a hydatidiform mole

(2) it causes elevated serum human chorionic gonadotropin (HCG) levels

(3) it can be treated by chemotherapy

(4) it can be treated by radiation therapy

9. Adenosis of the vagina is the presence of benign mucinous epithelium of the endocervical type in an area that is normally covered by stratified squamous epithelium. True statements concerning vaginal adenosis include

(1) it occurs in individuals who were exposed to diethylstilbestrol (DES) in utero

(2) it can be associated with anatomic deformities of the vagina

(3) it can be associated with clear cell carcinoma of the cervix

(4) the cells in adenosis stain positively with application of Lugol's solution

ANSWERS AND EXPLANATIONS

1. The answer is A. (*V B 6*) Cervical intraepithelial neoplasia is an inclusive term covering dysplasia and carcinoma in situ. Epidemiologic studies have shown an association between cervical intraepithelial neoplasia and papilloma virus infections of the cervix and vagina. Papilloma infection of the cervix causes a condylomatous cervicitis. These infections are more frequent in women with multiple sex partners.

2. The answer is C. (*VI B 3 a*) Benign cystic teratoma, also known as dermoid cyst, is the most common ovarian tumor found in premenopausal women. A dermoid cyst orginates from the germ cell component of the ovary. The tumor can thus contain tissues that are characteristic of all three germ cell layers: endoderm, mesoderm, and ectoderm. The dermoid tumor is benign; the malignant counterpart is known as an immature teratoma.

3. The answer is D (4). (*V C 2*) Chronic endometritis is diagnosed by the presence of plasma cells in an inflamed endometrial stroma. The hormonal phase of the endometrium has little to do with the presence of the inflammation; however, the presence of a foreign body, such as an intrauterine device (IUD), is often the cause of chronic endometrial infection.

4. The answer is A (1, 2, 3). (*V C 4*) There are three histologic forms of endometrial hyperplasia: cystic, adenomatous, and atypical. Each form is associated with an increased risk for the development of endometrial cancer. Patients often present with unusual bleeding in the peri- or postmenopausal period of life. Among the causes of endometrial hyperplasia is increased estrogen produced by ovarian granulosa cell tumors.

5. The answer is A (1, 2, 3). (*VIII B 2*) Bowen's disease is carcinoma in situ of the vulva and thus cannot be invasive squamous cell carcinoma. Invasive squamous cell carcinoma of the vulva can appear as an ulcerated endophytic or exophytic lesion. The tumor progresses to involve the vulva, vagina, and cervix in some cases. Approximately 10 percent of the time this vulvar tumor is associated with other primary malignancies.

6. The answer is B (1, 3). (*VIII B 3*) Paget's disease of the vulva is a rare tumor. In many instances, the neoplasm begins as a tumor in the mucous or sebaceous glands in the skin of the vulva or perineum. The association between adenocarcinoma of Bartholin's glands and Paget's disease of the vulva is especially common. If the Paget's disease extends into the dermis, lymph node metastases are likely to occur.

7. The answer is A (1, 2, 3). [*VI A 3 b (2) (b)*] Borderline serous cystadenocarcinomas are characterized by the presence of complex branching papillae, which cover the serosal surface of the ovary as well as line the cavities of cystic spaces within the tumors. A clear yellow fluid fills the cysts. The fibrous cores of the papillae are covered by stratified epithelium with nuclear atypia, growing two to three cell layers thick. Stromal invasion is absent in borderline lesions.

8. The answer is A (1, 2, 3). (*III B 6*) Choriocarcinoma is a relatively rare tumor in the United States. Individuals who develop choriocarcinoma usually are found to have had a hydatidiform mole. Choriocarcinoma produces gonadotropins, so that the presence of elevated levels of serum human chorionic gonadotropin (HCG) can be used as a marker for the presence of the disease. Fortunately, the tumor is quite sensitive to chemotherapy, with nearly an 80 percent cure rate.

9. The answer is A (1, 2, 3). (*IX A 2*) In utero exposure of females to diethylstilbestrol (DES) taken by the mother before the eighteenth week of gestation has been linked with the appearance, beginning in adolescence, of vaginal adenosis and clear cell adenocarcinomas of the vagina and cervix. Adenosis may be found in association with anatomic deformities of the vagina known variously as ridges, hoods, and collars. Because adenosis is mucinous epithelium, it does not stain positively with Lugol's solution as does normal cervical epithelium, which contains glycogen.

14
The Breast

I. INTRODUCTION. This chapter deals with the most common benign and malignant lesions that affect the mammary gland.

II. DEVELOPMENT

    A. EMBRYOLOGY. The mammary gland is a modified sweat gland that develops from a primitive epidermal thickening of the ectoderm and remains rudimentary in males.

    B. HISTOLOGY

        1. The breast is composed of an epithelial parenchyma, supporting muscular and fascial elements, plus varying amounts of fat, blood vessels, lymphatics, and nerves.

        2. The epithelial component consists of ducts and acini, which together form lobules, the basic structural units of the mammary gland. The number of lobules varies in each mammary gland.

        3. The epithelial and mesenchymal elements are intermingled and are capable of responding to hormonal stimulation.

    C. NEUROENDOCRINE CONTROL. The development and function of the breast is controlled by the neuroendocrine system. The ovaries, the pituitary and adrenal glands, and the hypothalamus are essential members of this system. At puberty, a complex mechanism involving the central nervous system, pituitary gland, and hypothalamus initiates ovarian function and estrogen production. The estrogens act upon the breast, stimulating the acini and duct proliferation until the breast reaches maturity.

III. CONGENITAL ABNORMALITIES

    A. Supernumerary breast is the most common congenital anomaly; accessory glands can occur at any site along the embryonal milkline.

    B. Congenital absence of the breast, "amastia," although rare, may be unilateral or bilateral and occurs in males as well as females.

IV. PHYSIOLOGIC CHANGES

    A. CHANGES WITH AGE

        1. The infantile breast consists of small ducts scattered in fibrous tissue. At puberty, the main lactiferous ducts proliferate and lobules and acini form.

        2. After menopause, hormonal stimulation stops and there is involution of the glandular portion of the breast, with an increase of fat tissue and hyalinization of the intervening connective tissue. These changes are accompanied by atrophy of acini and ducts.

    B. PREGNANCY AND LACTATION. During pregnancy and postpartum, the breast proliferates and new ducts and acini are formed. The epithelial cells show marked vacuolization with luminal secretion of colostrum and milk. The changes are stimulated by the secretion of the hormone **prolactin**, but the mechanism is not completely understood.

    C. GYNECOMASTIA

        1. Gynecomastia is hypertrophy of the male breast, chiefly ductal and periductal, with stromal proliferation. There are no lobules in the male breast. Gynecomastia is more common unilaterally than bilaterally.

2. Hormonal imbalance with an increase of estrogenic substances appears to be the cause. The condition is found most frequently either at puberty or in old age. Patients with testicular tumors and cirrhosis of the liver commonly have gynecomastia.

V. INFLAMMATORY PROCESSES

A. ACUTE MASTITIS

1. This process is almost always a complication that occurs during lactation (puerperal mastitis). The producing agent, usually *Staphylococcus* or *Streptococcus*, becomes invasive through fissures in the nipple. The breast is swollen, erythematous, and painful.

2. Histologically, there is diffuse infiltration by acute inflammatory cells that destroy ducts, lobules, and surrounding stroma.

B. CHRONIC MASTITIS is commonly a granulomatous inflammation, in most instances secondary to a systemic disease such as tuberculosis or sarcoidosis.

C. DUCT ECTASIA occurs predominantly in postmenopausal women. The condition is characterized by dilatation of the collecting ducts in the subareolar region with periductal fibrosis and the presence of chronic inflammatory cells. In the lumina of the ducts, inspissated amorphous material is present. Clinically, the condition can be misdiagnosed as carcinoma.

D. FAT NECROSIS

1. This is an unusual lesion produced by injury or trauma to the breast. It produces tumoral masses that clinically can simulate carcinomas.

2. Histologically, the adipose tissue is inflamed and necrotic, with areas of saponification and calcification. Chronic inflammatory cells and lipid-filled macrophages are present.

VI. PROLIFERATIVE LESIONS. The discussion in this section is limited to **fibrocystic disease.**

A. Incidence. Fibrocystic disease is the most common disorder of the breast and is the reason for more than one-half of all operations on the female breast.

B. Etiology.
1. This common disorder is believed to be the result of estrogenic hormonal imbalance because it does not become clinically evident until ovarian function is fully evolved, and it regresses after menopause.
2. Women with cystic disease are said to have up to four times the average risk of developing breast cancer. It is believed that microscopic cysts not visible grossly are commonly found at autopsy and represent no risk for the patient. Gross cysts (larger than 3 mm) are considered higher risks for the development of carcinoma.

C. Clinical Data.
1. The lesions are commonly bilateral and multiple. Typically, the upper outer quadrant is most commonly involved.
2. The disorder is clinically characterized by dull, heavy pain and tenderness on palpation. These symptoms increase premenstrually.

D. Pathology.
1. The **gross appearance** is that of fine fibrofatty tissue with cystic spaces, some of which are bluish in color and are called **"blue-domed" cysts.**
2. The **microscopic findings** include
  a. Microcysts—cysts that are not visible to the naked eye
  b. Ductal epithelial proliferation—which, if severe, may form a lace-like pattern filling the ducts
  c. Apocrine metaplasia—the normal cuboidal epithelium being transformed into columnar epithelium with abundant eosinophilic cytoplasm
  d. Adenosis—proliferation of acini and ducts in a lobular pattern
  e. Fibrosis

E. Treatment. There is no adequate treatment for this condition; however, careful follow-up by the clinician is recommended.

VII. BENIGN NEOPLASMS

A. FIBROADENOMA

1. **Incidence.** Fibroadenoma is the most common benign tumor of the female breast. It is a disease of youth, and the tumor may develop at any time after puberty, most frequently before the age of 30 years. Fibroadenoma develops as the result of increased sensitivity of a focal area of the breast to estrogens.

2. **Clinical Data.** The lesions are usually solitary but occasionally may be multiple. The tumor is easily movable, and neither the overlying skin nor the adjacent axillary lymph nodes show significant changes.

3. **Pathology.**
   a. **Grossly,** the tumor is sharply demarcated from the surrounding breast tissue, seemingly encapsulated, although it does not have a true capsule. The tumor is often 2 cm to 4 cm in size or larger and has a gray-white firm surface on cut section (Fig. 14-1).
   b. **Microscopically,** the tumor consists of two components: a proliferation of the connective tissue stroma and an atypical multiplication of ducts and acini. Both components are histologically benign.

4. **Treatment.** Complete surgical excision of the tumor is curative.

B. INTRADUCTAL PAPILLOMA

1. **Clinical Data.** These neoplasms appear as small masses located in the region of the nipple. Often the lesion is not palpable and is called to a patient's attention by the passage of **bloody fluid** from the nipple. Nipple discharge is more common in benign than in malignant lesions; and intraductal papilloma is the most common cause. Intraductal papilloma occurs in women at or shortly before menopause.

2. **Pathology.**
   a. **Grossly,** the papillomas appear as small raspberry-like growths attached to the wall of a dilated duct.
   b. **Histologically,** the duct has a thick wall. Within the dilated duct, the intraductal papilloma is recognized by its broad stalk of connective tissue covered by two layers of benign

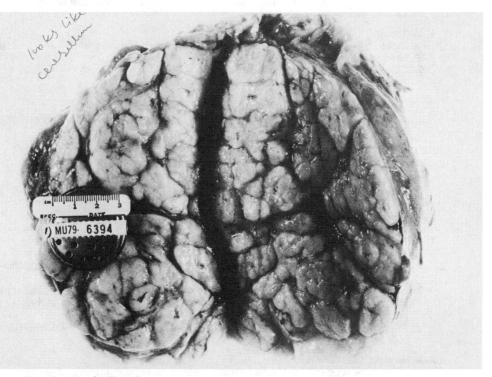

Figure 14-1. Section of a fibroadenoma. Notice the prominent lobulation and the surrounding pseudocapsule.

epithelial cells. The connective tissue stalk of one papilla may fuse with the fibrous stalk of an adjacent papilla, trapping the epithelium in the process and forming duct-like spaces within the lesion.

3. Treatment is surgical resection of the lesion.

VIII. MALIGNANT NEOPLASMS

A. GENERAL CONSIDERATIONS

1. Incidence.
   a. Breast cancer is the leading cause of death in women over 40 years of age. Approximately 1 out of 13 women (about 7 percent) will develop breast cancer during her lifetime.
   b. The incidence of a contralateral breast cancer in those patients with a known breast cancer is greater than the incidence of a primary breast cancer in the general population.

2. Etiology. Although the etiology of breast cancer is unknown, epidemiologic studies indicate certain **risk factors**.
   a. Age over 40 years
   b. Familial history of breast cancer
   c. Nulliparity or late age of first pregnancy
   d. Previous cancer in one breast
   e. History of certain benign breast diseases (e.g., fibrocystic disease)
   f. An adverse hormonal milieu

3. Clinical Data.
   a. Clinically, the chief complaints of patients with breast cancer are
      (1) Palpable lump or mass
      (2) Pain
      (3) Skin symptoms such as edema, redness, and dimpling
      (4) Nipple retraction
      (5) Axillary masses
   b. Carcinomas involve the left breast more frequently than the right, and they arise most commonly in the upper outer quadrant, probably because this area contains the greatest volume of mammary tissue.

4. Pathology.
   a. Eighty percent of breast cancers arise from the ductal epithelium and are therefore adenocarcinomas.
   b. Classification of Malignant Neoplasms.
      (1) Ductal carcinomas include
         (a) Intraductal (in situ)
         (b) Infiltrating
         (c) Medullary
         (d) Mucinous
         (e) Papillary
      (2) Lobular carcinoma
      (3) Paget's disease
      (4) Sarcomas—cystosarcoma phyllodes and angiosarcoma
      (5) Metastasis from other tumors

B. DUCTAL CARCINOMAS can be classified according to their activity.

1. Intraductal (In Situ) Carcinoma.
   a. The tumor is confined to the duct system. It represents 5 percent to 10 percent of all mammary cancers. Grossly, the ducts are thick-walled, dilated, and, in some instances, filled with necrotic material (Fig. 14-2).
   b. Histologically, the epithelial lining has proliferated and there is marked cellular pleomorphism with hyperchromatic nuclei and mitotic figures. Necrotic debris and histiocytes are present in the lumina (Fig. 14-3).
   c. Approximately 20 percent to 25 percent of these in situ tumors will break through the duct wall and become invasive.

2. Infiltrating Carcinoma.
   a. This tumor accounts for the majority of breast carcinomas and originates from the ductal epithelium (adenocarcinoma).
   b. The tumor cells vary in size and shape, are pleomorphic, and have prominent nucleoli.

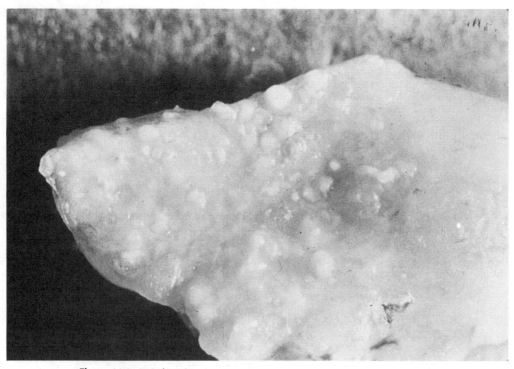

Figure 14-2. Intraductal carcinoma of the breast showing areas of focal necrosis.

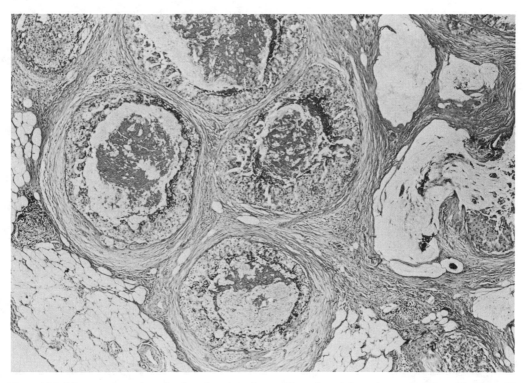

Figure 14-3. Microscopic section of an intraductal carcinoma. The enlarged ducts show epithelial proliferation with central areas of necrosis.

Frequently they form glandular structures.Necrosis may or may not be present. This tumor produces a severe desmoplastic reaction with abundant connective tissue in which tumor cells can be identified (Fig. 14-4).

c. The prognosis for this tumor depends upon the prognostic factors discussed under IX.

3. Medullary Carcinoma.

a. This tumor accounts for approximately 5 percent of all breast carcinomas. Grossly, the lesion is soft and well circumscribed, with a homogeneous gray, moist, cut surface. Focal hemorrhagic areas are present.

b. Histologically, the tumor is recognized by the large pleomorphic cells and marked lymphocytic infiltration. This lesion is believed to behave in a less aggressive fashion than infiltrating ductal carcinoma.

4. Mucinous Carcinoma.

a. This lesion is a well-circumscribed, soft, glistening tumor characterized by a gelatinous appearance.

b. Histologically, there are large pools of mucin separated by bands of connective tissue. Suspended in the mucin are clumps of tumor cells. This tumor has a better prognosis than the ordinary ductal cancer, probably because it has less tendency to metastasize.

5. Papillary Carcinoma.

a. This tumor is a very rare form of cancer that can be difficult to differentiate from benign papilloma. It may first appear as a lump, or an affected patient may complain of hemorrhagic nipple discharge. The lesion is frequently located close to the nipple.

b. Grossly, the tumor is confined within the wall of a duct and appears as a reddish, friable, polypoid mass. Histologically, the diagnosis is made because the lesion shows varying degrees of pleomorphism, mitosis, and necrosis. Clinically, the tumor behaves in a benign fashion, unless it occurs in association with intraductal carcinoma.

C. LOBULAR CARCINOMA

1. Lobular Carcinoma In Situ.

a. **Clinical Data.** Lobular carcinoma in situ is a rare variant of breast cancer that occurs in younger (premenopausal) women. The tumors are bilateral in up to 20 percent of cases

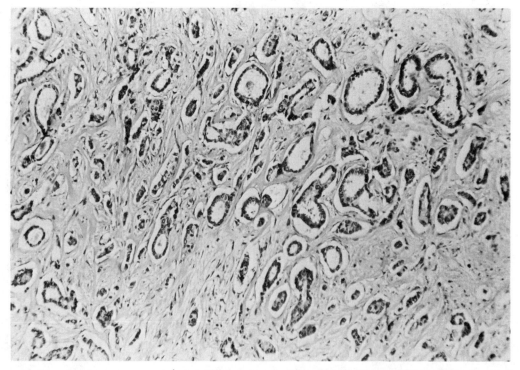

Figure 14-4. Microscopic section of an infiltrating duct carcinoma with glandular differentiation. Abundant desmoplastic stroma surrounds the epithelial glands.

and are frequently multifocal, involving several areas within the same breast. They do not form a palpable tumor mass and are often discovered as an incidental finding when a breast biopsy is performed for other reasons.

    b. Pathology. The lesion is confined to the lobules, which appear distended and filled with uniform cells with abundant cytoplasm. The basement membrane of each acinus is intact. These tumors do not metastasize but predispose to the development of invasive carcinomas.

2. Infiltrating Lobular Carcinoma.

    a. Clinical Data. The age of affected patients is older than that of patients with lobular carcinoma in situ, and the tumor's presentation is similar to that of other forms of carcinoma.

    b. Pathology. The tumor is composed predominantly of small cells, which individually infiltrate the stroma and have a linear arrangement known as Indian filing. In approximately 30 percent of cases, there is evidence of an in situ lobular component. The tumor has the same prognosis as infiltrating duct carcinoma.

D. PAGET'S DISEASE

    1. Paget's disease is an eczematous, excoriated lesion that involves the nipple and adjacent skin. The lesion is accompanied in almost all cases by a carcinoma arising within the ducts (intraductal or infiltrating carcinoma).

    2. Histologically, Paget's cells can be recognized singly or in groups within the epidermis and in the adjacent portions of the mammary duct (Fig. 14-5).

E. SARCOMA.
This tumor arises from the specialized mesenchyma of the breast and accounts for less than 1 percent of all breast neoplasms.

    1. Malignant Cystosarcoma Phyllodes.

        a. Clinical Data. This type of sarcoma occurs in older women who complain of a rapidly growing tumor mass.

        b. Pathology.

            (1) The **gross features** of the tumor are not characteristic, but in some instances the tumor has a fleshy, leaf-like appearance. The gross appearance can be confused with fibroadenoma.

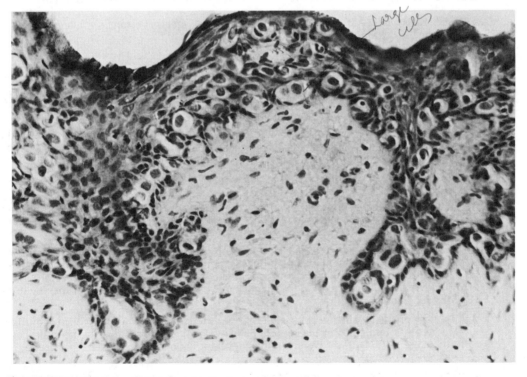

Figure 14-5. Paget's disease of the breast. Notice the large cells with abundant cytoplasm present within the epidermis.

(2) **Histologically,** the hallmark is the presence of a very cellular stroma composed of atypical spindle cells and abundant mitotic figures. Epithelium lines the leaf-like processes but is essentially benign.

(3) The behavoir of cystosarcoma cannot be predicted on the basis of a single feature, but in general it is accepted that these tumors are locally aggressive and that some have the capacity to metastasize through blood vessels. Large tumors with a high mitotic index and nuclear pleomorphism have the worst prognoses.

  c. **Treatment** should be directed towards surgical resection of the mass. Since cystosarcomas metastasize through the blood stream, axillary lymph node resection is not necessary.

  2. **Angiosarcoma.**

    a. **Clinical Data.** This tumor is a highly aggressive neoplasm that accounts for less than 0.5 percent of breast tumors. Most affected patients are in their second or third decade of life. The usual clinical history is that of a lesion that grows rapidly to form a bulky breast tumor.

    b. **Pathology.** Grossly, the lesion consists of an ill-defined infiltrative hemorrhagic mass. Histologically, there is a rich network of communicating vascular channels with prominent endothelial cells that vary in size and shape. Mitoses are frequently encountered.

    c. **Treatment.** These tumors are associated with a poor prognosis and a high mortality rate. Mastectomy is recommended in order to resect the primary tumor mass. Metastases can occur to any organ.

 F. METASTASES TO THE BREAST. The most common tumors to involve the breast secondarily are leukemia, lymphoma, melanoma, lung carcinoma, and endometrial cancer. In general, however, metastases to the breast are rare.

IX. PROGNOSTIC FACTORS.
In general, the 5-year survival rate for patients who have breast cancer is about 53 percent. However, certain factors influence the prognosis of these patients.

 A. EARLY DIAGNOSIS correlates with a better than average prognosis.

 B. HISTOLOGIC FEATURES. Some tumors, such as medullary, papillary, and mucinous ones, seem to have a better prognosis, a lower incidence of lymph node metastasis, and a longer survival rate than other histologic types.

 C. AGE AT ONSET. The younger the patient, the worse the prognosis is believed to be.

 D. STAGE OF THE DISEASE. Advanced cancers that have metastatic spread to lymph nodes or other organs at the time of diagnosis have poor prognoses.

 E. HOST RESISTANCE

  1. The growth and spread of breast cancer depends upon the results of the interaction between cancer cells and the host. The tumor-host relationship in these tumors is not readily assayed, but the fact that breast cancer usually has obtained a significant size before it becomes clinically apparent may be a sign of inadequate host resistance.

  2. Certain histologic features, such as an increased number of histiocytes in lymph nodes or the presence of plasma cells and lymphocytes bordering a tumor, are interpreted as favorable signs, related to a better prognosis.

 F. ESTROGEN RECEPTOR STATUS

  1. About 50 percent of breast carcinomas contain estrogen-receptor proteins, specifically binding estradiol. These proteins are detected by performing steroid-receptor assays. Currently, the most reliable method appears to be sucrose density gradient sedimentation analysis.

  2. Few patients whose breast cancers lack estrogen receptors respond to endocrine therapies, while more than 50 percent of patients whose tumors contain estrogen receptors obtain objective remissions from such treatments. Therefore, the results of estrogen-receptor assays provide valuable information for making clinical decisions as to the type of therapy to be employed and the prognosis.

  3. Tumors in premenopausal women have been reported to have a lower incidence of estrogen receptors than tumors occurring in postmenopausal women. This finding has been attributed to the presence in younger women of high levels of endogenous estrogens that occupy the receptor sites.

  4. At the present time, there is no histopathologic feature that can predict the estrogen-receptor status of a cancer, although it is believed that well-differentiated tumors may have a higher proportion of estrogen receptors than poorly differentiated ones.

G. METASTASES FROM THE BREAST. Carcinoma of the breast has a high tendency to metastasize to regional lymph nodes. The presence of four or more positive lymph nodes at the time of diagnosis is associated with a poor prognosis. Visceral metastases are commonly found, predominantly in the lungs, liver, bones, and brain, but any organ can be involved.

X. TREATMENT. Surgical excision of the breast (mastectomy) is the treatment of choice, followed by radiation, chemotherapy, or both, according to the stage of disease and the estrogen-receptor status. Recently, some surgeons have been using a new modality of treatment, lumpectomy, or local resection of the tumor mass followed by radiation therapy.

STUDY QUESTIONS

Directions: Each question below contains five suggested answers. Choose the **one best** response to each question.

1. The primary structural unit of the mammary gland is known as the

(A) duct
(B) ligament
(C) nipple
(D) lobule
(E) quadrant

2. What is the most common benign tumor encountered in the breasts of premenopausal women?

(A) Cystic fibroma
(B) Fibroadenoma
(C) Lipoma
(D) Intraductal papilloma
(E) Hemangioma

3. A woman who presents clinically with a bloody discharge from one nipple is most likely to have

(A) Paget's disease of the nipple
(B) intraductal papilloma
(C) medullary carcinoma
(D) mucinous carcinoma
(E) intraductal carcinoma

Directions: Each question below contains four suggested answers of which **one or more** is correct. Choose the answer

A   if **1, 2, and 3** are correct
B   if **1 and 3** are correct
C   if **2 and 4** are correct
D   if **4** is correct
E   if **1, 2, 3, and 4** are correct

4. Complications most often occurring during lactation and breast feeding include

(1) chronic mastitis
(2) duct ectasia
(3) fat necrosis
(4) acute mastitis

5. Histologic changes typically seen in fibrocystic disease of the breast include

(1) the presence of microcysts
(2) epithelial hyperplasia
(3) fibrosis
(4) adenosis

6. Of the following pathologic conditions that affect the breast, those linked with the development of breast carcinoma include

(1) acute mastitis
(2) fat necrosis
(3) fibroadenoma
(4) fibrocystic disease

7. True statements concerning gynecomastia include

(1) it is caused by hormonal imbalance
(2) the unilateral pattern is most common
(3) it is associated with cirrhosis
(4) it is associated with some testicular tumors

8. Lobular carcinoma in situ is characterized by which of the following findings?

(1) A high incidence of bilateral occurrence
(2) Premenopausal occurrence
(3) Multifocal origin
(4) Impalpability

9. Invasive lobular carcinoma of the breast is distinguished by which of the following criteria?

(1) Pools of mucinous material
(2) Its arrangement in pseudoglands
(3) Papillary outgrowths
(4) Individual cell infiltration of stroma

10. Clinical characteristics of malignant cystosarcoma phyllodes include

(1) rapid growth as a palpable mass
(2) occurrence in elderly women
(3) hematogenous metastasis
(4) metastasis to regional lymph nodes

ANSWERS AND EXPLANATIONS

1. The answer is D. (*II B 2*) Clusters of epithelial cells formed into acini are arranged about a ductule to create the lobule, which is the basic structural unit of the breast. Each lobule empties into epithelial-lined ductules and larger ducts, which drain toward the lactiferous sinuses at the nipple. Cooper's ligaments are the fibrous supports of the breasts.

2. The answer is B. (*VII A, B*) Fibroadenoma is the most common benign breast tumor. It frequently appears in young women sometime between puberty and 30 years of age. A fibroadenoma is composed of proliferated connective tissue and ductal and acinar elements. Cystic fibroma, lipoma, intraductal papilloma, and hemangioma are all much less common in occurrence.

3. The answer is B. (*VII B 1*) Nipple discharge is encountered more frequently in benign conditions of the breast than as a sign of malignant tumors. Intraductal papilloma is the most common cause. This papilloma is a discrete tumor of the connective tissue; it is covered by two layers of benign epithelial cells. Minor trauma to the delicate, well-vascularized papilloma may be the reason for the intermittent serous or serosanguineous discharge through the nipple.

4. The answer is D (4). (*V*) Acute mastitis is usually produced by a strain of *Staphylococcus* or *Streptococcus*, which enters the breast through fissures in the nipple produced by the minor trauma of breast feeding. This inflammation is thus termed puerperal mastitis. The infection can usually be controlled with antibiotics before severe destruction of breast tissue occurs.

5. The answer is E (all). (*VI A 4*) Fibrocystic disease is the most common disorder of the breast, accounting for a significant number of unnecessary mastectomies. The histopathologic criteria used for diagnosis of fibrocystic disease include the presence of microcysts, epithelial hyperplasia, fibrosis, and adenosis. Apocrine metaplasia with characteristic cell changes is the fifth important sign.

6. The answer is D (4). (*VI A; VIII A 2 e*) Fibrocystic disease of the breast with evidence of epithelial hyperplasia is often related to the development of breast carcinoma. Fat necrosis as a result of trauma and breast infections has not been linked with increased likelihood of malignant tumor occurrence. Fibroadenoma is a benign tumor of the breast and has no association with malignant cancers.

7. The answer is E (all). (*IV C*) Gynecomastia is hypertrophy of the male breast. Since the male breast does not contain lobules, enlargement occurs because of proliferation of ductal and stromal elements. Hormonal excesses, particularly of estrogen-like products, are linked with gynecomastia.

8. The answer is E (all). (*VIII C 1*) A high incidence of bilateral occurrence, premenopausal occurrence, multifocal origin, and impalpability are all possible descriptions for lobular carcinoma in situ, which is a rare form of breast malignancy occurring in young women. Nearly one-fifth of the patients have involvement of both breasts, and within an involved breast, multiple tumor foci are often found. Lobular carcinoma is a carcinoma in situ and thus is not palpable because no mass is present.

9. The answer is D (4). (*VIII C 2*) Invasive lobular carcinoma is hallmarked by a pattern of linear, single-file, invading cells of the stromal tissues, which is termed "Indian-filing." These invasive cells have moderate amounts of eosinophilic cytoplasm and large hyperchromatic nuclei.

10. The answer is A (1, 2, 3). (*VIII E 1*) Malignant cystosarcoma phyllodes is a rapidly growing, locally invasive malignancy of the breast, which behaves like other sarcomas. It metastasizes via the bloodstream, often to the lungs. Surgical resection of the tumor mass is therapeutic, but axillary lymph node dissection is not useful.

15
The Endocrine System

I. INTRODUCTION

A. The endocrine system is dispersed throughout the body; its major function is regulation. Endocrine regulation occurs at three sites: the hypothalamus, the pituitary gland, and the endocrine or target organs.

B. Negative and positive feedback systems stabilize the action of the individual target organs and the interaction among the endocrine glands, hypothalamus, and pituitary gland. Lesions (i.e., disturbances of these intricate and delicately balanced feedback systems) lead to over- or undersecretion of various hormones and clinical syndromes or endocrinopathies.

C. Not only will lesions of the endocrine system lead to endocrine disease, but disturbed functional states (e.g., chemically abnormal neurotransmitters or overabundant or insufficient amounts of hypothalamic releasing factors) without morphologic abnormalities can upset this system to such a degree that they create a pathologic lesion.

II. HYPOTHALAMIC AND PITUITARY LESIONS AND DYSFUNCTIONS. The hypothalamus serves as the center for regulation between itself and the pituitary with its many connections to the rest of the nervous system. Thus, the hypothalamus integrates incoming neural signals from the body and environment and requests specific endocrine responses via regulatory systems (releasing or inhibiting factors) on the pituitary.

A. HYPOTHALAMIC LESIONS that can destroy or replace this vital area include hamartomas, neoplasms, trauma, and inflammatory conditions (sarcoidosis). The result of any of these is interference with the delicate feedback balance and control of the pituitary.

B. PITUITARY DYSFUNCTION can be divided into **hyperfunction** (hormone overproduction) and **hypofunction** (hormone deficiency).

1. Hyperfunction. Intrinsic hypersecretion of one of the pituitary trophic hormones is almost always the result of either a neoplasm (an adenoma or microadenoma) or a localized area of hyperplasia. There are three common syndromes associated with these conditions.
  a. Acromegaly results from excess production of growth hormone by an **acidophil cell (eosinophilic)** pituitary adenoma.
   (1) Clinical Data. The manifestations of this syndrome vary with a patient's age. Such a lesion in a growing child leads to **gigantism**, whereas in an adult whose skeletal epiphyses are closed, the change in appearance consists of a gradual **coarsening** of the facies, enlargement and swelling of the hands and feet, and thickening of the lips. Because of the influence of growth hormone on glucose tolerance, diabetes often is found in affected patients.
   (2) Pathology. The pituitary lesion usually is slow growing, leading to a gradual change in an affected individual's appearance.
  b. Hyperprolactinemia—Amenorrhea-Galactorrhea Syndrome.
   (1) Clinical Data. An elevated serum prolactin level associated with spontaneous or inducible galactorrhea recently has been recognized as a cause of female infertility and secondary amenorrhea. This symptom complex has been noted in young women following cessation of oral contraceptives after prolonged use.
   (2) The **pathologic** lesion may be one of a variety of abnormalities ranging from grossly and radiologically visible adenomas to microscopic foci of hyperplasia (microadenomas).

c. **Hypercorticism (Cushing's Syndrome).**
   (1) **Clinical Data.** This symptom complex consists of a variety of electrolyte and glucose-tolerance abnormalities, obesity, edema, hypertension, and psychiatric disturbances associated with an excess of circulating corticosteroids.
   (2) **Pathology.** The causes include excess hypothalamic corticotropin-releasing factor, pituitary tumors producing adrenocorticotropic hormone (ACTH), primary adrenal lesions, and ectopic ACTH production by nonendocrine tumors (see below). The pituitary lesion most frequently found is a **basophilic adenoma** or **microadenoma.** Such tumors usually are quite small and thus difficult to detect.
   (3) **Prognosis.** Follow-up studies indicate that the majority of affected patients probably have primary pituitary pathology. After bilateral adrenalectomy, some patients develop **Nelson's syndrome**, in which a basophilic pituitary adenoma is found. This lesion often is locally invasive and difficult to treat. Patients who have Nelson's syndrome have extremely high serum ACTH levels and hyperpigmentation.

2. **Hypofunction.** Although decreased or absent production of one pituitary hormone occurs, **panhypopituitarism**, in which a lesion destroys the pituitary gland, is more commonly encountered.
   a. **Clinical Data.** Because of decreases or depletion of tropic hormones and resultant nonstimulation of target endocrine organs, affected patients show symptoms of hypothyroidism, hypogonadism, and hypoadrenalism (lethargy, infertility, and susceptibility to infection). If pituitary hypofunction occurs in children, **dwarfism** results because of a lack of growth hormone.
   b. **Pathology.** Destruction of the pituitary gland may result from
      (1) Tumor
         (a) A primary adenoma compressing the rest of a normal gland
         (b) A tumor of a neighboring structure
         (c) Metastasis to the pituitary
      (2) Infarction, especially in the peripartum period (Sheehan's syndrome)
      (3) Irradiation to the area
      (4) Granulomatous disease, especially sarcoid
      (5) The mysterious **empty sella syndrome**, in which the pituitary is absent or has been destroyed, although the sella turcica is enlarged by radiologic evaluation. The etiology is unknown.

C. **PITUITARY LESIONS** (tumors) may produce symptoms by their size, location, and infiltrative growth.

   1. Although in some cases multihormonal production is found, **clinically,** a symptom complex associated with one hormone usually predominates.

   2. The **histology** of pituitary tumors is shared by endocrine tumors in general. They usually are composed of groups or nests of uniform, cytologically bland cells, encompassed by a delicate vascular network. **Immunohistologic techniques** are useful in elucidating the predominant hormone produced by such tumors.

D. **THE NEUROHYPOPHYSIS (POSTERIOR PITUITARY GLAND)** secretes vasopressin, a hormone regulating the maintenance of serum osmolality. Deficiency of vasopressin secretion leads to **diabetes insipidus**, clinically manifested by polyuria (the excretion of large volumes of dilute urine, even in the presence of body dehydration). Causes of vasopressin deficiency include compression or destruction of the neurohypophysis by tumors of the pituitary gland or brain, radiation, trauma, or previous surgery in the area.

III. THE THYROID GLAND

A. **THE NORMAL THYROID GLAND** is soft, red, and weighs between 25 g and 50 g. On cut surface, the gland glistens because of the colloid contained in the follicles. The follicle is the functional unit of this endocrine organ and is composed of a sac lined by epithelium containing colloid—thyroid hormones and thyroglobulin.

B. **GOITER** is a nonspecific term denoting thyroid enlargement. Such increase in gland size and weight may have a variety of causes (Table 15-1).

   1. **Inborn Defects of Thyroid Hormonogenesis (Absent or Deficient Enzyme Synthesis).** When insufficient thyroid hormone is produced by the thyroid gland, the pituitary responds with increased thyrotropin secretion, which stimulates the thyroid follicular epithelium, which then undergoes hyperplasia.

Table 15-1. Causes of Goiter

Dyshormonogenesis with glandular hyperplasia

Nutritional (iodine) deficiency

Goitrogenic drugs

Nontoxic nodular goiter

Diffuse toxic goiter

Thyroiditis

Neoplasms

2. **Iodine deficiency** due to dietary or environmental causes also can reduce thyroid hormone concentrations and act by a similar mechanism on the pituitary to increase thyrotropin and spur the thyroid gland to hyperplasia. In certain areas of the world, usually those distant from the sea (and hence iodine), **endemic goiter** is very common, occurring in up to 50 percent of the population.

3. **Goitrogens** (certain drugs and naturally occurring substances) can interfere with thyroid hormone production and lead to goiter.

4. **Nontoxic nodular goiter** is an enlargement of the thyroid gland due to repeated or continual hyperplasia in response to a relative deficiency of thyroid hormone.
   a. **Clinical Data.** The thyroid can reach huge size (up to 250 g or more), extend substernally, and produce **respiratory embarrassment**. Although nodular goiter involves the entire gland, the nodules may be asymmetrical or one nodule may dominate the clinical picture and be mistaken for a thyroid neoplasm.
   b. **Pathology.** In regions of the world where goiter is not endemic, the initial stimulus to nodular formation is unknown. Once an area of hyperplasia is formed, however, relative intrathyroidal iodine trapping (relative iodine deficiency) may occur, promoting the process. As hyperplasia continues over years, nodules are formed by follicles distended with colloid, which lie next to zones of microfollicles lined by hyperplastic columnar cells, which contain little colloid. Eventually, some of the huge follicles rupture and extrude colloid, inciting an inflammatory reaction. The combination of nodularity, focal hyperplasia, and degenerative changes comprises the entity of nodular goiter. Sometimes, the foci of hyperplasia are relatively large and circumscribed, resembling a neoplasm (adenoma), and the terms **adenomatous goiter** or **adenomatous hyperplasia in nodular goiter** are used.

5. **Diffuse Toxic Goiter (Graves' Disease).**
   a. The **causes of hyperthyroidism** are varied and include functioning thyroid adenomas or carcinomas, pituitary tumors secreting thyrotropin, and choriocarcinomas secreting thyrotropin-like substances. However, the most common condition associated with hyperthyroidism is diffuse toxic goiter.
   b. **Clinical Data.** Affected patients are usually young females who exhibit nervousness, tachycardia, sweating, and weight loss. Often exophthalmos also is present.
   c. **Pathology.** The thyroid shows a diffuse, severe hyperplasia of the follicular epithelium. The overactivity of the thyroid is caused by excessive stimulation of the gland by substances not yet clearly defined.
      (1) **Grossly**, diffuse toxic goiter is a symmetrical enlargement of two to four times normal size.
      (2) **Microscopically**, the follicles are small and contain little colloid. The follicular cells are tall, columnar, and their nuclei are enlarged. Because there are increased numbers of cells that cannot be accommodated in the follicle in the usual way, **papillary infoldings** occur (Fig. 15-1). The stroma shows marked vascularity, and lymphocytic infiltrates are common.
      (3) This condition is a systemic disorder of unknown etiology, which presumably is caused by immunologic mechanisms. Autoimmune diseases are found commonly in patients who have Graves' disease or in their close relatives.

6. **Thyroiditis.**
   a. **Acute** suppurative thyroiditis is a bacterial infection of the thyroid gland, usually occurring in young children or debilitated patients. It is very rare.

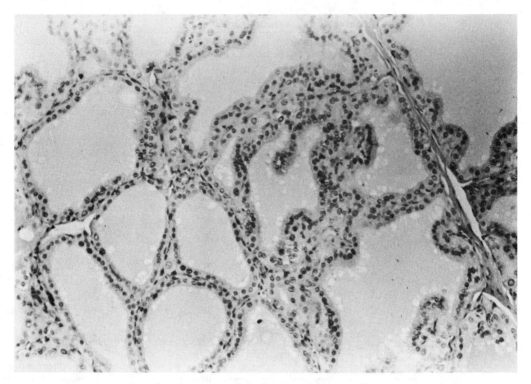

Figure 15-1. Diffuse hyperplasia (Graves' disease) of the thyroid gland. Focal papillary ingrowths into follicles can be seen. Individual cells are enlarged, and their number is increased [low power, hematoxylin and eosin (H and E) stain].

    b. Subacute (granulomatous) thyroiditis is a self-limited disorder, lasting 1 to 3 months, characterized by swelling of the thyroid gland, transient hypothyroidism, and recovery. The incidence is unknown, although classic forms comprise about 2 percent of all thyroid disease. The etiology is unknown, although a viral causation is suspected.

        (1) Clinical Data. In the classic form of subacute thyroiditis, **neck pain** is found, radiating to the jaw or ear. Fever and malaise may be present.

        (2) Pathology.

            (a) Grossly, the gland is slightly enlarged. The involved areas are firm and poorly defined, resembling carcinoma.

            (b) Histologically early in the disease, the follicular epithelium degenerates. Colloid leakage from disrupted follicles initiates an inflammatory response, which becomes granulomatous.

        (3) Prognosis. Eventual regeneration of follicles occurs, usually from the edges of the most severely affected areas, and clinical recovery follows.

    c. Chronic thyroiditis (struma lymphomatosa, Hashimoto's disease, autoimmune thyroiditis) is a classic example of autoimmune disease and represents a group of disorders sharing some clinical and pathologic characteristics. Although the pathogenesis of the disease is unknown, both humoral and cell-mediated immunity are postulated to be involved. Affected patients and their close family members have circulating antibodies to thyroid antigens as well as to other organs. The antibodies are directed against thyroid cell components or surface receptors. Different concentrations and types of antibodies may account for the different clinical manifestations of this form of thyroiditis.

        (1) Clinical Data. Patients who have chronic thyroiditis may be euthyroid or, more often, hypothyroid. Hypothyroid (myxedematous) patients often are lethargic, intolerant of cold, sluggish, and have thick skin, slow pulses, and a low body temperature.

        (2) Pathology.

            (a) Grossly, the gland is moderately enlarged, from two to four times normal size, and firm. On cut surface, the lobulation of the normal thyroid gland is accentuated and the individual lobules bulge. In the end stage of Hashimoto's thyroiditis, the gland is very small and fibrotic (idiopathic myxedema).

(b) Microscopically, the thyroid follicles are small and atrophic with sparse or absent colloid. Oxyphilic (Hürthle cell) metaplasia of much or all of the follicular epithelium is recognized (Fig. 15-2). The most prominent characteristic is infiltration by lymphocytes with formation of germinal centers. Fibrosis, which varies in extent, is found.

d. Riedel's struma (Riedel's disease) is not a disorder of the thyroid gland per se but a connective tissue proliferation that involves the gland.

   (1) Clinical Data. Association of this disorder with fibrosing processes in the retroperitoneum, orbit, and mediastinum suggests that it is a systemic collagenosis. Vasculitis, usually involving veins, is found in the neck and elsewhere in the body of affected patients.

   (2) Pathology. Grossly, the gland is woody or iron hard, and the abnormal tissue is adherent to surrounding structures; tissue planes are obliterated.

7. Neoplasms.

  a. Adenomas. All benign tumors of the thyroid gland arise from glandular follicular epithelium and are designated as adenomas. The most common type is the follicular adenoma.

   (1) Grossly, follicular adenomas have the usual well-circumscribed appearance of a benign tumor. They usually are solitary, demarcated from the adjacent normal thyroid tissue, and encapsulated (Fig. 15-3).

   (2) Microscopically, the encapsulation and the sharp demarcation from the adjacent thyroid tissue are evident. The adjacent thyroid tissue is compressed from the expansile growth of the adenoma.

  b. Carcinomas.

   (1) Papillary adenocarcinoma is the most common type of thyroid cancer and accounts for approximately 70 percent to 80 percent of all malignant tumors arising in the thyroid.

    (a) Clinical Data. The majority of affected patients are bimodally rather evenly distributed between the third and the seventh decade of life. As with all thyroid cancers, this tumor is more common in women than men. It has been related to head and neck irradiation.

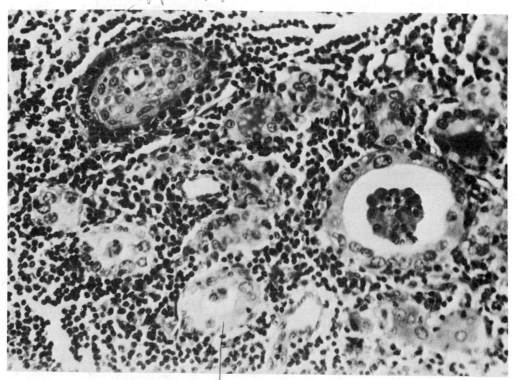

Figure 15-2. Chronic (Hashimoto's) thyroiditis showing follicular atrophy and lymphocytic infiltration [low power, hematoxylin and eosin (H and E) stain].

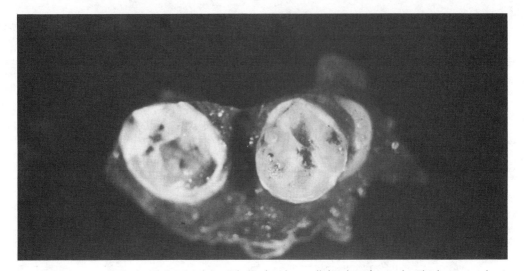

Figure 15-3. A circumscribed nodule of the thyroid gland with a well-developed capsule. The lesion is a benign follicular adenoma.

(b) Pathology.
   (i) The **gross** appearance varies considerably with the size of the tumor. Small tumors, often called sclerosing or occult carcinomas, resemble minute scars. Large tumors have ill-defined borders, although some show at least partial encapsulation. Cyst formation is common; papillae may project from the cyst lining, or the tumor may be solid. Fibrosis and calcification sometimes are extensive.
   (ii) Microscopically, the single-layered and well-differentiated tumor epithelium is arranged on fibrovascular stalks. Nuclei show characteristic clearing ("ground-glass"). About 40 percent of papillary carcinomas contain laminated calcific spherules known as **psammoma bodies**. Lymphatic invasion by papillary carcinoma is extremely common and probably accounts for the frequency of multiple intrathyroidal foci of the tumor. Metastasis to cervical lymph nodes is so common that 50 percent of patients already have lymph node involvement at the time of diagnosis. Papillary carcinomas are characterized by their extremely slow growth. Many of these tumors show follicular differentiation, and some pathologists prefer the term **mixed papillary and follicular carcinoma**. The biologic behavior is similar. The 10-year survival rate is about 95 percent.
(2) Follicular carcinoma accounts for about 10 percent of all malignant thyroid carcinomas.
   (a) Clinical Data. It affects adults, with a slight predominance in females. It presents as a nodule. Invasion of blood vessels is common and is responsible for metastases to brain, bones, or lungs. Not uncommonly, the metastatic tumor calls initial attention to the thyroid tumor.
   (b) Pathology.
      (i) Some follicular carcinomas are indistinguishable **grossly** from follicular adenomas because their invasive nature is not extensive enough to be seen grossly. With other follicular carcinomas, the invasion is obvious both grossly and clinically.
      (ii) Microscopically, some tumors are nearly solid with only abortive attempts at follicle formation; others show neoplastic follicles so well-developed that they are indistinguishable individually from normal thyroid tissue.
   (c) Prognosis depends largely upon the extent of invasion at the time of initial treatment. If the invasion is so minimal that the cancer looks grossly like an adenoma and only microscopically shows limited capsular or vascular invasion, the prognosis is very good (85 percent survival at 5 years). Such tumors may take up radioiodine and can be stimulated by thyrotropin to take up additional radioiodine; this characteristic of the tumor is useful both in diagnosis and in therapy.

(3) Medullary Carcinoma.

(a) **Clinical Data.** These tumors usually affect patients over 40 years of age but occasionally are seen in younger adults and children. Medullary carcinomas occur in both sporadic and familial forms. Both forms arise in the areas of the thyroid gland where parafollicular cells are found in highest concentration—upper two-thirds lateral aspects of the thyroid. Parafollicular cells normally secrete calcitonin, and the tumors derived from these cells retain the capacity to secrete this hormone. Thus, measurement of calcitonin in serum is useful as a diagnostic tool and prognostic indicator in affected patients. In the familial form, medullary carcinoma is associated with pheochromocytomas and parathyroid hyperplasia (**Sipple's syndrome**); in this case, the tumor tends to be multifocal and bilateral.

(b) **Pathology.**

(i) **Grossly**, the tumor typically is a hard, gray-white to yellow-tan mass, usually well demarcated.

(ii) **Microscopically**, it contains clusters of tumor cells growing in solid or irregular groups, which are separated by a hyaline, **amyloid-containing** stroma.

(c) **Prognosis.** Medullary carcinoma can metastasize both by lymphatics and blood vessels. Its prognosis is not as good as that of the papillary-follicular carcinoma group but is, however, better than that for undifferentiated carcinomas. The overall survival rate is 50 percent.

(4) Anaplastic (undifferentiated) carcinoma usually is a rapidly growing tumor with a poor prognosis. It is one of the most malignant of all cancers in the body and comprises about 3 percent to 5 percent of thyroid carcinomas.

(a) **Clinical Data.** Anaplastic carcinoma almost exclusively occurs in individuals over 60 years of age and is preceded by a long history of goiter (either benign adenoma or low-grade carcinoma) in over 50 percent of patients.

(b) **Pathology.**

(i) The **gross** appearance is that of a typical cancer with invasion into adjacent areas of the thyroid gland and structures of the neck. Remnants suggesting a preexisting adenoma are frequently present.

(ii) **Microscopically**, the tumor cells are large, often of giant size, and pleomorphism is common.

IV. THE PARATHYROID GLANDS

A. NORMAL DEVELOPMENT

1. In up to 90 percent of individuals, four parathyroid glands are found, usually located at the inferior and superior poles of the thyroid gland and together weighing 120 mg to 150 mg. In 10 percent of individuals, the number of glands found varies from three to ten (usually five).

2. The upper parathyroids are derived from the fourth branchial pouch (as is the thymus) and the lower glands from the third pouch. This embryonic fact explains the presence of mediastinal thymic-associated parathyroid tissue and the occasional discovery of intrathymic parathyroid adenomas.

3. Ectopic locations of normal parathyroid glands are found in about 5 percent of the population, the most common areas being intrathyroidal, retroesophageal, and intrathymic.

4. The cellularity of the glands normally decreases with age, and in a normal middle-aged adult the ratio of cells to fat should be 1:1.

B. HYPERCALCEMIA. The normal range for serum calcium is 9 mg/100 ml to 10.5 mg/100 ml.

1. The most important **causes** of hypercalcemia are
   a. **M**alignancy (myeloma)
   b. **I**ntoxication (vitamin D)
   c. **S**arcoidosis
   d. **H**yperparathyroidism
   e. **A**lkali (mild alkali syndrome)
   f. **P**aget's disease of bone

2. **Clinical Data.** Symptoms of hypercalcemia can be divided according to the systems affected: gastrointestinal, musculoskeletal, cardiovascular, neuropsychiatric, or urinary. In general, there is a poor correlation between the severity of the clinical manifestations and the degree of hypercalcemia. At levels above 18 mg/100 ml, a patient is very ill and may die.

C. HYPERPARATHYROIDISM

1. **Primary Hyperparathyroidism.**
   a. **Clinical Data.** One or more symptoms of hypercalcemia may be present, but many asymptomatic patients who have hypercalcemia and primary hyperparathyroidism now are identified because of the recent advent of mass screening techniques.
   b. **Pathology.** From 40 percent to 80 percent of patients have solitary parathyroid adenomas, (Figs. 15-4 and 15-5), and 10 percent to 50 percent have primary hyperplasia. The hyperplasia and adenomas usually are of the chief cell type. Frequently the histologic distinction between adenoma and hyperplasia is difficult, if not impossible, to determine, resulting in the wide range of percentages listed above.
   c. **Primary therapy** consists of surgical removal of the enlarged parathyroid gland or glands.

2. **Secondary hyperparathyroidism** may be caused by renal disease or, more rarely, by malabsorption.
   a. **Clinical Data.** Soft tissue calcification and osteosclerosis are prominent. The end stage of secondary hyperparathyroidism may, however, be impossible to distinguish from the primary form of the disease.
   b. **Pathology.** The parathyroid glands usually show diffuse hyperplasia (chief cell or clear cell).

3. **Carcinoma of the parathyroid glands** is very rare, accounting for approximately 1 percent of primary cases of hyperparathyroidism. Mitoses, local invasion, and metastases (usually functional) characterize the lesion. Clinically, these tumors are frequently large enough to be palpable and result in severe hypercalcemia.

4. **Ectopic hyperparathyroidism.** Neoplasms (usually carcinomas) may produce substances that mimic the actions of parathyroid hormone and hence produce hypercalcemia.

D. HYPOPARATHYROIDISM is a failure of the parathyroid glands to maintain a normal concentration of ionized calcium in the plasma, either under normal conditions or in response to deliberate attempts to decrease the calcium level.

1. **Clinical Data.** All affected patients have hypocalcemia and hyperphosphatemia, with associated neuromuscular irritability, malabsorption, anxiety, depression, and functional psychoses. These symptoms are related to the degree and duration of the hypocalcemia.

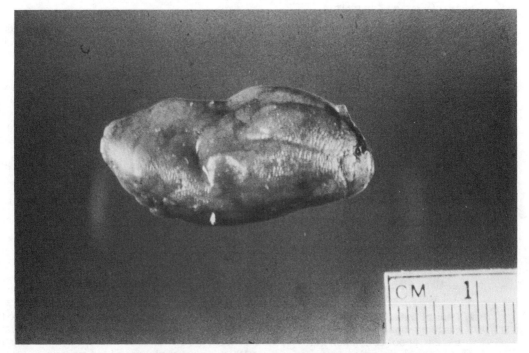

Figure 15-4. A 1.3 cm parathyroid adenoma removed from a patient. The patient's other three parathyroid glands were atrophic.

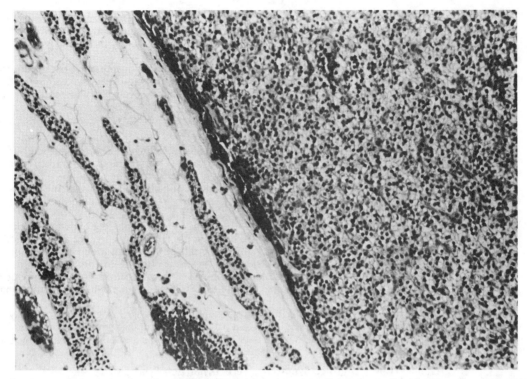

Figure 15-5. Microscopic view of a parathyroid adenoma. Note the cellular area (*right*) abutting upon the rim of residual parathyroid tissue containing few cells and fat (*left*) [low power, hematoxylin and eosin (H and E) stain].

2. The condition may be familial, idiopathic (? autoimmune), or may be caused by
   a. Thyroidectomy
   b. Radioactive iodine therapy for Graves' disease
   c. Metastatic carcinoma to the parathyroids
   d. Infiltration of the glands by iron in long-standing iron-storage disease

3. **Therapy** includes dietary supplements of calcium and vitamin D.

V. PANCREATIC ISLETS are rounded masses of cells that are scattered throughout the pancreas but are most numerous in the distal portion (tail). The beta cells produce insulin, the alpha cells produce glucagon, and a variety of other cells secrete vasoactive intestinal peptides, gastrin, somatostatin, and other hormones. The assignment of particular cell morphology to particular hormone secretion is difficult and is most reliably done by immunohistochemical localization of a hormone in a cell.

A. **ISLET CELL TUMORS** are relatively uncommon compared to adenocarcinoma of the pancreas and may be benign or malignant, functioning or nonfunctioning. Most islet cell tumors make themselves known clinically by some type of **functional abnormality**.

   1. Benign **nonfunctional islet cell adenomas** do not produce clinical problems and therefore usually are found incidentally at autopsy.

   2. **Insulin-producing islet cell tumors** (insulinomas) are of **beta cell origin**. They most commonly are found in the distal two-thirds of the pancreas but may be seen in the head of the pancreas or in ectopic locations such as the duodenal wall.
      a. These tumors produce large quantities of insulin, most often intermittently. The **clinical symptoms** are related to **hypoglycemia** and include dizziness, weakness, bizarre behavior, seizures, and coma. Some patients learn to avoid attacks by eating, which leads to obesity.
      b. **Pathology.** Ninety percent of insulin-producing islet cell tumors are benign (including ten percent morphologically suspicious for malignancy), thus ten percent are malignant. Most of these tumors are solitary, but approximately 5 percent are associated with diffuse hyperplasia and multiple tumors (**multiple endocrine adenomatosis**).

(1) These tumors have an endocrine or organoid pattern, with nests and cords of cells supported by fibrovascular stroma (Fig. 15-6). Evidence of malignancy includes blood vessel and capsular invasion, numerous mitoses, and metastases to regional lymph nodes and liver.

(2) In general, the tumors grow much more slowly than adenocarcinomas of the pancreas. Patients may have a metastatic tumor in the liver for many years before enough liver tissue is sufficiently replaced to produce hepatic failure. Typically, patients die because of the effects of the hypoglycemia produced by an unresectable tumor.

c. **Therapy** consists of surgical resection of the tumor; sometimes liver metastases also are resected if technically feasible.

3. **Gastrin-Producing Islet Cell Tumors (Gastrinomas)—Zollinger-Ellison Syndrome.** These tumors lead to stimulation and hyperplasia of the **parietal cells** of the gastric fundus, resulting in 10 to 20 times the normal amount of **gastric acid** being produced.

a. **Clinical Data.** Patients present with **intractable peptic ulcer** disease, which is unresponsive to ordinary medical treatment. The ulcers are frequently multiple and may be in atypical locations.

b. **Pathology.** Most recent reports indicate that 60 percent to 70 percent of gastrin-producing islet cell tumors are malignant (Fig. 15-7), thus approximately 30 percent are benign. Five to ten percent of affected patients also have diffuse hyperplasia and multiple tumors **(multiple endocrine adenomatosis)**. Gastrinomas are found in the pancreas or the duodenal wall. On **gross** and **histologic** examination they are similar to insulin-producing neoplasms and present the same difficulties in differentiating benign from malignant tumors.

c. **Treatment.** Gastrin-producing tumors frequently are slow-growing lesions, even when they are in the liver. The major threat to a patient's life is not the tumor itself but complications of peptic ulcer disease. Patients with unresectable tumors are treated by **total gastrectomy** to remove all acid-producing parietal cells.

4. **VIPoma—Watery Diarrhea Syndrome, Verner-Morrison Syndrome.**

a. **Clinical Data.** Excess pancreatic and intestinal secretions or decreased intestinal absorption of these secretions characterize the condition produced by this tumor. The hormone responsible for the condition, which also is called **pancreatic cholera**, is believed to be

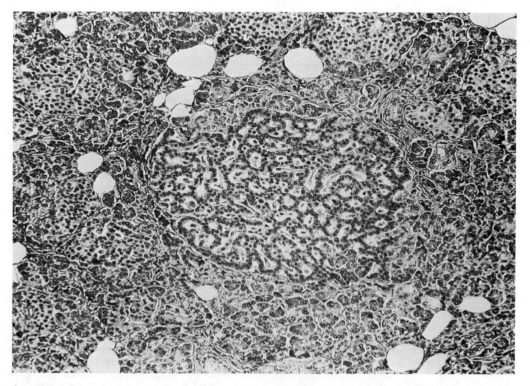

Figure 15-6. A tiny islet cell adenoma of the pancreas found in a patient with hypoglycemia [low power, hematoxylin and eosin (H and E) stain].

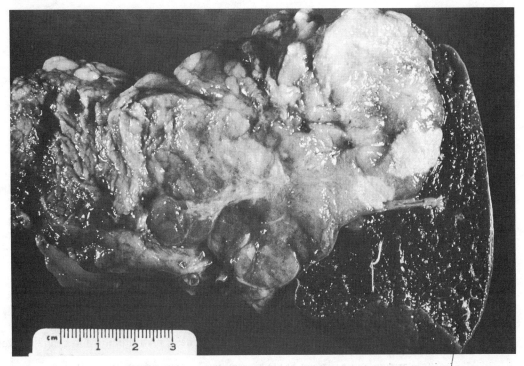

Figure 15-7. A malignant islet cell tumor (carcinoma), which produced Zollinger-Ellison syndrome. Note invasion of the spleen.

spleen

vasoactive intestinal polypeptide, hence the term VIPoma. The electrolyte imbalance produced, which is severe, can prove fatal.

    b. Pathology. About 80 percent of these lesions have been classified as malignant.

5. Glucagonoma is an alpha cell tumor that produces an excess of glucagon. It is responsible for an unusual clinical syndrome characterized by hyperglycemia (often manifest as diabetes) and a necrotizing skin lesion, which is called the **glucagonoma syndrome**. Most of these tumors are malignant.

6. Nonfunctional islet cell carcinomas produce no hormones and thus make themselves known clinically by their **malignant behavior**, simulating adenocarcinomas. Affected patients may present with obstructive jaundice, metastases to the liver, or a large mass in the abdomen. **Histologically**, an endocrine or organoid pattern may be seen in these tumors, as opposed to the glandular or ductal pattern of adenocarcinoma.

7. Nesidioblastosis is a condition usually found in newborn infants who present with uncontrollable hypoglycemia. Cells similar in morphology to islets are found as nodules close to the pancreatic exocrine ducts. Subtotal pancreatectomy often is needed for cure.

8. Malignancy of Islet Cell Tumors (Table 15-2).

    a. Islet cell tumors are considered benign if they are circumscribed or encapsulated and if no metastases are demonstrated. Neoplasms without metastases but with infiltrative borders, mitoses, or vascular invasion are considered borderline lesions. To diagnose an islet cell carcinoma, metastases to nodes or liver are needed. Malignant behavior may be noted many years after the initial diagnosis because these lesions usually follow a prolonged course.

    b. Therapy for malignant or unresectable tumors often is directed at the hormonal effects produced rather than at the tumor, because many patients succumb to the hormonal problems (e.g., hypoglycemia) before there is replacement of vital organs by the tumor. This situation is very different from that produced by adenocarcinoma of the exocrine pancreas.

B. HYPERGLYCEMIA. Islets can be destroyed or ablated, leading to hyperglycemia, and permanent diabetes can occur following surgical resection of the pancreas, severe pancreatitis, exten-

Table 15-2. Malignancy of Islet Cell Tumors (Estimates)

Tumor	Benign (%)	Malignant (%)
Insulinoma	70	30
Gastrinoma	25	75
VIPoma	20	80
Glucagonoma	rare	98
Nonfunctional islet cell tumor	40	60

sively infiltrating carcinoma of the body or the tail of the pancreas, and hemochromatosis (bronze diabetes). The pathogenesis of most cases of diabetes is not, however, known.

   C. DIABETES MELLITUS affects many organs and is characterized by glucose intolerance and abnormalities of insulin secretion or metabolism.

   1. Clinical Data.
   a. The diabetic state includes polyuria, polyphagia, and polydipsia.
   b. The diabetic patient may experience
   (1) Increased susceptibility to infection
   (2) Polyneuropathy
   (3) Impotence
   (4) A progressive proliferative and destructive retinitis, often causing blindness
   (5) Precocious vascular disease involving the kidneys, myocardium, and central nervous system
   (6) Infarction and gangrene of the extremities, often requiring amputation
   (7) (Iatrogenic) hypoglycemia, which can produce serious intellectual impairment and neurologic deficits
   (8) A progressive focal or diffuse nodular glomerulosclerosis, which can lead to renal failure
   c. There are two principal forms of diabetes mellitus: juvenile-onset and maturity-onset.
   (1) Juvenile-onset diabetes (often occurring before the age of 15 years) is characterized by abrupt onset, insulin dependence, weight loss, ketoacidosis, a less conspicuous genetic background than maturity-onset diabetes, and brittleness or instability. Only 20 percent of diabetic patients have the juvenile-onset type. The onset may follow a viral illness.
   (2) In the **maturity-onset** diabetic patient, the principal problem may be in the delivery of insulin rather than in its synthesis. The maturity-onset diabetic may exhibit insulin resistance, especially in association with obesity. Over 80 percent of diabetic patients have the maturity-onset type.

   2. Pathology.
   a. Islets. Histologic changes in the islets range from complete hyalinization and fibrosis with occasional lymphocytic infiltration to no discernible changes.
   b. Small Blood Vessels. Diabetic microangiopathy affects the small arteries and capillaries. Its main early morphologic features are the disappearance of pericytes and a thickening of the basement membrane in muscle, skin, retina, kidney, and other tissues.
   c. Kidneys. The most characteristic lesion of the diabetic glomerulus is a nodular change, which represents focal thickening of the capillary basement membrane and an exudative accumulation of hyaline material.
   d. Eyes. Diabetic retinopathy is the most common cause of blindness in the United States. The microcirculation exhibits leaky microaneurysms, new formation of capillaries, and hemorrhage into the vitreous.
   e. Generalized Arteriosclerosis. Precocious development of arteriosclerosis in medium-sized arteries is almost invariably encountered. Lesions are especially common in the coronary, cerebral, mesenteric, renal, and femoral arteries.

VI. THE ADRENAL GLAND

A. GENERAL INFORMATION

   1. The adrenal **cortex** may be affected either by lesions that produce an **excess of steroid hormone** (Table 15-3) or by lesions that produce a deficiency.

Table 15-3. Adrenocortical Hyperfunction

	Adrenal Lesion		
Disease	Bilateral Hyperplasia (%)	Adenoma (%)	Carcinoma (%)
Cushing's syndrome	53	5	5
Hyperaldosteronism	8	25	1
Adrenogenital syndrome	2.5	2.5	4

2. The adrenal **medulla** may undergo hyperplastic or neoplastic changes, producing catecholamine excess.

B. **ADRENOCORTICAL EXCESS: CUSHING'S SYNDROME.** Cushing's syndrome is defined as the symptom complex associated with prolonged exposure to elevated plasma corticosteroids. In this condition, the normal diurnal variation of corticosteroid levels (high in the morning and low in the evening) is lost.

1. **Clinical Data.** Adrenocortical hyperfunction produces truncal obesity, redistribution of truncal fat with a characteristic buffalo hump, rounded facies, striae, mild glucose intolerance, mild hypertension, alterations in immune function (rendering a patient more susceptible to infection), plethora, thinning of the skin, and osteoporosis. Mild hypokalemia is not uncommon, and other mild electrolyte abnormalities also occur.

2. Cushing's syndrome may be divided into two main groups depending on whether or not the condition results from exposure to excessive ACTH.
   a. **ACTH-Dependent Causes.**
      (1) **Iatrogenic**—administration of excessive quantities of ACTH or its synthetic analogs
      (2) Pituitary-dependent bilateral **adrenocortical hyperplasia**, conventionally called Cushing's disease
      (3) **Ectopic** ACTH syndrome—secretion of ACTH by malignant or benign tumors of nonendocrine origin
   b. **Non-ACTH-Dependent Causes.**
      (1) Iatrogenic—administration of supraphysiologic doses of corticosteroids
      (2) Adenomas or carcinomas of the adrenal cortex

3. **Adrenal Pathology in Cushing's Syndrome.** Three lesions may be identified in the adrenal cortex (Table 15-4).
   a. **Bilateral hyperplasia** with widening of the zona reticularis is found in most cases.
   b. **Adrenal adenomas** are responsible for the development of Cushing's syndrome in about 10 percent of cases. These tumors affect women more commonly (80 percent of cases) than men.
   c. **Adrenal carcinomas** are responsible for the syndrome approximately as often as adrenal adenomas in adults, but they are the most common cause of Cushing's syndrome in children.
   d. Malignancy cannot be diagnosed morphologically because the usual criteria—mitotic activity and vascular or capsular invasion—frequently are absent and also can occur in benign growths. The only accepted criterion is the demonstration of distant metastases. In the presence of a functioning adenoma or carcinoma, the contralateral adrenal gland becomes grossly and functionally atrophic.

Table 15-4. Incidence of Adrenal Lesions in Cushing's Syndrome

	Incidence (%)	
Adrenal Lesion	Adults	Children
Hyperplasia	81	35
Adenoma	9	14
Carcinoma	10	51

4. **Ectopic ACTH Syndrome.**
   a. A substance similar to ACTH functionally and immunologically may be secreted by nonendocrine tumors, usually oat cell carcinomas of the lung (accounting for 60 percent of cases), thymic tumors, or islet cell tumors of the pancreas.
   b. Most tumors producing the ectopic ACTH syndrome are rapidly growing malignancies. Often an affected patient does not manifest the typical clinical features of Cushing's syndrome because these require time to develop. The major abnormalities found are electrolyte disturbances, which may be severe and difficult to control.

C. **HYPERALDOSTERONISM WITH LOW PLASMA RENIN**

1. **Definition.** This syndrome, commonly referred to as **Conn's syndrome**, accounts for approximately one-third of all cases of hypercorticalism. In primary aldosteronism there is an increased secretion of aldosterone, which produces sodium retention, increased total plasma volume, increased renal artery pressure, and inhibition of renin secretion.

2. **Clinical Data.** Most patients are women in the age range of 30 to 50 years who present with essential hypertension. Alkalosis and hypokalemia are almost always present.

3. **Pathology.** The most common lesion in Conn's syndrome is a single, benign adrenal adenoma (Fig. 15-8). Typically, this tumor is a circumscribed, encapsulated lesion with a distinctive golden-yellow cut surface. Histologically, the most common cellular pattern consists of large lipid-laden clear cells similar to those of the normal zona fasciculata. Rarely, bilateral adrenal hyperplasia will be responsible for the hyperaldosteronism syndrome.

D. **ADRENOGENITAL SYNDROMES.** The adrenal cortex normally secretes a number of androgenic (masculinizing) compounds. The action of these androgens may be divided into their anabolic effects on the synthesis of protein and their effects on secondary sex characteristics.

1. **Defects** (inborn errors of metabolism) involving deficiency of one of these enzymes results in a series of syndromes (Table 15-5). Each of these inborn errors of metabolism appears to be caused by an autosomal recessive gene, which is manifested only in the homozygous state, albeit with varying degrees of expression.

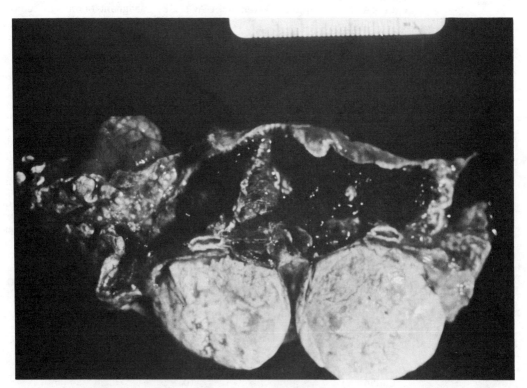

Figure 15-8. An adrenal cortical adenoma, which produced hyperaldosteronism.

Table 15-5. Adrenogenital Syndromes

Syndrome	Defect	Symptom Complex
Lipoid hyperplasia	Conversion of cholesterol to pregnenolone	Pseudohermaphroditism in males
Salt-losing syndrome	21-Hydroxylase defect	Precocious virilism in males, pseudohermaphroditism in females, salt loss
Eberlein-Bongiovanni syndrome	11-β-Hydroxylase defect	Virilism, hypertension

2. Pathology. Adrenal cortical hyperplasia (with weights of 15 g) is the usual lesion. Histologically, the cortical cells are eosinophilic with finely granular cytoplasm, reflecting the effect of elevated levels of circulating ACTH.

E. ADRENAL INSUFFICIENCY

1. Primary. Addison's disease (primary adrenocortical failure) results from destruction of the cortex. In recent years, 60 percent of cases have been due to idiopathic destruction, probably autoimmune in nature. Before effective control of active tuberculosis, over 50 percent of cases of adrenal failure were caused by tuberculous infection of the gland. Other causes, (e.g., metastatic tumors, amyloidosis, hemorrhage, arterial emboli, and fungal diseases) account for only a small proportion of cases.

2. Secondary. Reduced secretion of ACTH (due to destructive lesions of the pituitary gland or hypothalamus) produces adrenocortical insufficiency, which also may result from prolonged treatment with exogenous corticosteroids.

   a. Acute adrenal insufficiency is a rapidly progressive illness (over hours or days) presenting clinically as **shock**. Such an illness may occur in septicemia, especially meningococcemia (Waterhouse-Friderichsen syndrome). The septic state, with its associated **disseminated intravascular coagulation**, produces multiple vascular thrombi and hemorrhagic infarcts in many organs.

   b. Chronic adrenal insufficiency varies from a complete failure of hormone production to a minor impairment of adrenal reserve capacity. Symptoms develop insidiously and include
   (1) Malaise and weight loss
   (2) Skin pigmentation
   (3) Hypotension
   (4) Loss of body hair
   (5) Menstrual irregularity or amenorrhea

3. Pathology.
   a. In idiopathic Addison's disease, the pathology consists of loss of the three-layered architecture of the adrenal cortex. The adrenocortical cells are reduced to islets surrounded by an increased stroma of fibrous tissue, and lymphocytic infiltration is present.
   b. Adrenal destruction by infarcts, tuberculosis, fungi, or metastatic tumors is accompanied by the same pathologic patterns produced by such lesions elsewhere in the body.
   c. The autoimmune basis for Addison's disease is supported by finding antibodies to adrenal cells in most patients who have the idiopathic form of the disorder. In addition, dysfunctions of other organs associated with autoantibodies are known to coexist with Addison's disease, including
   (1) Schmidt's syndrome (chronic lymphocytic thyroiditis and Addison's disease)
   (2) Pernicious anemia and Addison's disease
   (3) Idiopathic hypoparathyroidism, gonadal failure (with antiovarian antibodies), and Addison's disease

F. ADRENAL MEDULLA

1. Pheochromocytoma, an unusual tumor of the adrenal medulla, is a treatable cause of hypertension. Approximately 10 percent of pheochromocytomas are malignant; 10 percent are bilateral; and 10 percent are extra-adrenal.
   a. Clinical Data. A neoplasm of chromaffin cells, this lesion causes paroxysmal or sustained hypertension, angina, cardiac arrhythmias, headache, and carbohydrate intolerance.

These features are related to the concentration of catecholamines released into the circulation. If the tumor goes untreated, a cerebrovascular accident (leading to death during one of the paroxysmal episodes), congestive heart failure with pulmonary edema, or ventricular fibrillation may result.

b. Typically, laboratory findings include elevated urinary vanillylmandelic acid and norepinephrine levels. Abnormal glucose tolerance also is common.

c. Recently defined adrenal medullary hyperplasia (bilateral or unilateral) has symptoms similar to those of a pheochromocytoma. Although this condition may occur sporadically, most affected patients are individuals from families with Sipple's syndrome [multiple endocrine neoplasia, type II] (see below).

2. Neuroblastoma.

a. Clinical Data. Neuroblastoma is the most common extracranial malignant **solid** tumor in infancy and childhood, comprising approximately 7 percent to 14 percent of childhood malignancies and 15 percent to 50 percent of neonatal malignancies. It has a slightly greater frequency in males than females. The most frequent sites are the adrenal glands and the cervical, thoracic, and abdominal sympathetic ganglia. Abnormal quantities of catecholamines are present in the urine of approximately 80 percent of affected patients, forming the basis of diagnosis.

b. Pathology.

(1) On **gross** examination, neuroblastomas usually are contained within a pseudocapsule, are nodular in appearance, and have a grayish surface when cut. Frequently, areas of necrosis, hemorrhage, and calcification are present within the tumor.

(2) On **microscopic** examination, a typical neuroblastoma is highly cellular, with cells arranged in broad sheets that in some areas form rosette patterns. Mitotic figures often are found in large numbers. The presence of rosette formations along with neurofibril formation is pathognomonic.

c. Prognosis. The most important determinants of survival are **age** at the time of diagnosis (younger patients having better survival rates) and **stage** of disease (survival rates ranging from 85 percent for localized disease to 30 percent for widely metastatic neuroblastoma).

VII. MULTIPLE ENDOCRINE NEOPLASIA SYNDROMES

A. Usually familial and genetically induced (autosomal dominant), multiple endocrine neoplasia (MEN) syndromes include several complexes characterized by neoplasia (benign and malignant), hyperplasia of one or more of the endocrine glands, or both. Because the tumors are often malignant, the old term multiple endocrine adenomatosis (MEA) has fallen into disuse and has been replaced by MEN.

B. The two most clearly defined of these syndromes are called **Wermer's syndrome (MEN, type I)** and **Sipple's syndrome (MEN, type II)** [Table 15-6]. In each of these, parathyroid abnormalities are prominent. Tumors may occur synchronously or asynchronously in the same patient, or some tumors may occur in some family members, while others occur in other members. Frequently multiple endocrine lesions are found at autopsy, although during life one particular tumor may have dominated.

C. Recently, it has been suggested that these two syndromes can be explained by theorizing a disorder of a ''second'' endocrine system based on the fact that the lesions all affect cells derived from the neural crest, which have certain electron-microscopic and histochemical characteristics in common. This system has been termed the **APUD** (amine precursor uptake and decarboxylation) **system**.

1. The importance of the APUD system lies in its conceptualization of a diffuse system of cells interrelated in certain derivative, structural, functional, and secretory aspects. These cells produce a variety of polypeptide hormones and neurotransmitters. Because of common relationships, it was assumed that the members of this system could respond similarly to various stimuli, including tumorigens. It was assumed further that these cells shared certain portions of a genome.

2. Although all APUD cells originally were considered to be derived from the neural crest, embryologic experiments have invalidated this hypothesis. Hence, this concept is no longer tenable.

Table 15-6. Components of Multiple Endocrine Neoplasia Syndromes

MEN, Type I (Wermer's)	MEN, Type II (Sipple's)	MEN, Type II (Variants)
Pituitary adenoma	Medullary carcinoma of the thyroid	Medullary carcinoma of the thyroid
Pancreatic islet cell tumors (Zollinger-Ellison, insulinomas, multiple tumors, or diffuse hyperplasia)		
Adrenal cortical adenomas	Pheochromocytoma (usually multiple and bilateral)	Pheochromocytoma
Parathyroid tumors (usually multiple discrete adenomas or adenomatous hyperplasia)	Parathyroid adenomas or adenomatous hyperplasia	Occasionally parathyroid hyperplasia
Occasionally carcinoid tumors	Occasionally carcinoid tumors	
Occasionally thyroid adenomas		
		Multiple mucosal and gastrointestinal tract neuromas
		Melanosis, myopathy, marfanoid habitus

STUDY QUESTIONS

Directions: Each question below contains five suggested answers. Choose the **one best** response to each question.

1. A 32-year-old woman was found to have a nontender nodule in the side of the neck. On routine examination she was asymptomatic. No other masses were identified. The thyroid felt normal. Thyroid function tests and scan were unremarkable. Biopsy of the mass was undertaken, and pathologically normal-appearing thyroid was found in an enlarged lymph node. This represents

(A) a lateral aberrant thyroid

(B) a metastatic thyroid papillary carcinoma

(C) a metastatic thyroid follicular carcinoma

(D) a thyroglossal duct remnant

(E) none of the above

2. Hypopituitarism may be produced by each of the following conditions EXCEPT

(A) pituitary irradiation

(B) chromophobe adenoma

(C) Sheehan's syndrome

(D) basophil adenoma

(E) breast cancer

3. Hypertension is found in all of the following endocrine disorders EXCEPT

(A) Cushing's syndrome

(B) pheochromocytoma

(C) adrenal medullary hyperplasia

(D) Addison's disease

(E) Conn's syndrome

Directions: The group of questions below consists of lettered choices followed by several numbered items. For each numbered item select **one** lettered choice with which it is **most** closely associated. Each lettered choice may be used once, more than once, or not at all.

Questions 4–8

Match the following eponyms with their characteristic symptom complexes.

(A) Postpartum pituitary failure

(B) Hypothyroidism and hypoadrenalism

(C) Hyperparathyroidism and hypoglycemia

(D) Gastrointestinal ulcers

(E) Familial medullary carcinoma

4. Sheehan's syndrome

5. Schmidt's syndrome

6. Sipple's syndrome

7. Zollinger-Ellison syndrome

8. Wermer's syndrome

ANSWERS AND EXPLANATIONS

1. The answer is B. (*III B 7 b*) Despite the follicular appearance, this case represents a papillary tumor in the primary site. Most papillary cancers have follicles; this fact does not make a papillary lesion a follicular cancer. The biology of these lesions is distinctive.

2. The answer is D. (*II B 2*) Pituitary irradiation, infarction as is characteristic of Sheehan's syndrome, and tumor replacement of the pituitary (chromophobe adenoma and breast cancer) can all produce signs and symptoms of hypopituitarism. Basophil adenomas are usually quite small and do not destroy or replace the pituitary gland, although they can lead to hyperpituitarism (Cushing's syndrome).

3. The answer is D. (*II B 1*) Cushing's syndrome is caused by either pituitary or primary adrenal lesions and by excessive glucocorticoid intake, resulting in hypertension. Similarly, Conn's syndrome (usually produced by an adrenal cortical adenoma) is associated with excessive production of aldosterone, which, via the renin-angiotensin system, produces hypertension. Both adrenal medullary lesions (pheochromocytoma and medullary hyperplasia) characteristically produce hypertension by excessive catecholamine release. Addisonian patients often are hypotensive because of destruction of the adrenal cortex and hence steroid deficiency.

4–8. The answers are: 4-A, 5-B, 6-E, 7-D, 8-C. [*II B 2; VI E 3; III B 7 b (3) and VII B; V A 3; VII B*] The presence of hypopituitarism in a woman shortly following pregnancy was described in detail by Sheehan, and the syndrome carries his name. It is believed that the pituitary is infarcted because of either excessive blood loss at delivery and hence shock or because of thrombosis of the veins or arteries feeding the pituitary, possibly due to coagulation abnormalities at term.

Autoimmune destruction of multiple endocrine glands can be seen in a variety of combinations. Thyroiditis is common; Addison's disease (hypoadrenalism) is unusual. Sometimes both occur in one patient (Schmidt's syndrome) and both pathological and clinical evidence indicate an autoimmune etiology.

The association of a thyroid carcinoma of a specific subtype (medullary) and adrenal pheochromocytomas and parathyroid hyperplasia has been called Sipple's syndrome, which is often familial.

Gastrointestinal ulcers are common in the duodenum and stomach and are usually solitary. If ulcers are found in several sites and in uncommon areas, the patient often has a gastrin-producing tumor (usually of pancreatic islet origin), which is called Zollinger-Ellison syndrome.

Polyendocrine neoplasia characterizes Wermer's syndrome; parathyroid abnormalities are prominent.

16
The Nervous System

I. INTRODUCTION. This chapter will review disorders of

A. THE CENTRAL NERVOUS SYSTEM

1. Common arterial disturbances

2. Occlusive diseases

3. Thrombosis of venous sinuses and cerebral veins

4. Infections

5. Metabolic disorders

6. Congenital abnormalities and heredofamilial diseases

7. Intoxications

8. Traumas

9. Degenerative and demyelinating diseases

10. Neoplasms

B. THE PERIPHERAL NERVOUS SYSTEM

1. Multiple neuropathies

2. Traumas

3. Intoxications

4. Vascular disorders

5. Infiltrative disorders

6. Neoplasms

C. THE MUSCULAR AND NEUROMUSCULAR SYSTEMS

1. Muscular dystrophy

2. Polymyositis

3. Myasthenia gravis

II. DISORDERS OF THE CENTRAL NERVOUS SYSTEM

A. COMMON ARTERIAL DISTURBANCES

1. **Clinical Manifestations.**

   a. **Cerebral Hemorrhage** (Cerebrovascular Accident, **"Stroke"**). The patient suddenly loses consciousness and falls. The head is thrown back, the face is congested, breathing is hard, and there is paralysis of limbs on one side (hemiplegia). Urinary and fecal incontinence may develop. If hemorrhage appears toward the surface of the brain, irritation of the cerebral cortex may give rise to convulsions. Coma may occur and deepen, and death may occur in a few hours or days. If the hemorrhage is small and is resorbed and the edema subsides, the patient may recover completely or have a defect, depending upon the site of the hemorrhage.

   b. **Thrombotic Stroke.** The clinical picture depends upon the portion of the brain affected.

Often permanent hemiplegia results. As a rule, symptoms appear much more slowly than those due to cerebral hemorrhage. Aphasia (difficulty in producing or in understanding speech) may also result.

2. The **classification** and **pathogenesis** of hemorrhagic disorders are based upon the natural partition of the intracranial space into four anatomic compartments: the brain parenchyma, the subarachnoid space, the subdural space, and the epidural space. Each has distinctive lesions.

   a. **Brain parenchyma intracerebral hemorrhage** is diverse in pathogenesis, size, and clinical expression. It produces lesions predominantly in three locations with the following approximate incidences: in the basal ganglia thalamus (65 percent); in the pons (15 percent); and in the cerebellum (10 percent). Minute lesions, or petechiae, are less harmful per se than the obstruction of the associated small vessel. Large hematomas, as masses, have the potential to produce focal neurologic deficits and to initiate lethal transtentorial herniation.

   (1) **Hypertension** is a prominent cause of intracerebral hemorrhage.

   (2) Hematomas accompany **leukemia**, particularly when the neoplastic cells engorge and obstruct the small vessels. The thrombocytopenia associated with leukemia and its therapy is also significant.

   (3) Saccular **aneurysms** and arteriovenous **malformations** (AVMs) may rupture and produce intracerebral hematomas.

   (4) Primary and metastatic **neoplasms** within the brain may bleed.

   (5) Intracerebral hemorrhages that result from **trauma** are usually multiple and are associated with adjacent superficial cortical contusions.

   (6) Other causes of intracerebral hemorrhage include coagulation disorders and vasculitis.

   b. **Subarachnoid hemorrhage** produces

   (1) Headache by increasing intracranial pressure

   (2) Nuchal rigidity by meningeal irritation

   (3) Alterations in mental status

   (4) Hydrocephalus by obstruction of the flow of cerebrospinal fluid (CSF)

   c. **Subdural hemorrhage,** with rare exceptions, results from trauma that shears the veins or small arteries that traverse the space between the arachnoid and the dura. Most vulnerable to hemorrhage are the superior cortical veins that lead to the superior sagittal sinus.

   (1) In the **acute** phase, signs and symptoms are expressions of mass effect, with increasing intracranial pressure and transtentorial herniation.

   (2) The **chronic** lesion may follow a seemingly insignificant head injury and, after a latent period of several months, may produce nonlocalizing and diagnostically confusing signs, such as deterioration of mental capacity.

   d. **Epidural hemorrhage.** A skull fracture can shear the middle meningeal artery, and the resultant bleeding dissects the dura from the inner table of the skull. The expanding mass increases intracranial pressure, produces herniation, and must be evacuated promptly to save life.

3. **Pathology.**

   a. **Malformation.**

   (1) AVM is one of the most significant aberrations of angiogenesis (Fig. 16-1). Fundamental to this lesion are congenital, low-resistance arteriovenous (AV) shunts that siphon blood from the adjacent parenchyma. In time, this tangle of abnormal vessels enlarges.

   (2) AVM favors the cerebral hemispheres that lie within the distribution of the middle cerebral artery. The clinical manifestations include seizures, neurologic deficits, chronic mass effects, and acute hemorrhages. Three additional vascular malformations are recognized entities (none of which generally are symptomatic).

   (a) Telangiectasis

   (b) Venous angioma

   (c) Cavernous angioma

   b. **Aneurysms.**

   (1) **Saccular aneurysms** or "berry" aneurysms originate from a structural weakness at the branch point of a large cerebral artery on, or within several centimeters of, Willis' circle. More than 90 percent of saccular aneurysms occur within the carotid supply. They are multiple in about 20 percent of cases.

   (a) Rupture of a saccular aneurysm is the most common cause of nontraumatic symptomatic subarachnoid hemorrhage in adults.

   (b) The pathogenesis is thought to be due to a congenital defect of the media at the bifurcation (branching) of an artery with superimposed degeneration of the

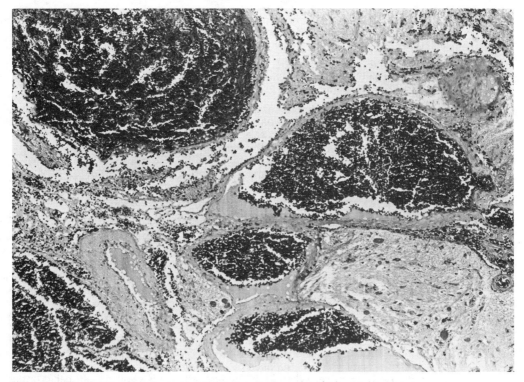

Figure 16-1. Arteriovenous malformation (AVM) of the brain showing large, blood-filled, thin-walled vessels. Brain tissue at *lower right* (low power).

internal elastic membrane. The wall gives way under arterial pressure at such a weak point and a saccular aneurysm occurs.

(2) **Mycotic (septic) aneurysms**, though infrequent, are most common in subacute bacterial endocarditis and are due to weakening of the walls of both large but more often small arteries by infected emboli. These aneurysms may cause single large or multiple small hemorrhages anywhere in the brain. Complications of septic aneurysms include the spread of infection into the subarachnoid space, which produces **leptomeningitis**, and extension into the parenchyma, which may cause an **abscess**.

(3) **Arteriosclerotic aneurysms** are fusiform and are typically situated on the internal carotid, vertebral, or basilar vessels. The complications are those of mass effect or thrombosis.

B. OCCLUSIVE DISEASES

1. **Atherosclerosis** appears first in the carotid artery (at origin, bifurcation, and distal segments), in the vertebral artery (at origin and distal segments), and in the basilar artery and later in the middle, posterior, and anterior cerebral arteries, usually in that order.

   a. **Gross examination** shows patches of yellow or yellowish-orange discoloration in arterial walls, often near points of branching.

   b. The **histology** is similar to that in atherosclerosis in other parts of the body (see Chapter 4, "The Heart").

   c. **Consequences.** Atherosclerosis often leads to thrombosis. If this occurs in small arteries, multiple areas of destruction in the brain may be seen as microscopic or small lesions, which appear most often in the basal ganglia, in the central white matter of the cerebrum, and in the cerebral cortex. If the thrombosis involves large arteries, encephalomalacia resulting from infarct and necrosis occurs.

2. **Hypertension.**

   a. Twenty percent of patients with systemic hypertension develop cerebral lesions. Most of these patients develop nervous system lesions in the latter half of life and also have atherosclerosis.

   b. Pathology. Changes in the brain parenchyma result from hemorrhage and ischemic necrosis. The arterial changes resemble those seen in the vascular system in general (see Chapter 5, "The Vascular System").

3. Embolism. Either in bacterial endocarditis or in conditions associated with thrombi in the left cardiac chambers, portions of thrombotic material travel to the cerebral circulation and produce often multiple arterial occlusions with areas of encephalomalacia.

4. Rare Conditions Involving Arteries of the Nervous System. Periarteritis nodosa (which more often produces lesions in the peripheral nervous system), thrombotic thrombocytopenic purpura, lupus erythematosus, giant cell arteritis, and other possibly allergic vascular diseases may affect the CNS circulation and produce ischemic changes.

5. Effects of Vascular Diseases on Nerve Tissue.
   a. Acute massive hemorrhage in the brain usually occurs in hypertension, embolism, or vasculitis and is due to the rupture of an abnormal vessel wall.
      (1) Gross Appearance (Fig. 16-2). When the hemorrhage is fresh, the affected cerebral hemisphere is swollen and its gyri are flattened. The mass of recent thrombus and fluid blood disrupts and distends the basal ganglia. The mass may rupture into the lateral ventricles, filling the ventricular system with blood. Structures around the area of hemorrhage are compressed and edematous. If the patient survives, the clot shrinks and becomes chocolate colored and the edema disappears.
      (2) Histological Appearance. In a fresh hemorrhage, masses of erythrocytes replace the destroyed tissue. Within 3 days, microglial phagocytes begin to ingest degenerating red blood cells, and within 6 to 10 days, hemosiderin begins to appear. The central area of destruction is cleared out by this phagocytic activity (within 3 to 6 weeks after the initial event), leaving a cystic space.
   b. Encephalomalacia occurs due to atherosclerosis, arterial occlusion (thrombic or embolic), and other causes of inadequate blood flow. Encephalomalacia is most common in the area of the cerebrum that is supplied by the middle cerebral artery.
      (1) Gross Appearance. When fresh, the affected area is swollen, soft, pallid or dusky, and peppered with petechial hemorrhages. Normal architectural markings are obscured, and there is considerable edema of surrounding brain tissue. The area becomes increasingly yellow, soft, finely cystic, and shrunken. Eventually, in a period

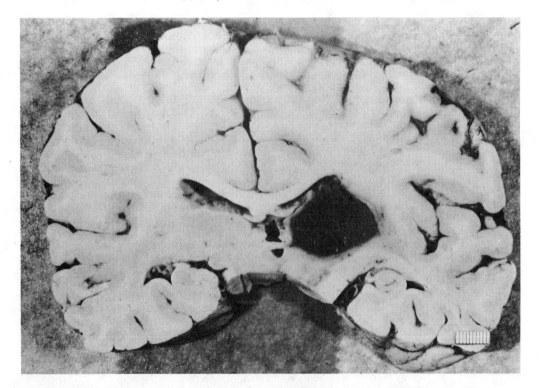

Figure 16-2. Cross section of the brain from a 70-year-old man with hypertension showing a large hemorrhage in the area of the basal ganglia.

from 6 weeks to several months, a roughly rounded or stellate cystic space appears wherever tissue was destroyed.

(2) **Histological Appearance.** In the acute stage, nerve cells undergo ischemic necrosis in the gray matter and axons swell enormously in the white matter. Marked edema is seen, with greatly widened perineuronal and perivascular spaces. Many polymorphonuclear leukocytes enter the zone within the first 24 hours and disappear in 3 to 6 days. Marginal astrocytosis begins in about 3 days and reaches its height in about 4 to 6 weeks.

C. THROMBOSIS OF VENOUS SINUSES AND CEREBRAL VEINS. Cerebral venous disorders are much rarer than arterial disorders. They reflect either venous wall defects or coagulation abnormalities.

1. **Clinical Data.** Spontaneous thrombosis is rare in adults but common in poorly nourished, anemic children and in those with severe (acute or chronic) infections. Of adults, postpartum women are the most likely victims. The superior sagittal sinus and superior cerebral veins usually are affected.

2. **Pathology.**
   a. **Gross Appearance.** Veins are distended and firm. Hemorrhages and marked congestion of the leptomeninges and cerebrum are seen.
   b. **Microscopic Appearance.** Multiple, pericapillary hemorrhages are seen associated with changes described under **Encephalomalacia** above.

D. INFECTIONS

1. **Bacterial Infections.**
   a. **Suppurative infection** chiefly occurs secondary to diseases of the middle ear and its related cavities, to diseases of the accessory nasal sinuses, and to diseases of the throat and thoracic organs. Less commonly it follows trauma to the head, and it rarely results from the hematogenous spread of other infections.
   (1) **Acute suppurative meningitis (leptomeningitis)** is the most frequent pyogenic infection of the nervous system.
      (a) **Clinical Data.** It may occur at any age but is most common in children. Intense headache, vomiting, increased intracranial pressure, fever, and stiff neck are found. Convulsions and motor disabilities may be seen also. CSF under increased pressure is clouded and reveals an abnormal increase of cells (polymorphonuclear leukocytes), increased protein, absence of sugar, and the presence of pathogenic organisms.
      (b) **Pathogenesis.** The most frequently encountered microorganisms are meningococcus, pneumococcus, streptococcus and hemophilus. Staphylococcus and gram-negative bacteria are seen less often. The organisms may invade the meninges directly from an infected sinus or ear, or they may "seed" the meninges in a septicemic patient.
      (c) **Gross Appearance.** The subarachnoid space contains an exudate, which invariably is present over the base of the brain and spinal cord and which varies considerably in amount.
      (d) **Microscopic Appearance.** The subarachnoid space contains bacteria and pus; the underlying brain and cord are edematous and moderately congested. The exudate contains considerable numbers of lymphocytes and large mononuclear cells. The exudate as a rule remains confined to the leptomeninges. If a patient recovers, the subarachnoid space is cleared completely by the activity of phagocytes. If infection persists in low-grade form for a time, trabeculae form across the subarachnoid space, followed by progressive fibrosis with narrowing or localized obliteration of the subarachnoid space. When such changes are localized to basilar leptomeninges near the foramina, the blockage of outflow of CSF from the ventricular system results in **hydrocephalus.**
      (e) **Prognosis.** Recovery with complete resolution is common. Permanent disabilities may occur, for example, localized paralysis, speech defect, and mental deficiency.
   (2) **Brain Abscess.**
      (a) **Clinical Data.** This condition, encountered with 20 percent the frequency of suppurative meningitis, occurs at any age. Symptoms and signs are those of a rapidly expanding intracranial lesion. The CSF is under increased pressure; lymphocytes are found, and protein is increased; there is no change in sugar content; no pathogenic organisms are seen (unless rupture of the abscess with

meningitis occurs). The source of infection is usually evident, for example, middle ear disease.

(b) **Pathogenesis.** Common causative microorganisms include staphylococcus, pneumococcus, streptococcus; rarely are gram-negative bacilli the causative agents. Sources of brain abscess are otitis media, mastoiditis, frontal sinusitis, lung abscess, empyema, and bacterial endocarditis. These may spread from adjacent cephalic structures by direct extension or by infected emboli in the bloodstream.

(c) **Gross Appearance.** If solitary, the abscess is located most often in the temporal lobe or cerebellum. If multiple, abscesses are seen in the cerebrum at the junction of the gray and white matter (most multiple abscesses are embolic). The abscess is a cavity in the brain containing thick exudate, surrounded by a narrow, marginal band of intensely congested tissue; there is marked edema of surrounding brain tissue with swollen white matter.

(d) **Microscopic appearance** is that of necrotic tissue.

(e) **Complications.** If infection breaks beyond the abscess wall due to virulence, poor resistance of the patient, or inadequate development of the abscess wall, a spreading suppurative **encephalitis** may ensue.

(3) **Septic thrombosis (thrombophlebitis)** occurs in transverse sinuses from infection in the middle ear or in the mastoid cells or from localized osteomyelitis and epidural abscess. It may occur in the cavernous sinus following infections of the face, particularly of the upper lip with retrograde thrombophlebitis of the angular and ophthalmic veins.

b. **Tuberculous Infections. Tuberculous meningitis (leptomeningitis)** is the most common form of tuberculous infection in the nervous system.

(1) **Clinical Data.** There is an insidious onset, with 2 to 3 weeks of anorexia, loss of weight, and change of disposition. Drowsiness with occasional delirium is followed by characteristic lucid intervals. Spinal fluid contains **lymphocytes**, increased protein, decreased sugar, and tubercle bacilli.

(2) **Pathogenesis** is secondary to infection in the mediastinal or mesenteric glands, bones, joints, lungs, or genitourinary tract. It is usually, but not always, the result of miliary dissemination.

(3) **Gross Appearance.** There is a delicate, white or gray-white, lacy exudate in the leptomeninges at the **base of the brain**. The exudate tends to pool in all basilar cisterns and particularly in the sylvian fissure. At the margins of this thin exudate, sharply outlined, white, round nodules (tubercles) are seen.

(4) **Microscopic Appearance.** The subarachnoid space is filled (and in places is distended by exudate) with **granulomas** composed of lymphocytes and large mononuclear cells. Tubercle bacilli are present.

2. **Syphilis, Toxoplasmosis, and Fungal and Viral Infections.**
   a. **Syphilis.** Neurosyphilis is one form of the tertiary stage of syphilis, with approximately 2 percent of infected individuals developing nervous system lesions. Two types of neurosyphilis are recognized.

   (1) **Meningovascular Syphilis.**
      (a) The neural parenchyma may be involved secondarily. Meningovascular syphilis may occur a few years after initial infection.
      (b) **Clinical Data.** There is great variability in symptoms, depending on the predominance of spinal or cerebral meningitis. The cerebrospinal fluid usually has a normal pressure, few cells (20 to 100, chiefly lymphocytes), increased protein, and a positive serology in 90 to 100 percent of affected patients.
      (c) **Gross Appearance.** There is a yellowish opaque exudate in the meninges, at times containing tiny, firm nodules.
      (d) **Microscopic examination** shows infiltration of the subarachnoid space and pia by plasma cells and lymphocytes, followed by extension of the exudate into the perivascular spaces of the superficial parenchyma. Proliferation of fibroblasts and capillaries give rise to syphilitic granulomas **(gummas)**. Spirochetes rarely are demonstrable in the leptomeninges and blood-vessel walls. **Syphilitic arteritis** is often associated with meningitis in meningovascular syphilis.

   (2) **Parenchymatous Syphilis.**
      (a) **Tabes Dorsalis.**
         (i) **Clinical Data.** The onset, insidious 8 to 12 years after initial infection, is most often in males in the fourth and fifth decades of life. About 2 to 3 percent of persons with syphilis develop tabes. Signs and symptoms include **lightning pains** constricting the chest, abdominal pains, and **ataxia** with a

wide stride. There is sensory loss, analgesia, loss of vibratory sense, diminution and loss of deep tendon reflexes. There are also "trophic changes" (Charcot's joint, leg ulcers) of unknown etiology. The spinal fluid is abnormal (70 percent shows a positive serology), with increased protein and lymphocytes.

(ii) **Gross Appearance.** The posterior columns of the spinal cord are reduced in size.

(iii) **Microscopic examination** in the early stages shows localized changes around the dorsal roots in the lumbar region with granulation tissue formation as occurs in meningovascular syphilis. Spirochetes are present in these radicular leptomeningeal sheaths. Degeneration of axons and myelin sheaths in the dorsal roots also occurs.

(b) **General Paresis** (Paralysis).

(i) **Clinical Data.** The onset, 10 to 15 years after the initial infection, is most often in males in the fourth and fifth decades of life. General paresis comprises less than 10 percent of neurosyphilis. Because the cerebral cortex is involved, the earliest symptoms are mental: impairment of intellectual efficiency, memory, and judgment. Until they die, the patients are bedridden and incontinent. **CSF serology is positive** 95 to 100 percent of the time, and there is an increase in protein and lymphocytes.

(ii) **Gross Appearance.** There is atrophy of cerebral gyri, most marked in the frontal lobes. + in Alzheimer disease

(iii) **Microscopic examination** shows mild-to-marked leptomeningeal infiltration by lymphocytes and plasma cells. Gradual degeneration of nerve cells may result from syphilitic capillary changes and consequent anoxia.

b. **Toxoplasmosis.**

(1) **Clinical Data.** Occurring predominantly as a congenital infection, the onset of toxoplasmosis is at birth or shortly thereafter; hydrocephalus is common, as are bilateral focal chorioretinitis, intracerebral calcification, convulsions, and ocular palsies. The spinal fluid shows an increase in cells and protein. Mothers of affected children are apparently healthy.

(2) **Pathogenesis.** The causative protozoon is *Toxoplasma gondii*. *Toxoplasmae* enter the bloodstream and are carried to many organs, producing the most severe lesions in the CNS.

(3) **Gross Appearance.** Depressed, soft, sharply circumscribed, yellowish areas are seen on the surfaces of the cerebral hemispheres; stenosis of the aqueduct of Sylvius with internal hydrocephalus is noted in most cases.

(4) **Microscopic Appearance.** These lesions are sharply outlined, inflammatory, necrotizing lesions in the brain, with associated secondary leptomeningitis. *Toxoplasma* cysts are plentiful in the lesions and cause intense destruction of all neural and glial structures.

(5) **Prognosis.** Affected infants may die within a few days or a few months after birth, or they may survive with apparently arrested infection but with defects due to neural destruction: mental deficiency, chronic hydrocephalus, blindness, and seizures.

c. **Fungal infections** occur in immunocompromised hosts, especially in patients with malignant lymphoma and leukemia. Cryptococcosis (Fig. 16-3), with extraneural lesions occurring most frequently in the lungs, actinomycosis, and coccidioidomycosis may also infect the nervous system. Clinically and pathologically each resembles tuberculous meningitis.

d. **Viral Infections.** When viruses involve the nervous system, they invade both neural and meningeal areas, producing a **meningoencephalitis**.

(1) Infection may occur via an insect bite (equine encephalitis), by gastrointestinal route (polio), via skin or mucosa (herpesvirus), by ascending via the peripheral nerves (rabies), or occasionally by hematogenous spread.

(2) **Nervous system response** to viral infection may be reflected as **neuron degeneration**, with associated gliosis; a perivascular inflammatory response (chiefly in mononuclear cells) often is seen. In some infections, such as cytomegalovirus, **inclusion bodies** in nervous and glial cells are seen. The latter may be nuclear (herpes) or cytoplasmic (rabies, indicated by the presence of Negri bodies).

(3) **Specific Infections.**

(a) **Poliomyelitis.**

(i) This small RNA virus is transmitted by sewage (water) contamination and is introduced into the gut. It has a neurotropism and chiefly affects the spinal cord and brain stem.

(ii) **Clinical Data.** Patients may or may not manifest gastrointestinal symptoms,

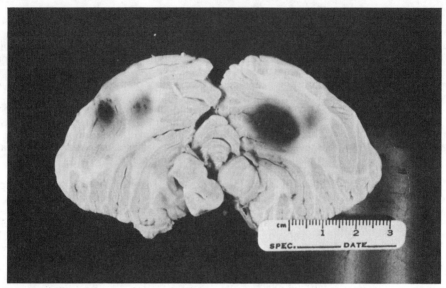

Figure 16-3. Cerebellum with several hemorrhagic foci. These are embolic septic foci (abscesses) containing cryptococcal organisms. Cryptococcal endocarditis was the presumed source of these emboli. Thirty-year-old woman with leukemia and extensive chemotherapy-related immunosuppression.

but within a few weeks of infection they show lower motor neuron paralysis, usually affecting the lower limbs. The brain-stem neurons may become affected with resultant respiratory paralysis and death if not treated. If the patient survives, significant neurologic sequelae result, especially affecting the legs.

   (iii) **Pathology.** Grossly, the spinal cord may show small hemorrhages and congestion. The anterior horn cells of the spinal cord are affected predominantly with an initial polymorphonuclear leukocytic infiltration. Later, gliosis takes place.

(b) **Rabies.**
   (i) In an infected animal (predominantly dogs but wild animals also may be affected), the virus is secreted in the saliva and is transmitted to man by bite.
   (ii) **Clinical Data.** The classic form of rabies follows the bite by about 1 month, and the patient exhibits restlessness and **hydrophobia**. These symptoms may progress until death occurs. Autopsied cases have shown myocarditic lesions in addition to the neuropathologic changes.
   (iii) **Pathology.** The virus may infect neurons throughout the nervous system. These cells are destroyed, and a reactive gliosis is found. **Negri bodies** (intracytoplasmic inclusions) are diagnostic of the disease.

(c) **Herpes.**
   (i) **Clinical Data.** Herpes simplex encephalitis frequently presents an acute course of fever, somnolence, and then coma. If the disease is not fatal, neurologic and mental deficiencies often result.
   (ii) **Pathology.** Grossly, the brain may show zones of necrosis and softening. This is reflected microscopically by demonstrations of perivasculitis, neuronal destruction, and glial proliferation. Intranuclear inclusions are characteristic.

(d) **Subacute Sclerosing Panencephalitis (SSPE).**
   (i) **Clinical Data.** This progressive disorder affects children and is associated with **prior measles infection**. A rare disease of involuntary muscular movements and dementia, SSPE is fatal within 1 to 2 years and at present is unresponsive to any known treatment.
   (ii) **Pathology.** The brain shows multifocal areas of neuronal destruction and gliosis. Occasional intranuclear inclusions are seen.

E. METABOLIC DISORDERS

1. **Pernicious Anemia.**
   a. **Clinical Data.** Dorsolateral degeneration of the spinal cord occurs in 30 to 50 percent of untreated cases of pernicious anemia. The first neurological symptom is paresthesia in the distal parts of the extremities, which is followed by unsteady gait (ataxia) and an impaired sense of both position and vibration. **Vitamin B$_{12}$** administration may arrest the degenerative process but cannot restore those nerve fibers that already have been destroyed.
   b. **Gross examination** shows gray discoloration of the posterior and lateral columns.
   c. **Microscopic examination** shows degeneration of myelin sheaths and axons, characteristically in the posterior columns and lateral pyramidal tracts (hence the term "dorsolateral degeneration") and usually most severe in the middle and upper thoracic segments of the cord.

2. **Wernicke's Syndrome (Wernicke's Encephalopathy).**
   a. **Clinical Data.** It is a complication of **chronic alcoholism** and symptoms develop rapidly: severe ataxia with mental confusion, delirium, and restlessness. Severe cases are fatal.
   b. **Pathology.** Lesions are strikingly localized to periventricular gray matter around the third ventricle, the aqueduct of Sylvius, and sometimes the floor of the fourth ventricle.
      (1) **Gross Appearance.** There is marked congestion of periventricular gray matter usually with many petechial hemorrhages.
      (2) **Microscopic Examination.** Capillaries are more prominent than usual due to endothelial hypertrophy and hyperplasia. Dependent nerve cells undergo acute ischemic necrosis.

F. CONGENITAL ABNORMALITIES AND HEREDOFAMILIAL DISEASES

1. **Congenital malformations** are common lesions that vary from minor asymptomatic defects to gross malformations incompatible with life. These are assumed to be due to a transient pathologic state during pregnancy (metabolic, nutritive, toxic, or infective or faulty implantation of placenta) or to genetic abnormalities.
   a. **Failures or Abnormalities of Growth** (Ageneses and Dysgeneses).
      (1) **Anencephaly.** The vault of the skull is usually missing, and the cerebral hemispheres, diencephalon, and midbrain are absent. There is an exposed mass of undifferentiated vascular tissue. This condition is incompatible with life.
      (2) **Agenesis of the corpus callosum** may be complete or partial; hemispheres are connected only at the brain-stem level. Affected patients may have no symptoms or only minor psychiatric dysfunction.
      (3) **Tuberous Sclerosis** (Bourneville's Disease).
         (a) **Clinical Data.** Patients have epileptic seizures, mental retardation, and facial eruptions ("adenoma sebaceum"). This is a genetically determined disorder.
         (b) **Pathology.** Smooth nodules composed of glial fibers, malformed astrocytes, and nerve cells are found in the walls of the ventricles and cerebral gyri. These grow slowly, producing mass effects. Neoplasms of heart, liver, kidney, or pancreas may also occur.
   b. **Hydrocephalus** is defined as CSF under increased pressure in the ventricles of the brain with dilatation of these cavities (internal hydrocephalus).
      (1) **Clinical Data.** In late prenatal life and early infancy, before the bony sutures of the skull close, hydrocephalus leads to abnormal enlargement of the head. The sutures are widely separated, and the fontanelles are large and tense.
      (2) **Pathology and Pathogenesis.**
         (a) **Noncommunicating hydrocephalus** is due to partial or complete **obstruction** of the flow of fluid at the following points with **dilatation** of the entire ventricular system **proximal to the block**: intraventricular or in the subarachnoid space above the exit from the fourth ventricle. **No communication** remains between the ventricles and the spinal subarachnoid space.
         (b) In **communicating hydrocephalus**, no point of obstruction is found, and hence free communication exists between the ventricles and the spinal subarachnoid space. The cause of interference with CSF flow is not always known but may be due to malformation of subarachnoid spaces, overproduction of fluid by the choroid plexus, or deficient filtration through the arachnoid granulations.
         (c) **Effects of Hydrocephalus.** The brain is large with dilated ventricles, flattened gyri, and narrowed sulci. The walls of the cerebral hemispheres are thinned, and the central white matter is atrophied with compression of the basal ganglia and thalamus.

    c. **Defective closure of dorsal midline structures** may involve the skin, soft tissues of the back, vertebrae, meninges, and the neural tube.

        (1) The most common single defect is **spina bifida** in which there is absence of the arches and dorsal spines of one or more vertebrae.

        (2) **Meningocele,** herniation of spinal arachnoid and dura through the vertebral defect, is a soft sac-like swelling palpable beneath the skin in the midline of the back. If the spinal roots or part of the spinal cord are included in this herniated meningeal sac, it is called **meningomyelocele.**

        (3) **Arnold-Chiari malformation** is the caudal displacement of the medulla and cerebellum into the cervical region of the vertebral canal; it is associated with lumbar spina bifida and hydrocephalus.

        (4) **Symptoms** resulting from dorsal closure defects vary with the severity of the defect. Spina bifida may lead to difficulty in walking or the inability to walk. Meningomyelocele can be associated with ulceration of overlying skin with leakage of CSF, followed by entry of bacteria and suppurative leptomeningitis.

  2. Heredofamilial disorders comprise a large uncommon group of diseases in which the clinical course is chronic, with **progressive deterioration** of motor and mental functions and finally death in months or years. Pathologically, all heredofamilial disorders show degeneration and disappearance of nerve cells and fibers in various parts of the nervous system.

    a. Huntington's chorea is an autosomal-dominant familial dementia in which psychopathic disorders, involuntary movements, and grimacing are common. The average age at onset is about 50 years, with a fatal course lasting 10 to 15 years.

    b. Wilson's disease, an autosomal-recessive disease, is associated with a biochemical abnormality of copper metabolism, with accumulation of copper in the brain, the eyes **(Kayser-Fleischer rings)**, and the liver; the normal copper-carrying protein **ceruloplasmin**, is decreased, absent, or defective.

        (1) Clinically, the disease begins in adolescence with movement disorders and hepatic dysfunction.

        (2) Treatment with copper-chelating agents has dramatically improved the outlook.

    c. Storage Diseases. These disorders, Tay-Sachs disease and Niemann-Pick disease, are discussed in Chapter 17, "The Hematopoietic System." In the nervous system, accumulation of the abnormal lipid in nerve cells results in diffuse dysfunction, with mental retardation and early death.

    d. Friedreich's ataxia is a recessive genetic disorder involving degeneration of the spinal cord, kyphosis, and optic atrophy.

G. INTOXICATIONS

  1. Exogenous Toxins.

    a. Drugs, beneficial in proper amounts, are injurious in overdoses, which may be accidental or suicidal.

        (1) Some agents such as phenobarbital, ether, and chloroform produce depression of respiratory centers and cause death without organic neural damage.

        (2) Some drugs (e.g., morphine) produce nerve cell degeneration, especially if taken chronically.

    b. Alcohol.

        (1) Acute Ethyl Alcoholism. If the patient dies, the brain and leptomeninges are edematous and congested; occasionally petechial hemorrhages are noted in cerebral white matter. There are mild, diffuse, and degenerative changes in nerve cells, especially in those of the cerebellar cortex.

        (2) Methyl Alcohol Intoxication. More severe degenerative changes in the brain stem and cerebral cortex are produced. Petechial hemorrhages and degeneration of nerve cells of the retina and fibers of the optic nerve occur. Blindness is common.

    c. Carbon Monoxide.

        (1) Clinical Data. Headache, visual disturbances, nausea, vomiting, convulsions, coma, and respiratory paralysis occur, with symptoms growing more severe as the concentration of the gas or length of exposure to it increases.

        (2) Pathologically, in the acute state, the brain is hyperemic and edematous with scattered petechial hemorrhages.

  2. Bacterial Toxins.

    a. Tetanus toxin affects chiefly motor neurons of the spinal cord and brain stem.

    b. Botulism. The toxin affects the brain-stem nuclei. Death from respiratory paralysis occurs.

H. TRAUMAS. Head and spine injuries may be caused by vehicular accidents, falls, blows on the chin, birth, or by instrumental delivery during birth.

1. **Head injuries** result in intracranial hemorrhage (epidural, subdural, and subarachnoid), concussion, contusion, or laceration of the brain.
   a. **Epidural hemorrhage** is the least common of traumatic hemorrhages and is due to laceration of the middle meningeal artery and vein with fracture of the skull.
      (1) **Clinical Data.** Loss of consciousness follows the injury, often with apparent recovery and then relapse. Signs of increased intracranial pressure are noted, followed by depressed respiration and death, unless the hemorrhage is evacuated.
      (2) **Pathology.** The hemorrhage is external to the dura, which is firmly attached to the skull and limits the spread of the hemorrhage. Many small vessels between the dura and skull are torn incidentally as the dura is dissected away by the hemorrhage. The dura is pressed inward in a localized area, with focal compression of the brain, increased intracranial pressure, and finally herniation.
   b. **Subdural Hematoma.**
      (1) **Clinical Data.** Trauma to the head produces a tear of a meningeal vein, commonly one of the superior cerebral veins that lie relatively unprotected in the subdural space. The trauma is most often a blow to the frontal or occipital region or a birth injury.
      (2) **Gross Appearance.** A hematoma forms between the dura and leptomeninges. After 3 days, transparent membranes line the inner and outer surfaces of the hematoma, encapsulating it.
      (3) **Microscopic Examination.** Outgrowth of fibroblasts and capillaries from the inner surface of the dura forms the inner and outer membranes encapsulating the hemorrhage.
   c. **Subarachnoid hemorrhage**, although common, usually is not the major result of a head injury but accompanies some other, more serious lesion.
   d. **Concussion** is widespread paralysis of **functions** of the brain without visible organic changes and with a strong tendency to spontaneous recovery. It may follow a blow to the head or result from another head injury.
      (1) **Clinical Data.** In mild cases, the patient is momentarily dazed or unconscious, with subsequent temporary impairment of higher mental functions. In severe cases, there is prolonged unconsciousness, low blood pressure, slowed pulse and respiration, and flaccid muscles. Vomiting, headache, and delirium are common upon return of consciousness. Complete recovery is usual.
      (2) The **pathogenesis** of a concussion is not established but is possibly due to acceleration effects or shearing (rotational) strains on the brain.
   e. **Contusion** is essentially a bruise on the brain consequent to a blow on the calvarium. It is due probably to stress upon the vascular network with tearing of capillaries. It may be located directly beneath the area of impact or opposite it **(contrecoup)**. Most contusions affect the frontal and temporal poles of the cerebrum.
      (1) **Clinical Data.** Unconsciousness, which may lead to coma (death in a severe injury) is the common clinical presentation.
      (2) **Gross Appearance.** Recent contusions show swollen, edematous gyri studded with petechial hemorrhages. Old contusions are sunken areas, which may be finely cystic.
      (3) **Microscopic examination** of fresh contusions shows an edematous area of cortex and subcortical white matter containing many fresh pericapillary hemorrhages. In old contusions, areas of gliosis are seen.
   f. **Laceration** or tear of the brain is caused by **penetrating wounds**. Symptoms depend on the site of the lesion in which complete destruction of all neural, glial, and vascular elements in the line of the tear is found.

2. **Spinal Injuries.**
   a. **Hemorrhages in meninges** are relatively uncommon in the spinal canal but may result from the spread of a cranial subdural hemorrhage. Epidural hemorrhages associated with fractures of vertebrae may occur.
   b. **Concussion of the spinal cord** is much less frequent than concussion of the brain. The patient is paralyzed below the level of the injury. Complete return of function generally occurs.
   c. **Hematomyelia.**
      (1) **Clinical Data.** The patient experiences loss of perception of pain and temperature with paralysis of extremities below the level of the lesion. This occurs as a result of flexion of the spine or a severe blow to the back.
      (2) **Pathology.** Hemorrhage is seen grossly and microscopically in the spinal cord with a tendency to extend longitudinally in cephalad and caudad directions.
   d. **Compression-contusion of the cord** (cord-crush) follows dislocation of a vertebra.
      (1) **Clinical Data.** The patient is paralyzed and loses sensation below the level of the crush. If the patient survives, permanent disability results.

       (2) Etiology. Cord-crush occurs commonly in the lower cervical region following a sudden, forcible flexion of the head, as occurs in an automobile accident, or in the lower dorsal and lumbar region due to a heavy blow across the lower back or a fall.

    e. Laceration of the Spinal Cord.

       (1) In stab wounds, a knife usually enters obliquely, **hemisecting** or completely transecting the cord.

       (2) Bullet wounds can partially or completely tear the cord.

3. Herniation of Nucleus Pulposus: Extrusion of the Intervertebral Disc.

    a. Clinical Data. This disorder is common in males 30 to 50 years of age. It may follow mild-to-moderate trauma to the back and presents with low-back pain (sciatica).

    b. Pathology. There is extrusion of the center of the intervertebral disc (nucleus pulposus) through a tear in the annulus fibrosus, usually occurring at L4-5 or L5-S.

I. DEMYELINATING AND DEGENERATIVE DISEASES make up a group of conditions in which the white matter is primarily affected and myelin sheaths are injured. Myelin destruction is dominant but is associated with a lesser degeneration of axons and rarely with delayed necrosis of other neural and glial elements. There is no general agreement on causation of these diseases, but most now are considered to be autoimmune in etiology.

1. Multiple Sclerosis.

    a. Clinical Data. This condition affects young adults principally, with onset between the ages of 20 and 40 years. Symptoms are varied because of the widespread dissemination of lesions and the variability in their situation, size, and number. The onset can be sudden or slow, and remissions and relapses are common. Since a few axons probably are destroyed in each lesion, and since later lesions frequently strike the same tract, a **cumulative effect** of axonal loss leads to eventual permanent symptoms.

    b. Gross Appearance. The basic lesion is a discrete locus of demyelination, or **"plaque,"** the emergence of which produces an acute focal neurologic deficit in accord with its anatomic location. Plaques vary in size from a few mm in diameter to 5 to 6 cm (an average of 0.5 to 2.0 cm). Lesions are found scattered throughout the brain and spinal cord, with the white matter most severely affected.

    c. Microscopic examination shows localized edema, congestion, and microglial activation, followed by perivascular astrocytosis and infiltration by lymphocytes. There is progressive astrocytosis, which becomes increasingly fibrillar and forms a scar or sclerotic "plaque."

2. Leukodystrophies are disorders in which the formation of myelin or its composition is abnormal and in which the myelin tends to break down. All syndromes in this group are familial, with infantile or childhood demise. The prototype is **Krabbe's disease**, wherein defective myelin cerebroside is found with its accumulation in various parts of the neuraxis.

3. Progressive Multifocal Leukoencephalopathy.

    a. Clinical Data. Progressive multifocal leukoencephalopathy (PML) is a rare subacute disorder of adults that usually occurs in patients with an antecedent and debilitating disease, usually a malignancy and most often lymphoma or leukemia. The symptoms of hemiparesis, intellectual impairment, blindness, and aphasia reflect the predominant cerebral involvement. The disease is progressive and, within 3 to 6 months, contributes to the death of a patient already compromised by systemic illness.

    b. Pathology. The basic lesion of PML is a well-defined focus of demyelinization associated with viral infestation by oligodendroglia. Between the area of demyelinization and the intact white matter are prominent oligodendroglia, containing intranuclear inclusions. A papovavirus has been confirmed as producing the lesion.

4. Amyotropic lateral sclerosis (ALS) is a chronic disease that involves both upper and lower motor neurons of the brain stem and spinal cord.

    a. Clinical Data. Occurring mostly in males in the fourth to fifth decades of life, ALS presents as weakness and atrophy of various muscle groups, commonly the intrinsic muscles of the hand and muscles of the arm and shoulder. **Fasciculations** (spontaneous twitches of small groups of muscle fibers) are visible through the skin. The outcome is fatal, often within 2 to 3 years, due to respiratory paralysis or intercurrent infection.

    b. Pathology. The motor cells in the anterior horns progressively diminish in number with eventual total disappearance and associated degeneration of the ventral nerve roots. The disease is most severe in the cervical cord.

5. Werdnig-Hoffmann Disease (Infantile Spinal Muscular Atrophy).

    a. Clinical Data. This degeneration of the lower motor neurons of the spinal cord and medulla is the most common neuromuscular cause of profound weakness during child-hood. An autosomal-recessive inheritance is noted in many cases, but the etiology is obscure, and there is no effective therapy. Respiratory insufficiency and superimposed infection are usually the causes of death.

    b. Pathology. The diagnosis often is established through muscle biopsy by the presence of large numbers of small, round, atrophic fibers. In the spinal cord, anterior horn cell loss is apparent grossly. The spinal and lower cranial motor neurons are reduced markedly in number.

6. Syringomyelia is the development of an abnormal cleft or cavity in cord tissue.

    a. Clinical Data. Symptoms of this chronic disease usually begin in early adult life. The classic sign is "dissociated" sensory impairment; pain and temperature sensation are diminished or absent, while touch, position, and vibratory perceptions are retained.

    b. Gross Examination. The cavity most often is in the cervical spinal cord but may extend through almost the entire length of the cord. At the level of the cavity, the cord appears distended or fusiform or it may be collapsed and flattened. The syrinx is filled with colorless or amber-tinged fluid.

    c. Microscopic examination of the wall of the syrinx shows that it is made up of glial tissue. Cavity formation usually starts near the center of the cord; hence, early compression or destruction of pain fibers is found.

    d. Pathogenesis is unknown. It may represent reactive astrocytosis secondary to unknown injury.

7. Parkinson's Disease (Paralysis Agitans).

    a. Clinical Data. This slowly progressive disorder of unknown cause usually affects elderly males. Tremors, slow, labored muscular activity, and rigidity are found. Speech is unclear, but mental processes are normal.

    b. Pathology. Gradual degeneration and loss of nerve cells with gliosis is found especially in the substantia nigra. Some cells contain spherical, eosinophilic, cytoplasmic inclusions ("Lewey bodies"), often with peripheral clear halos representing a degenerative change.

8. Creutzfeldt-Jakob Disease.

    a. Clinical Data. This rapidly fatal dementia occurs in the fifth to sixth decades of life. Pyramidal, extrapyramidal, and sometimes abnormal reflexes and bladder dysfunction (signs of lower motor neuron dysfunction) are found.

    b. Pathology. The gross severe atrophy of the brain is manifested histologically by marked loss of nerve cells and intense astrocytosis in the cerebral cortex, caudate nucleus, and putamen.

9. Alzheimer's Disease.

    a. Clinically similar to senile psychosis, this condition occurs between the ages of 40 to 60 years and runs a more rapid course.

    b. Gross Examination. There is widespread atrophy of gyri, usually more intense in the frontal lobes. *+ Tabes Dorsalis 2 syphilis*

    c. Microscopic Examination. Diffuse loss of nerve cells in all cortical layers is associated with diffuse fibrillary astrocytosis. A very frequent but unspecific form of nerve cell degeneration is seen—Alzheimer's **neurofibrillary change**, wherein intracellular neuro-fibrils are thickened.

J. NEOPLASMS

1. General Considerations.

    a. Primary CNS tumors account for about 9 to 10 percent of all cancer deaths. Approximately 10 percent of all nervous system disorders are neoplasms.

    b. All age groups are affected by brain tumors, but there are important differences in not only the distribution of tumors but also in the histologic types encountered in the child and in the adult.

        (1) In the child, about 70 percent of all brain tumors are found below the tentorium; in the adult, 70 percent are found above it.

        (2) In the child, brain tumors account for a major proportion of all neoplasms (about 20 percent), trailing the leukemias. In the adult, tumors of the lung, breast, gastrointestinal system, and hematopoietic system exceed neural tumors in occurrence.

        (3) The most prevalent brain tumors in the adult are the astrocytic tumors (including glioblastomas), followed by metastatic tumors and meningiomas. In the child, the astrocytic tumors are also the most common but are followed by medulloblastomas, ependymomas, and craniopharyngiomas.

    c. The distribution of tumors by sex is rather consistently biased against the male.

d. Tumors may interfere with CSF circulation, with the added hazard of internal hydro-cephalus.

e. The location of tumors is of prime importance, with varying functional significance.

2. **Growth and Spread of Brain Tumors.**

a. Neoplasms derived from virtually every cell type in the nervous system have been reported, with many malignant and some benign varieties among them. The definitions of benign and malignant, however, require special clarification for tumors of the CNS. In most organ systems, there is a clear correlation between the histologic classification of tumors and the clinical outcome. With brain tumors this correlation is often obscure.

b. Brain tumors are divided conveniently into those of glial and nonglial origin. The glial tumors tend to grow by infiltration. This infiltrative quality and the sponge-like quality of the brain makes these tumors biologically malignant and makes their complete removal usually impossible. The nonglial tumors generally grow by expansion and therefore offer the surgeon a better opportunity for total removal.

c. An enigmatic and unique property of most brain tumors is that, regardless of their degree of histologic malignancy, they only rarely metastasize outside the CNS.

d. Tumors of the brain produce symptoms by interfering directly with local neurologic function in the tumor area by deafferentating neurons, thereby rendering them electrically unstable and liable to epileptiform discharges.

e. Tumors may produce pressure on nearby vital structures indirectly because of edema formation.

3. **Clinical Data.** Edema is probably the most important factor in the symptoms of brain tumors and is the ultimate determinant of the level of neurologic function that can be expected in the presence of the tumor. Common symptoms of brain tumors are headache, nausea, and vomiting—often of the projectile type. Lethargy, seizure activity, paralysis, aphasia, blindness, deafness, or abnormal behavior also may be seen. Another consequence of brain swelling and herniation is the **Duret** herniation hemorrhage in the midbrain and pons. This lesion results from rapid, unilateral brain swelling in which pressure is unevenly transmitted to the brain stem, resulting in shearing of midline vessels and destruction of the median portions of the upper brain stem. This destruction of reticular formation results in loss of consciousness, respiratory failure, and death.

4. **Specific Tumors.**

a. **Tumors of Astrocytic Origin.** Astrocytes in the presence of injury generally react by forming glial fibrils and expanding their cytoplasm, becoming greatly swollen or bloated (gemistocytic astrocytes). Neoplastic astrocytes may take on many forms, recapitulating normal cells or reactive processes and generally displaying the characteristics of normal astrocytes in that a close vascular relationship is maintained. The nucleus, however, reveals the changes that are associated with any neoplasm.

(1) **Astrocytomas** comprise about 30 percent of all gliomas. There are two major subtypes—protoplasmic and fibrillary, depending upon which type of astrocyte predominates.

(a) **Clinical Data.** Astrocytomas occur most often in the central white matter of the cerebrum in adults and in the cerebellar hemispheres in children and young adults.

(b) **Gross Appearance.** They are white or gray-white, firm, poorly demarcated tumors, the margins of which are extremely difficult to determine. They may contain tiny cysts or large cavities filled with clear yellowish fluid.

(c) The **microscopic appearance** varies from highly to sparsely cellular, and the tumors are highly fibrillar. Mitoses are rare or absent, and the architecture is uniform. Tiny cysts are due to the gradual degeneration of small numbers of astrocytes.

(d) **Prognosis.** They are slow growing, occasionally becoming more malignant with transformation into glioblastomas. The survival rate is 1 to 10 years.

(2) **Astrocytomas of the cerebellum** are very distinctive lesions both clinically and pathologically. These tumors, which may account for 30 percent of all posterior fossa tumors in children, are almost limited to individuals under the age of 20 years. Treatment consists of operative removal of the tumor. When adequately removed, the prognosis of cerebellar astrocytoma is excellent; 90 percent or more of patients survive. Of the survivors, probably less than 10 percent suffer any continued neurologic deficit.

(3) **Glioblastomas** (Fig. 16-4). Glioblastomas multiforme (astrocytomas) grade IV are the most common of all gliomas, comprising 40 percent.

(a) **Clinical Data.** Glioblastomas occur more commonly in males and are rapidly

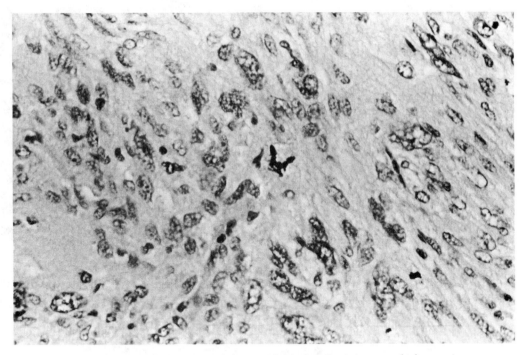

Figure 16-4. Glioblastoma multiforme with tripolar mitosis in *center* (high power).

multiple mitosis

growing lesions with a variety of symptoms reflecting rapidly increasing intracranial pressure.

    (b) **Gross examination** shows a usually massive, well-demarcated, soft, multico-
lored, highly vascular tumor growing in the central white matter of the cerebrum.
Rapid expansion of the tumor plus edema produce marked compression, distortion, and displacement of nearby structures. Not infrequently the tumor invades the corpus callosum, crossing to the opposite cerebral hemisphere.

    (c) **Microscopic examination** shows a highly cellular and vascular neoplasm, which
varies in appearance from area to area, and shows extensive necrosis and
multiple mitoses. The numerous capillaries commonly show intense endothelial
hyperplasia.

    (d) **Prognosis** is dismal, although it is somewhat better with aggressive modern
radiotherapy.

  (4) Oligodendrogliomas (Fig. 16-5).

    (a) **Clinical Data.** Oligodendrogliomas account for between 5 and 8 percent of all
intracranial tumors and most commonly occur in the cerebral hemispheres of
adults. The outstanding clinical feature of oligodendrogliomas is their slow
course.

    (b) **Gross Examination.** They are generally well-circumscribed tumors of the white
matter but often break through into the cortex.

    (c) **Histologically,** oligodendrogliomas are composed of small, rather uniform cells
that display a "fried egg" or honeycomb appearance. The small rounded nuclei
are surrounded by clear spaces. Calcification is prominent.

    (d) **Prognosis.** With operative removal when possible, it is estimated that about half
of the patients survive 5 years.

b. Ependymomas are derived from the ependymal lining cells of the ventricles of the brain
and of the central canal of the spinal cord.

  (1) Clinical Data. Fifty percent of ependymomas are located below the tentorium, and
forty percent are located above it. A few are located in the spinal cord or filum
terminale. The tumors can be seen in all age groups, with the highest percentage
occurring at about 3 to 4 years of age.

  (2) Pathology. The histologic appearance varies, but in nearly every tumor there is a
typical perivascular **pseudorosette pattern**. By special staining, ependymomas may

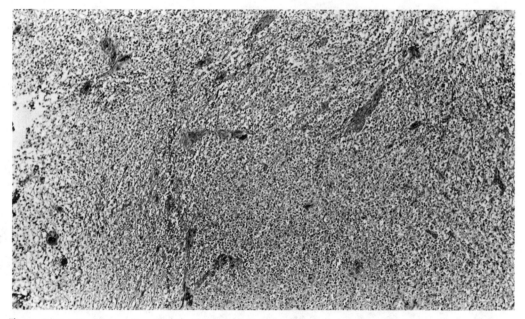

Figure 16-5. Oligodendroglioma with clear perinuclear halos around the cell ["fried egg" appearance] (low power).

be identified precisely by the presence of **blepharoplasts** in the cytoplasm near the nucleus.

(3) The **prognosis** varies with location of the ependymoma. Supratentorial tumors carry a more guarded prognosis than those in the posterior fossa. The average survival is 4 years or more.

c. **Medulloblastomas.**

    (1) **Clinical Data.** Medulloblastomas are clinically and pathologically malignant tumors that occur mostly in children under the age of 14 years. The cerebellum is the major site of occurrence. Fifty to eighty percent of the tumors usually arise in the midline posteriorly. There is a propensity for them to spread along the CSF pathway.

    (2) **Gross Appearance.** Medulloblastomas are homogeneous, reddish-gray, finely granular, well-defined neoplasms arising from the roof of the fourth ventricle and extending into and filling much of this cavity.

    (3) **Microscopic examination** shows highly cellular, uniform, relatively avascular tumors whose component cells tend to cluster.

    (4) **Prognosis.** Most patients survive between 1 and 2 years after the first onset of symptoms.

d. **Meningiomas** (Fig. 16-6).

    (1) **Clinical Data.** These common tumors account for 15 to 20 percent of all intracranial tumors in adults, usually women; however, they are uncommon in children. Symptomatology may be minimal. The tumors may produce slowly evolving deficits. About 50 percent of meningiomas are situated near the vertex in a paramedial location. Spinal meningiomas are among the most common intraspinal tumors but are rare compared to the intracranial tumors.

    (2) **Gross Appearance.** Meningiomas are firm-to-rubbery tumors that have a white or red gritty appearance. They are usually clearly demarcated from the surrounding brain, where they push inward but do not truly invade. They can be shelled out, leaving the depressed brain beneath.

    (3) **Histologically,** there is uniformity of the cells, which contain ovoid nuclei, often with intranuclear vacuoles. The cells often form whorls, and **psammoma bodies** are common.

    (4) **Prognosis.** Meningiomas are slowly growing tumors. Depending upon their location and the adequacy of surgical removal, they may be incompletely excised. Such lesions may recur.

e. **Hemangioblastomas.**

    (1) **Clinical Data.** These tumors of blood vessel origin are most often found in the

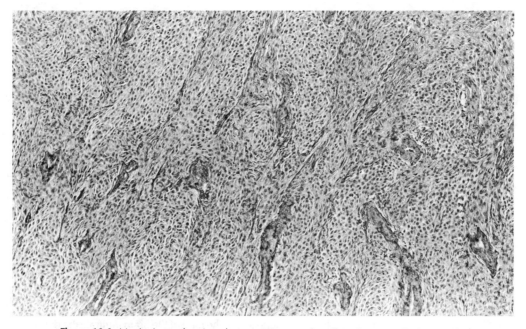

Figure 16-6. Meningioma showing characteristic wavy bundles of tumor cells (low power).

cerebellum of young adults and constitute 7 percent of primary posterior fossa tumors. Occasionally, polycythemia has been reported. Upon analysis of the cyst fluid, **erythropoietin** has been found. The patients present with gait and locomotion difficulties.

(2) **Gross appearance** is that of sharply outlined, spongy, purplish-red or brown neoplasms, which may be solid or cystic (sometimes a large cyst is present with a small mural nodule of tumor).

(3) **Microscopic appearance** varies from almost purely vascular, with capillaries or large cavernous channels, to highly cellular tumors in which the many capillaries are overshadowed by large polygonal cells containing lipids.

(4) **Prognosis.** Solitary hemangioblastomas can be easily shelled out, and the patient can enjoy an excellent prognosis.   *tumor of blood vessel*

(5) **Lindau's disease** is a rare familial disorder in which multiple hemangioblastomas of CNS and retina are associated with malformations, tumors of other organs (the kidney and adrenal gland), and cysts of the pancreas, liver, and kidney.

f. **Tumors of Nerve Sheath Origin.**

(1) **Schwannomas** are common intracranial tumors occurring mostly in middle-aged adults and accounting for 8 to 10 percent of all intracranial tumors. The most common location is the eighth cranial nerve.

(a) **Clinical Data.** Patients present with symptoms of hearing loss, disequilibrium, dizziness, headache, and ataxia. The tumors are often missed entirely or misdiagnosed as sensorineural deafness. Treatment is resection of as much of the tumor as possible. If total resection is not accomplished, the tumor often recurs. Overall, the prognosis is good.

(b) **Gross Appearance.** The tumors usually occur in conjunction with a nerve but grow external to it in most cases. The tumors may appear as spherical or oblong and, on a cut section, either as homogeneous or variegated. They are granular or cystic in consistency.

(c) **Histology.** (See Chapter 21, "Soft Tissues.")

(2) **Neurofibromas** occur in connection with peripheral nerves and grow intimately with and within them. (See Chapter 21, "Soft Tissues.")

(3) **Neurofibromatosis** (von Recklinghausen's disease) is a heredofamilial autosomal-dominant disease in which neurofibromas and schwannomas may occur in multiplicity in association with large **café au lait spots** on the skin and with hamartomatous or neoplastic lesions of not only the nervous system but of other organs as well. Malignant transformation of neurofibromas may occur.

g. **Miscellaneous Tumors.**
  (1) **Craniopharyngiomas.**
    (a) **Clinical Data.** Craniopharyngiomas mostly affect children between the ages of 4 and 16 years. These tumors are classically calcified suprasellar lesions that produce visual disturbances and hypothalamic syndromes.
    (b) **Gross Appearance.** The tumors are usually several cm in size, are multiloculated, and may be encapsulated by the surrounding brain into which they push. The cysts of the tumors contain a "machine oil" material in which there are suspended cholesterol crystals. Solid portions of the tumors are granular or crumbly.
    (c) **Microscopic Appearance.** The tumors are variegated in appearance and are usually multicystic. The solid regions contain foreign-body reactions, fibrous tissue, mineralization, and even bone formation in reaction to the degeneration products of the tumors. The tumor cells themselves may be epithelial in appearance or resemble tooth bud or squamous epithelium. Some resemble jaw tumors (ameloblastomas).
    (d) **Prognosis.** The treatment is total removal. If any tumor is left, recurrence is the rule. Survival for many years is common.
  (2) **Chordoma.**
    (a) **Clinical Data.** These slow-growing, persistent tumors affect men more often than women, and their occurrence peaks during the third and fourth decades of life. About 60 percent occur in the sacrococcygeal region, and about 30 percent occur in the region of the clivus at the base of the skull. The tumors aggressively invade bone and at the base of the brain infiltrate the basal structures of the skull. Most patients die of locally aggressive disease after a prolonged course.
    (b) **Gross Appearance.** The tumors are gelatinous, gray-white, friable, and lobulated.
    (c) **Microscopic Appearance.** The tumors are composed of clear cells in an amphophilic matrix that resembles cartilage. The large, water-clear, **physaliphorous** cells are characteristic but sometimes can be confused with cartilaginous tumors, metastatic renal cell cancer, or liposarcomas. The tumors are thought to arise in notochordal remnants.
h. **Tumors of the Pineal Body.**
  (1) **Clinical Data.** The pineal body gives rise to a series of tumors, most of which are "teratoid" in character. These tumors are identical to germ cell tumors of the ovary and testis. Characteristically they affect younger men generally under the age of 20 years. The tumors present with signs of increased intracranial pressure due to obstruction of the aqueduct or posterior third ventricle.
  (2) **Gross Appearance.** The tumors may vary in their cellular composition, appearing variegated in color and consistency, with cyst formation common.
  (3) **Histologically**, the typical teratomas have an appearance that does not set them apart from other teratomas that arise in the gonads. (See Chapter 12, "The Male Reproductive System," and Chapter 13, "The Female Reproductive System.")
  (4) The **prognosis** varies, with the pure seminoma types having the best (an average patient survival of 5 to 10 years) because of their radiosensitivity. Others show a corresponding lesser patient survival as a direct consequence of their failure to respond to irradiation and the difficulty of operative removal.
i. **Lymphomas of the Brain (Microgliomatosis).**
  (1) **Clinical Data.** Primary neoplasms of the reticuloendothelial system in the brain are uncommon. These tumors are most common during the sixth and seventh decades of life and present in a subtle fashion as disorders of higher neural functioning and mentation, with headache and seizures. The average duration of symptoms prior to diagnosis is a few months.
  (2) **Gross Appearance.** The tumors most often arise in the cerebrum and are usually multifocal in character. They appear to arise in the perivascular spaces of many vessels and in some cases resemble encephalitis rather than tumors.
  (3) **Histologically**, lymphomas of the brain may resemble the classic forms of lymphomas elsewhere.
  (4) **Prognosis.** The treatment is irradiation and chemotherapy. Survival of 1 to 2 years is common, and apparent total cures have been seen. The prompt, often dramatic, response to irradiation therapy is characteristic of the lesion.
j. **Metastatic Tumors.** Probably between 20 and 25 percent of all brain tumors represent metastatic lesions. The tumors most commonly producing metastatic disease in the CNS

are lung carcinomas, in which 40 to 50 percent of patients who die from this disease show brain involvement. Other tumors that commonly spread to the brain are carcinomas of the large intestine, the kidney, and the breast as well as the leukemias. Less common tumors, which have a high incidence of brain metastases, include malignant melanomas (in which nearly 50 percent of patients have brain lesions), follicular carcinomas of the thyroid, and the sarcomas. Some tumors metastasize to the dura mater and skull. Carcinomas of the breast are the most common examples of this.

(1) **Clinical Data.** Signs and symptoms of metastatic tumors of the brain are varied but generally are typical for any brain tumor.

(2) **Gross Appearance.** The phenomenon of metastases of the brain is usually an intravascular process, but direct invasion and diffuse spread by a paracranial tumor may also occur. Most metastatic tumors are at the junction of the gray and white matter, where the circulation is slower and the numbers of vessels diminish.

(3) **Histologically**, metastatic tumors generally display an intimate relationship with vessels, are discrete from the surrounding brain, and show the typical characteristics of the primary tumor.

(4) **Secondary Effects of Tumors of the CNS** include the following.

  (a) **Circulatory effects:** compression of the brain and cord with collapse of veins and capillary beds, producing edema, ischemia, and degeneration of neural tissue

  (b) **Compression, distortion,** and **displacement** of structures

  (c) **Herniations** of the brain and cerebellar tonsils

  (d) **Interference** with **CSF circulation**

  (e) **Papilledema:** swelling due to edema of optic nerve papilla with engorgement of retinal veins

III. DISORDERS OF THE PERIPHERAL NERVOUS SYSTEM.

Polyneuropathy and polyneuritis indicate widespread degeneration of the peripheral nerves. Predisposing causes are extremely varied. Neuropathy may be associated with a chronic focal infection or complicate almost any acute infectious disease (e.g., typhoid fever, pneumonia, malaria, and measles). It may result from poisoning by heavy metals (e.g., lead, arsenic, mercury, and thallium), alcohol, or other chemicals (e.g., carbon tetrachloride). It may occur in metabolic and deficiency disorders (e.g., diabetes mellitus, hematoporphyrinuria, beriberi, and pellagra) or may be associated with pregnancy, prolonged vomiting, or diarrhea.

Any combination of peripheral nerves, including the cranial nerves, may be affected by multiple neuropathies. Nerves supplying the extremities, especially the distal parts, are involved most often.

Grossly, abnormalities are not seen in multiple neuropathies. Microscopically, the myelin sheaths are swollen, fragmented, and form droplets and globules that lie in groups along the course of degenerating fibers. They stain progressively poorly and disappear. Axons also become swollen, fragmented, and disappear.

A. TRAUMAS of peripheral nerves occur by means of the three ways listed below. After injury, degeneration and regeneration of affected peripheral nerves proceed concomitantly. Regeneration is affected by the nerve involved, by the degree of separation of the severed nerve ends, by the state of the blood supply, and by any complicating infections. The traumas happen through

1. **Compression** by a neoplasm, callus, aneurysm, prolonged pressure against a hard surface, necrosis, inebriation, or bandages

2. **Tension** or stretching by abnormal movements (e.g., overextension of limbs) or by bone fracture, with wide separation of fragments

3. **Severance** by knife, bullet, or jagged edge of fractured bone

B. INTOXICATIONS

1. Arsenic poisoning leads to a polyneuropathy about 1 to 2 months after acute exposure or may be very delayed if there is low-grade chronic ingestion. The symptoms include numbness, tingling, pain, and weakness, especially of the legs.

2. **Lead** intoxication results chiefly in a motor neuropathy with a predilection for the wrist, fingers, and arms.

3. **Alcoholic** intoxication results in a neuropathy with usually a severe sensory loss problem with sparing of the motor nerves.

C. VASCULAR DISORDERS

1. Vasculitis such as polyarteritis can produce clinical neuropathy by what is presumed ischemic injury to specific nerves or nerve groups.

2. Diabetic neuropathies are due presumably to focal ischemic changes in small vessels, such as microangiopathy.

D. INFILTRATIVE DISORDERS. The prototype is **amyloidosis** wherein amyloid is deposited within nerves, leading to focal degeneration. Most instances of infiltrative disorders of the peripheral nerves are seen with primary amyloidosis.

E. NEOPLASMS. These include benign schwannomas and neurofibromas or their malignant counterparts. (See Chapter 21, "Soft Tissues.")

IV. DISORDERS OF THE MUSCULAR AND NEUROMUSCULAR SYSTEMS

A. MUSCULAR DYSTROPHY (Duchenne Muscular Dystrophy)

1. **Clinical Data.** This sex-linked recessive disorder affects children, chiefly boys, and becomes evident through weakness and falling when the child begins to walk. Early on, the muscle involvement is mainly of the pelvic girdle; therefore, the legs are weak and the child tends to use his arms and shoulders. As the disease progresses, all muscles are involved. Most children die before the age of 20 years, often of pneumonia associated with respiratory muscle weakness. The diagnosis is confirmed by the marked elevation of muscle enzymes, especially creatinine phosphokinase.

2. **Pathology.**
   a. **Gross Appearance.** The muscles appear atrophic and yellowish.
   b. **Microscopic Appearance.** Variation in fiber size is seen, with some degenerated and some hypertrophied fibers. In older patients, there is replacement of muscle tissue by fat.

B. POLYMYOSITIS

1. **Clinical Data.** This is a diffuse inflammatory disease of unknown origin affecting mostly women that causes symmetrical muscle weakness (more marked in proximal muscle groups—shoulder and pelvic girdles) and pain. Some patients show an associated inflammatory skin lesion (dermatomyositis).

2. **Pathology.** Muscle biopsy shows variation in fiber size and muscle degeneration with vacuolization and necrosis. An inflammatory infiltrate is seen. Muscle enzymes are elevated.

3. **Prognosis.** In 15 to 50 percent of affected adults, an associated visceral malignancy (for the most part, carcinoma of the lung, breast, or colon) is found or develops shortly after recognition of the myositis. In cases not associated with malignancy, the course and prognosis are variable. Children fare better than adults.

C. MYASTHENIA GRAVIS

1. **Clinical Data.** This common disorder usually affects women in the third or fourth decades of life. It presents as weakness relieved by rest and worsened by exercise. Often cranial and extraocular muscles are involved. Electromyographic studies show decremental responses to repeated nerve stimulation, and this is characteristic. Associated abnormalities are common: 75 to 80 percent of patients have thymic hyperplasia; 10 to 15 percent have a **thymoma** (epithelial tumor of the thymus).

2. **Pathogenesis.** Eighty percent of myasthenic patients have antibodies directed against neuromuscular acetylcholine receptors. Immunoglobulin G (IgG) and complement on the muscle receptor sites probably interfere with neural transmission.

3. **Pathology.** In the muscle, the characteristic findings are **lymphorrhages** (lymphocytic infiltrates around degenerating myofibers). By electron microscopy (EM), abnormal myoneural junctions are seen with widened clefts.

4. **Prognosis.** The course of the disease is variable, with partial remissions often seen. Relapse and progression are found. Death, usually due to intercurrent infection (pneumonia associated with respiratory muscle weakness), occurs in most cases after several years. In some individuals, especially those with thymoma, complete resection of the thymic lesion results in remission of the myasthenia. Removal of the nontumoral hyperplastic thymus as therapy for myasthenia remains controversial; only young women seem to benefit from this therapy.

STUDY QUESTIONS

Directions: Each question below contains five suggested answers. Choose the **one best** response to each question.

1. For 6 months a 45-year-old woman complained of increasingly severe headaches, which then became associated with right-arm weakness and an unsteady gait. Evaluation and subsequent surgery disclosed a lesion in the left occipital area; pathologic examination showed a meningioma. The major prognostic determinant in this woman's condition is

(A) the histologic subtype of the meningioma

(B) the mitotic index of the tumor

(C) the completeness of surgical removal

(D) tumor vascularity

(E) her amenability to radiation therapy

2. A 39-year-old man noted slowly progressive hearing loss over a 2-year period. Except for occasional headaches, he had no other complaints. Evaluation disclosed severe sensorineural hearing loss on the left side. X-rays showed a 1.5-cm mass at the left cerebellopontine angle. The mass is most apt to be a

(A) meningioma

(B) schwannoma

(C) metastatic tumor from the lung

(D) tuberculous abscess

(E) glioblastoma

3. Acoustic neuroma is most likely to be found in which of the following patients?

(A) A 16-year-old boy with multiple endocrine neoplasia, type 3 (MEN III)

(B) A 49-year-old woman with pigmented macules of the axillary skin

(C) A 28-year-old man with malignant melanoma of the scalp

(D) A 46-year-old woman who received radiation for pituitary adenoma

(E) A 3-month-old boy with ventricular septal defect

4. An 18-year-old woman presented with progressive generalized weakness and a recent onset of diplopia. Examination disclosed weakness of the eyelids and all extraocular muscles as well as generalized muscle weakness, which is greater in the proximal than in the distal groups. The suspected diagnosis is

(A) systemic lupus erythematosus

(B) myasthenia gravis

(C) Hodgkin's disease

(D) Duchenne muscular dystrophy

(E) polymyositis

5. A 27-year-old woman presents with a sudden onset of right-sided blindness and weakness in the left leg. There is no history of trauma; however, she experienced a similar episode 8 months ago and was diagnosed as having aseptic meningitis. The most probable diagnosis is

(A) meningeal carcinomatosis

(B) multiple sclerosis

(C) pernicious anemia

(D) meningioma of the falx

(E) tabes dorsalis

6. In viral encephalitis, the virus reaches the central nervous system via

(A) peripheral nerve spread

(B) Schwann cells

(C) lymphatics

(D) the olfactory system

(E) the bloodstream

7. Most viral infections of the brain produce all of the following histologic changes in the nervous system EXCEPT

(A) neuronal degeneration

(B) polymorphonuclear leukocytic infiltration

(C) glial cell proliferation

(D) perivascular lymphocytic infiltration

(E) production of intracytoplasmic inclusion bodies

8. Each of the following statements concerning Alzheimer's disease is true EXCEPT

(A) atrophic gyri and enlarged sulci are seen

(B) cerebellar atrophy is prominent

(C) neurofibrillary tangles are characteristic

(D) the disease course is prolonged and progressive

(E) it occurs in the fifth and sixth decades of life

Directions: The question below contains four suggested answers of which **one or more** is correct. Choose the answer

    A if **1, 2, and 3** are correct
    B if **1 and 3** are correct
    C if **2 and 4** are correct
    D if **4** is correct
    E if **1, 2, 3, and 4** are correct

9. Congenital malformations of the nervous system may result from which of the following conditions?

(1) Maternal irradiation

(2) In utero viral infections

(3) Maternal vitamin deficiency

(4) Maternal anoxia

Directions: The group of questions below consists of lettered choices followed by several numbered items. For each numbered item select the **one** lettered choice with which it is **most** closely associated. Each lettered choice may be used once, more than once, or not at all.

Questions 10–14

For each clinical history listed below, select the lesion from which it is most likely to result.

(A) Progressive multifocal leukodystrophy

(B) Microgliomatosis

(C) Ependymoma

(D) Meningioma

(E) Glioblastoma multiforme

10. A 4-year-old boy with papilledema and headache

11. A 20-year-old man with Hodgkin's disease and multifocal neurologic deficits

12. A 52-year-old man with a 2-month history of severe headache, double vision, and seizures

13. A 22-year-old renal transplant patient with a recent onset of visual disturbances and left-sided weakness

14. A 40-year-old woman with headache and right-sided weakness

ANSWERS AND EXPLANATIONS

1. The answer is C. [*II J 4 d (4)*] Completeness of removal at the initial surgery is the most important prognostic variable. Not one of the histologic parameters matters (histologic subtype, mitotic index, and vascularity); if surgery is incomplete, recurrence will follow. The need for radiation therapy implies inadequacy of surgery and hence a poorer prognosis.

2. The answer is B. [*II J 4 f (1)*] The history and findings are classic for a schwannoma (acoustic neuroma). Although a meningioma may occur at the cerebellopontine angle, it is unusual. The hearing loss symptoms point toward a tumor of cranial nerve VIII. All other possibilities are ruled out by the 2-year history in this case.

3. The answer is B. [*II J 4 f (3)*] Acoustic neuromas occur in middle-aged to elderly people, they affect women more often than men, and they are found commonly in patients with evidence of von Reck-linghausen's disease [manifested in the 49-year-old woman as café au lait spots (macules) of the axillary skin]. The patient with multiple endocrine neoplasia, type 3, (MEN III) has colonic ganglioneuromatosis, but he has no apparent increased chance of developing acoustic neuroma. The patient with melanoma (a tumor that is related to neural lesions) would not have an increased propensity for a central nervous system (CNS) tumor. Neither radiation nor congenital abnormalities of other systems are associated with increased frequency of acoustic neuroma.

4. The answer is B. (*IV C 1*) The symptoms and the age and sex of the patient lead to a diagnosis of myasthenia gravis. Lupus erythematosus and Hodgkin's disease, which occur in this age group, may be associated rarely with neurologic symptoms, but they are not so well-defined. Muscular dystrophy chiefly affects males and is of chronic duration. Polymyositis usually affects specific muscles and is not characterized by generalized weakness.

5. The answer is B. (*II I 1*) Multiple sclerosis is a strong possibility in a young patient with neurologic signs that remit and recur. Meningeal carcinomatosis is unlikely in this age group and in a patient with no known primary site. Pernicious anemia and tabes dorsalis would not remit and recur. Meningioma would not remit and would produce signs localized to one side of the body only.

6. The answer is E. (*II D 2 d*) Most viruses infect the central nervous system (CNS) in man via the bloodborne route. Lymphatics run in a centrifugal path away from the CNS. The olfactory, peripheral nerve, and Schwann cell routes may play minor roles in the spread of virus to the CNS, although this remains to be proven in naturally acquired human infections.

7. The answer is E. [*II D 2 d (2)*] Although virtually all viral infections cause neuronal degeneration, polymorphonuclear leukocytic and perivascular lymphocytic infiltration, and proliferation of glial cells, only a few, specific infections (e.g., cytomegalovirus) produce recognizable inclusion bodies.

8. The answer is B. (*II I 9*) The cerebral cortex, especially the frontal lobes, is involved most prominently in Alzheimer's disease; cerebellar disease does not occur or is minor in extent. The disease course and the age group that it affects describe the clinical aspects of the disease. The gross and microscopic features are described through the appearance of atrophic gyri and enlarged sulci and neurofibrillary tangles, respectively.

9. The answer is E (all). (*II F 1*) Irradiation of the pregnant mother, viral infections in utero, maternal vitamin deficiency, and maternal anoxia have all been associated with central nervous system (CNS) malformations in both humans and animals. In the United States, irradiation and viral infections account for most instances in which an etiology is known or suspected.

10-14. The answers are: 10-C, 11-A, 12-E, 13-B, 14-D. [*II J 4 b; II 1 2; II J 4 a (3); II J 4 i; II J 4 d*] Ependymoma is the most common central nervous system (CNS) tumor in the young child, and it characteristically presents with papilledema and headache.

The history of Hodgkin's disease has demonstrated an immunocompromised host. Multiple unusual neurologic abnormalities lead to a diagnosis of progressive multifocal leukodystrophy.

The relatively rapid course (2 months) and severity of symptoms in the 52-year-old man are strongly indicative of a malignant lesion; of the choices, glioblastoma multiforme is the most likely.

The history of renal transplantation leads to the suspicion of the unusual microgliomatosis in the case of the 22-year-old patient with recent visual disturbances and left-sided weakness.

Apparently slow, progressive symptoms in a middle-aged woman would be indicative of a benign process. Meningioma is the best choice.

17
The Hematopoietic and Lymphatic System

I. INTRODUCTION. Disorders of the hematopoietic system usually include those of the red blood cells (decreased amounts of red blood cells lead to anemia; increased amounts lead to polycythemia), coagulation and hemostasis, and white blood cells (decreased amounts of white blood cells lead to neutropenia; increased amounts lead to leukemia). Also included are disorders that affect the lymph nodes, thymus, spleen, and the entire immune system, such as malignant lymphomas, lymphatic leukemia, plasma cell neoplasms, and histiocytic tumors and mimickers of those tumors. This chapter will review

A. Disorders of red blood cells

B. Disorders of coagulation and hemostasis

C. Disorders of white blood cells

D. Disorders of undetermined cellular origin

E. Lymphadenopathies of non-neoplastic causes

F. Lymphadenitis of unknown causes

G. Reactive adenitis

H. Diseases of histiocytes

I. Disorders of the spleen

II. DISORDERS OF RED BLOOD CELLS

A. ANEMIA, defined as a reduction in the amount of circulating hemoglobin, red blood cells, or both, occurs when hematopoietic tissues are disturbed, malfunctioning, or replaced or when loss of red cells or hemoglobin from the circulation surpasses the body's ability to replace these elements.

   1. If red cells are destroyed too rapidly or lost (through bleeding), red cell production in the marrow is stimulated. The stem cells are transformed along erythroid lines.

   2. Symptoms of anemia vary with the **degree** of anemia and its **rate** of development. Common to all anemias are pallor of the skin and mucous membranes, increased pulse rate, shortness of breath, palpitations, dizziness, and fatigue. The symptoms result from a decreased oxygen supply to the affected organs. Heart failure may occur. If anemia develops slowly, compensation occurs and few symptoms and signs may be found.

   3. Classification of Anemias. The **morphologic categorization** of anemias into **macrocytic, microcytic, normocytic, hypochromic**, and **normochromic-normocytic** can lead the clinician to the appropriate etiology. Macrocytic, microcytic, and normocytic refer to red cell size, whereas hypochromic and normochromic-normocytic refer to hemoglobin content as determined by red cell color. Although cell size represents a more objective measurement, color differences are very subjective. Basically, the causes of anemia are two: excessive blood turnover and failure of blood production.

a. Excessive blood turnover occurs through hemorrhage (blood loss to the outside of the vascular system) and **hemolysis** (red cell destruction within the body). Acute blood loss usually results in a normochromic-normocytic anemia, which is dramatic and often traumatic. The dominant clinical picture is one of decreased blood volume and **shock**, with tachycardia, hypovolemia, and hypotension. Bleeding nearly always results in a deficiency of iron, which, when severe, is characterized by a hypochromic anemia.

(1) Common to hemorrhage and hemolysis is evidence of attempted compensation by the marrow: erythroid hyperplasia in the bone marrow and increase of reticulocytes in the peripheral blood.

(2) One can distinguish between hemorrhage and hemolysis through the aid of different tests.

(a) In **acute** situations of excessive blood turnover, one can measure serum **haptoglobin**, a plasma protein the usual function of which is to conserve the iron elaborated from the small amount of hemoglobin that is normally in the plasma. If there is acute hemolysis, haptoglobin binds the released hemoglobin in the plasma. The formed complex is cleared from the circulation by the reticuloendothelial system, and within a matter of hours after the acute hemolytic episode, serum haptoglobin is unmeasurable. Thus, if haptoglobin is present, the diagnosis is hemorrhage; if absent, acute hemolysis has occurred.

(b) In **chronic** excessive blood turnover, in order to differentiate hemorrhage from hemolysis, knowledge of **iron metabolism** is necessary. Iron, which is found predominantly in red cells, is decreased in the serum and in the reticuloendothelial cells of the marrow only if there is blood loss to the outside. In any other type of anemia, the marrow shows increased iron stores. The cause of chronic hemorrhage is usually a problem of the gastrointestinal (ulcer, cancer, or polyp), genitourinary (cancer or stone), or gynecologic (excessive menstrual flow) systems.

(3) Hemolysis, whether acute or chronic, can be of two types: an intrinsic erythrocyte defect or an abnormal marrow or systemic environment. An intrinsic red cell defect is **congenital**, whereas the abnormal environment is an **acquired** abnormality (the red cell itself is perfect). Congenital defects are manifested in childhood, and a family history of anemia is common. In acquired defects, the patient's family is normal and often the onset of the anemia can be pinpointed.

(a) **Congenital hemolytic anemias** can be produced by **abnormal hemoglobins, disturbances of red cell metabolism**, or **abnormal hemoglobin synthesis**.

(i) **Abnormal Hemoglobins (Hemoglobinopathies).** Hemoglobin A (Hb A), normal adult hemoglobin, consists of two α- and two β-chains and is written as $\alpha_2\beta_2$. Although α-chains are unique, both γ- and δ-chains can substitute for β-chains. Thus, Hb F is $\alpha_2\gamma_2$, and Hb A_2 is $\alpha_2\delta_2$.

Differences that can be demonstrated by electrophoresis in the hemoglobin molecule are in the globin portion. This type of hemoglobin is genetically controlled. When abnormal hemoglobin occurs in the heterozygous state along with normal adult hemoglobin, a nonsymptomatic "trait" condition usually results. When abnormal hemoglobin is present in the homozygous state or when an individual is heterozygous for two abnormal hemoglobin types, a clinical disease characterized by a hemolytic disorder usually occurs.

Sickle cell anemia is the prototype of these disorders. Inherited as a mendelian dominant, this disorder, which affects predominantly blacks, occurs as the **sickle trait** in 8 percent to 10 percent of black persons in the United States. The disease itself, which develops in the homozygous state (Hb SS), occurs in about 0.2 percent of blacks in the United States. Although sickle trait is usually asymptomatic, sickle cell anemia leads to severe disease. The genetically determined biochemical anomaly in the β-chain of hemoglobin produces an altered solubility. At low pH and with decreased oxygen tension, Hb S precipitates out of solution in the red cells, and the latter become sickle-shaped. Such red cells get stuck in small venules, arterioles, and capillaries, with vascular obstruction, occlusion, and then hemolysis of red cells.

Vascular occlusions account for most of the symptoms, which include leg ulcers, splenic autoinfarction, hepatomegaly, hepatic dysfunction, cholelithiasis, pulmonary thrombi, and stroke. Unusual infections (salmonella osteomyelitis and pneumococcal meningitis) are also found in these patients.

Sickle crisis is a painful and dramatic expression of vascular occlusion.

The initiating factor in the sickle crisis is not known. Febrile episodes seem to predispose a patient to crisis. Portal circulations in which oxygen tension is low, such as those in the liver and kidneys, seem to be at particular risk.

   (ii) **Disturbances of red cell metabolism** affect red cell membrane structure or are enzyme defects. The classic example of an intracorpuscular defect is **hereditary spherocytosis**, inherited as a mendelian dominant trait. Presumably, there is a genetically determined abnormality in a membrane polypeptide, which allows sodium to enter the erythrocyte passively at an enhanced rate. The red cells that have a decreased diameter and are abnormally shaped are sequestered selectively by the reticuloendothelial cells of the spleen and are destroyed.

   Glucose-6-phosphate dehydrogenase (G6PD) deficiency is another common red cell defect. It is especially common among people of Mediterranean heritage and makes affected patients susceptible to drugs or compounds having oxidative activity (e.g., fava beans and antimalarial drugs). The ingestion of such compounds leads to massive hemolytic episodes.

   (iii) **Abnormal Hemoglobin Synthesis.** Thalassemia (Cooley's anemia) is the prototype. This congenital abnormality, which occurs in patients predominantly from the Mediterranean region, is a failure of or a reduction in synthesis of the β-chain of hemoglobin, resulting in abnormal hemoglobins that are functionally inadequate. The erythrocytes are deformed and hypochromic. The homozygous form of the disease is fatal in early life due to intercurrent infection or hemosiderosis with liver or heart failure. Thalassemia minor, the heterozygous form of the disease, results in a mild anemia but is compatible with a normal life span.

   (iv) **Complications** of these various congenital defects include jaundice, bilirubinate gallstones, iron overload (hemosiderosis), and the effects of chronic anemia (fatigue, weakness, and cardiac enlargement and failure) on end-organs.

   (b) **Acquired Hemolytic Anemias.** Immunologically (autoimmune) mediated destruction of red cells provides the basis for these disorders. Antibodies, usually of the immunoglobulin G (IgG) class, are directed against red cells and may lyse the erythrocytes directly or react with red cell membrane antigens, altering their susceptibility to destruction in the spleen.

   The hemolytic process may be idiopathic or secondary to some underlying disease, such as lymphoma, carcinoma, sarcoidosis, or one of the collagen disorders.

   (c) **Other Examples of Immune Hemolysis.** Two classic examples of immune—not autoimmune—hemolysis illustrate the extent of the clinical variations of this condition.

   (i) In **fetomaternal incompatibility** at Rh locus D, the D-negative mother after contact with D-positive erythrocytes may produce an IgG anti-D antibody, which crosses the placenta, attacks fetal erythrocytes, and destroys them. The fetus is jaundiced.

   (ii) When a patient receives an **incompatible blood transfusion**, within minutes there is a devastating sequence of intravascular hemolysis.

   (d) **Microangiopathic (mechanical) hemolytic anemia** is characterized by the appearance on a peripheral smear of bizarre fragmented erythrocytes and by signs of hemolysis. The erythrocyte can withstand moderate deformation and twisting, but it breaks up when subjected to strong stretching or shearing forces. Stress of this magnitude occurs in jets produced by deformed aortic valves, arteriovenous shunts, ventricular septal defects, or older cardiac valvular prostheses.

b. **Failure of Blood Production.** These anemias can be divided into those caused by nutritional deficiencies, marrow aplasia, myelophthises (marrow replacement), and systemic disorders.

   (1) **Nutritional deficiencies**, decrease or absence of iron, folic acid, or vitamin B_{12}, are the most common types of deficiencies that produce nutritional anemias seen in clinical practice, although they may result also from severe protein malnutrition or deficient diets.

   (a) **Iron deficiency** results from chronic blood loss and may be caused by gastrointestinal tumors or ulcers, by parasites (e.g., tapeworms), or following extensive intestinal surgery.

   (b) **Folic acid** and **vitamin B_{12} deficiencies** produce megaloblastic anemia. Associated with this are neurological abnormalities, glossitis, and lingual atrophy.

   (c) **Pernicious anemia** is an autoimmune disorder characterized by absence of parietal cells in the gastric fundus, by achlorhydria, gastric mucosal atrophy, and by circulating antibodies to parietal cells. **Intrinsic factor**, produced by the fundus and necessary for the absorption of vitamin B_{12} from the diet, is absent, leading to vitamin B_{12} deficiency. A propensity to develop gastric cancer and the association of pernicious anemia with other autoimmune disorders, especially idiopathic hypoadrenalism (Addison's disease), characterize this disease.

   (2) Marrow Aplasia. Inciting or causative agents may be radiation, drugs (especially benzene derivatives), chemotherapeutic agents, certain antibiotics (especially chloramphenicol), viruses (especially hepatitis virus), or unknown agents. The agents act not only on the marrow but also on other sites of hematopoiesis, reflecting injury to the stem cells. The marrow spaces are occupied only by fat.

     Some cases of aplasia involve one hematopoietic line only, as in **Blackfan-Diamond syndrome**, a congenital defect involving erythroid hypoplasia, or as in certain tumors, such as **thymomas**, associated with **pure red cell aplasia.**

   (3) Myelophthisic Anemias. In these conditions, the marrow is replaced by foreign "invaders" (e.g., carcinomas, leukemias, fibrosis, and granulomas). Extramedullary hematopoiesis is seen.

   (4) Systemic disorders can produce anemia. Endocrine diseases such as hypothyroidism, hypopituitarism, and hypoadrenalism are associated with low blood counts. Poor marrow function and anemia can be seen in uremia, chronic low-grade infection, and malignancy. Whether or not these conditions produce anemia via deficiency states or whether or not there is production of specific substances that are toxic or depressive to marrow stem cells or their maturation remains unknown.

B. POLYCYTHEMIA. Increased red cell mass is termed polycythemia and may be primary polycythemia, a marrow-based disease, or secondary polycythemia, a reactive form of erythrocytosis caused by a variety of factors.

  1. Primary Polycythemia (Polycythemia Rubra Vera).

    a. Definition. This myeloproliferative disorder is characterized by **panmyelopathy** (proliferation of all bone marrow cell lines—red cells, white cells, and platelets). An absolute increase in red cell mass dominates the clinicopathological syndrome.

    b. Pathogenesis. Cytogenetic and karyotypic studies indicate that polycythemia vera is a **clonal** disorder, suggesting a **neoplastic transformation** in this disease.

    c. Clinical Data. Polycythemia vera is an uncommon disease, chiefly affecting individuals in the sixth to eighth decades of life. The disorder is often insidious in onset and may be diagnosed as an incidental laboratory finding. However, patients may present with symptoms of vascular occlusion, headache, and itching. Myocardial infarct, cerebrovascular accidents, bowel infarcts, or gangrene of the extremities may occur. The associated high platelet count (thrombocytosis) may produce local capillary or venule occlusion and ischemia. Some patients suffer hemorrhagic episodes, especially in the gastrointestinal tract and central nervous system (CNS).

    d. Pathology. The bone marrow demonstrates trilineage hyperplasia. Abnormal platelet precursors may be seen. Fibrosis with increased reticulin and collagen fibers in the marrow (myelofibrosis) is common and progresses during the course of the disease. Extramedullary hematopoiesis involving the spleen, liver, and lymph nodes is found.

    e. Course. The disease runs a chronic course with median survivals of 10 to 20 years. About 20 percent of patients develop myelofibrosis with spent marrows and anemia; a few patients develop acute leukemia. Both complications are considerably more common in individuals treated with alkylating-agent chemotherapy or radioactive phosphorus. Important causes of death include heart failure, cardiac infarction, stroke, hemorrhage, and the sequela of leukemia or myelofibrosis.

  2. Secondary Polycythemia. In this disease a variety of reactive changes may lead to elevations of red cell count. In such conditions, erythropoietin is elevated and stimulates marrow stem cells to produce erythrocytes. Other marrow elements are normal in number, function, and morphology; no marrow fibrosis is found.

III. DISORDERS OF COAGULATION AND HEMOSTASIS (HEMORRHAGE AND THROMBOSIS). Hemorrhagic disorders can be conveniently divided into three groups: vascular anomalies, wherein walls are fragile and do not withstand normal pressures, coagulation anomalies, and platelet defects or deficiencies. Patient histories are helpful in distinguishing among these disorders.

  A. VASCULAR ANOMALIES. Patients with **vascular fragility** give a history of purpura (**petechiae**, small hemorrhages or aneurysms in the skin or mucosae, usually of pinhead size, and ecchymoses, larger areas of hemorrhage). Tests of platelet number and function and tests of coagulation factors are normal.

1. **Hereditary hemorrhagic telangiectasia** is transmitted as an autosomal-dominant trait and appears clinically with epistaxis or gastrointestinal bleeding.

2. **Scurvy,** vitamin C deficiency, is very rare in the United States. It can cause skin, gingival, and mucosal bleeding with petechiae.

3. **Corticosteroid excess,** whether from endogenous or exogenous causes, produces cutaneous hemorrhages, which are probably due to corticosteroid-induced catabolism of the protein in vascular supportive tissues.

4. **Drug allergies** can produce a vasculitic purpura.

5. **Senile Purpura.** Patients have cutaneous hemorrhages on the dorsum of the hands, the wrists, the upper arms, and occasionally the calves. Serious bleeding does not occur. Presumably, this condition represents an age-dependent deterioration of the vascular supportive tissues.

B. **BLOOD COAGULATION DISORDERS.** Because the coagulation sequence is complex, defects in synthesis, function, or composition of or deficient amounts of any of the involved coagulation factors would interfere with proper clotting. Individuals with coagulation defects **must be injured before they bleed**.

1. **Hereditary disorders** in all of these coagulation factors are known. The prototype is hemophilia (due to defective or deficient factor VIII). This disorder occurs in about 1 in 20,000 live births. Since the gene for factor VIII is carried on the X chromosome, the disease is manifested in males. Diagnosis is made by the clinical picture, family history (positive in three-fourths of the cases), and the factor VIII coagulant level.

2. **Acquired clotting disorders** are more common than are hereditary clotting disorders. Clotting factors tend to be grouped into three classes by origin and behavior.
   a. Abnormalities in quantities of prothrombin, factors VII, IX, and X with normal levels of factors V, VIII, and fibrinogen are diagnostic of **vitamin K deficiency**. Vitamin K deficiency can result from malnutrition, malabsorption (e.g., sprue), and obstructive jaundice. Vitamin K-dependent factors can also be decreased by vitamin K antagonists (e.g., drugs such as warfarin and heparin).
   b. Abnormalities in the factors V, VII, IX, X, prothrombin, and fibrinogen point to **severe liver disease** in which the factors cannot be produced.
   c. The third pattern consists of decreases in the labile factors V and VIII, fibrinogen, and prothrombin. The diagnosis is defibrination syndrome or **disseminated intravascular coagulation**. This type of disorder is seen acutely in incompatible blood transfusion, in the peripartum period with premature separation of the placenta, and in endotoxic shock. Chronic disseminated intravascular coagulation is found usually in metastatic malignancies. In these conditions, fibrin is deposited widely in vessels, activation of the fibrinolytic mechanism ensues, and fragments of fibrin and fibrinogen are found in the plasma (fibrin split products). Platelets are decreased also because they are trapped in areas of clotting. This further perpetuates the bleeding tendencies.

C. **PLATELET DISORDERS**

1. **Thrombocytopenia** is a decreased platelet count or abnormal platelet function, leading to a hemorrhagic disorder.
   a. **Clinical Data.** The clinical features vary according to the etiology and the presence or absence of pancytopenia. The hallmark of thrombocytopenia is the presence of **petechiae**, but if the platelet count is very low, there may be a **purpura**, mucosal bleeding, and even deep tissue bleeding.

   Drug history is important since many classes of drugs can produce thrombocytopenia by idiopathic or allergic reactions. Patients may exhibit anemia, neutropenic infection, connective tissue disease, or a lymphoma.
   b. **Platelet Production Abnormalities.** A hypoplastic marrow in which the total cellularity is reduced implies aplastic anemia. A marrow that is fibrosed or infiltrated with leukemic or other malignant cells represents the syndrome of myelophthisis. A marrow showing normal cellularity and maturation with decreased numbers of apparently normal megakaryocytes suggests ingestion of a drug that specifically affects the megakaryocytic precursor cells.
   c. **Accelerated Removal of Platelets.**
      (1) When a patient has thrombocytopenia despite an abundance of normal megakaryocytes in the marrow, it is likely that the mechanism of thrombocytopenia is accelerated removal of platelets. Systemic lupus erythematosus, lymphoma, or Coombs'-positive acquired hemolytic anemia is usually the underlying problem.

(2) **Idiopathic thrombocytopenic purpura** typically appears in young women without a relevant history of drug ingestion. The marrow shows abundant megakaryocytes, many of which are young, and erythroid and myeloid precursors remain normal. In the serum of about 70 percent of these patients, there is an antiplatelet antibody, which coats and damages platelets, which are selectively removed by the spleen.

(3) **Platelet Sequestration.** Relatively modest thrombocytopenia (platelet counts of 40,000 to 80,000/mm³) is seen in patients with marked splenomegaly (hypersplenism).

(4) **Platelet function defects** have been in under the myeloproliferative diseases. Megakaryocytes frequently are abnormal. Abnormal platelet morphology is sometimes present.

(5) **Drug-Induced Disorders.** Aspirin, certain antibiotics, and antihistamines, among other drugs, can lead to hemorrhage because of interference with platelet function.

2. **Thrombocytosis and Thrombocythemia.**
   a. An elevated platelet count can occur in response to a variety of clinical disorders. Such elevation is referred to as reactive thrombocytosis (platelet count above 500,000/mm³).
   b. The platelet count can be increased autonomously in the myeloproliferative disorders. The platelet count can vary from 1,000,000 to 3,000,000/mm³ or more, and tests of platelet function are frequently abnormal. There appears to be enhanced propensity for hemorrhage and thromboembolism.

IV. DISORDERS OF WHITE BLOOD CELLS

A. NON-NEOPLASTIC DISEASES

1. **Decreased White Cells (Leukocytopenia).**
   a. **Neutropenia.** A decrease in the absolute neutrophil count below 500/mm³ is associated with a significant incidence of infection. The causes of neutropenia include inadequate production (aplastic marrow), toxic and drug effects, immune (autoimmune) diseases, and increased removal and redistribution of neutrophils as in hypersplenism.
   b. **Lymphocytopenia.** A decrease in the absolute lymphocyte count below 1500/mm³ is found in steroid-treated patients, in patients with certain malignancies after treatment with radiation therapy, in patients with uremia, and in those with marrow aplasia.

2. **Increased White Cells (Leukocytosis).**
   a. Non-neoplastic elevation of the white cell count usually reflects infection.
   b. In some severe infections, a very high **neutrophil** count **(leukemoid reaction)** is found. Specific elevation of **eosinophils** is found in parasitic infestations, especially with worms, and in allergic reactions (asthma, hay fever, and drug allergies).
   c. **Monocytosis** can be found in patients with infections eliciting a more chronic inflammatory response (e.g., tuberculosis, fungi, and listeriosis).
   d. **Lymphocytosis** can be found in tuberculosis and viral infections (e.g., infectious mononucleosis and measles).

B. NEOPLASMS OF THE WHITE CELL SERIES: LEUKEMIAS

1. **General Considerations.** Leukemia is a condition in which white blood cells (leukocytes) proliferate in an uncontrolled fashion in the bone marrow and in other lymphoreticular tissues (e.g., lymph nodes and the spleen) and may infiltrate any organ. The leukemic population of cells may arise from granulocytic, monocytic, or lymphocytic precursors.

   Leukemia is the proliferation of an abnormal hematopoietic cell clone that responds poorly to normal regulatory mechanisms. It has a tendency to diminished capacity for normal cell differentiation, the ability to expand at the expense of normal myeloid or lymphoid lines, and a possible ability to suppress or impair normal myeloid cell growth.

2. The **etiology** of leukemia is a subject of considerable study.
   a. Animal leukemias are caused by RNA viruses, but a **viral etiology** for human leukemias has not been proved.
   b. Human leukemias occur after **exposure** to ionizing irradiation or to radiomimetic agents (such as antimetabolites, chloramphenicol, and benzene) that produce marrow aplasia.
   c. The **genetic composition** of the host influences the incidences of both animal and human leukemias. Certain inherited chromosomal abnormalities, such as Down's syndrome (trisomy of chromosome 21), have been shown to increase the incidence of acute lymphocytic leukemia. The search for chromosomal changes in leukemic cell lines has led to the finding of a specific chromosomal abnormality for one type of leukemia. Bone marrow cells of 90 percent of patients with **chronic myelogenous leukemia** possess the

so-called Philadelphia chromosome, a translocation of part of chromosome 22 to chromosome 9.

3. The **pathophysiology** of the leukemias relates almost directly to the impact of the expanding cell number. The growing cell population infiltrates and renders the marrow functionally aplastic, leading to death by infection or hemorrhage through the depletion of normally functioning white cells and platelets. Leukemic cells also can infiltrate other areas, chiefly the liver, spleen, lymph nodes, and meninges, and cause organ dysfunction.

4. **Classification.**
    a. Leukemias are generally divided into **acute** and **chronic** types. The terms are predictive in that most chronic leukemias follow an insidious course and acute leukemias kill rapidly, unless there is aggressive therapeutic intervention.
       (1) **Acute leukemias** are comprised of precursor cells (blasts) that proliferate without undergoing the normal maturation process. Thus, the leukemic cells are large and primitive in appearance. Monoblasts, myeloblasts (the precursors of granulocytes), and lymphoblasts may be distinguished from one another by various morphological criteria and by cytochemical techniques. The primitive cells fill and replace the normal marrow and then spill over into the peripheral blood. They often comprise over 90 percent of the circulating leukocytes.
       (2) In **chronic leukemias** there are mature elements; the proliferating neoplastic cells are able to undergo normal and nearly normal maturation. However, the proliferative process advances without the normal control mechanisms operating to limit production. Thus, the abnormal cell line fills the bone marrow space.
    b. The second way of classifying leukemias is by their **cell of origin** (or the cell of the normal marrow that they most resemble). Hence, there are granulocytic or myelocytic leukemias, lymphocytic leukemias, monocytic types, and even combinations—myelomonocytic leukemias.

5. **Diagnosis.** The clinical diagnosis of leukemia rests on cytologic and morphologic groups: the finding of abnormal cells in the peripheral blood and the presence in a marrow smear of an infiltrate of abnormal cells replacing normal marrow elements. Biopsies of bone marrow, liver, spleen, or skin lesions also can provide the diagnosis through showing infiltration by the abnormal cells.

6. **Features of the Leukemias.**
    a. **Chronic granulocytic (myelocytic) leukemia** is a marrow-derived neoplasm composed principally of granulocytic cells in various stages of maturation. White blood cell counts are usually greater than 50,000/mm³. The Philadelphia chromosome is present in bone marrow cells in 90 percent of the cases.
       (1) **Clinical Data.** The typical patient is an adult with peripheral blood and marrow granulocytosis with a shift to the left. Fever, splenomegaly, and fatigue are common symptoms.
       (2) **Course and Prognosis.** Most patients with chronic granulocytic leukemia enter an accelerated phase of blast crisis in which the predominant cells resemble primitive myeloid, monocytic, or lymphoid cells. Almost all patients die as a result of a blast crisis.
    b. **Acute granulocytic (myelocytic) leukemia** is a marrow-derived neoplasm composed of blasts and cells differentiating into granulocytes. The marrow is infiltrated by blasts and promyelocytes (Fig. 17-1).
       (1) **Clinical Data.** Acute granulocytic leukemia affects adults and is preceded by a few days to weeks of weakness, bleeding, and fever. Physical examination shows petechiae, sternal tenderness, and sometimes adenopathy, splenomegaly, and hepatomegaly. There often is evidence of infection. Occasionally the leukemia will present as a mass lesion composed of blast cells (granulocytic sarcoma and chloroma) in the head, neck, and bowel.
       (2) **Laboratory Data.** The blood picture is characterized by anemia, thrombocytopenia, and an elevated white blood cell count, in which the predominant cell is a blast. Bone marrow shows a myeloblastic infiltrate replacing all marrow (Fig. 17-2).
       (3) **Course and Prognosis.** Untreated, this form of leukemia causes death within 1 to 3 months, usually as a result of infection or hemorrhage.
    c. **Lymphocytic Leukemias.** These common neoplasms, accounting for most of the acute leukemias of childhood, are better understood in the context of the recent knowledge of lymphocytes in general (as discussed below).

C. **LYMPHOMAS.** Whereas leukemias include bone marrow neoplasms originating from hematopoietic, histiocytic, and some lymphoid cell lines, most neoplasms of nodal or extramarrow

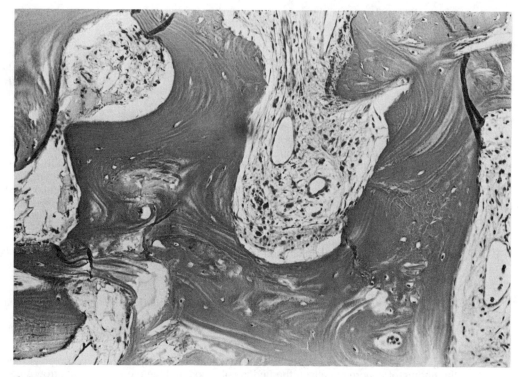

Figure 17-1. Agnogenic myeloid metaplasia with myelofibrosis. Bone marrow biopsy shows prominent fibrosis of marrow spaces with sparsely isolated residual marrow elements [hematoxylin and eosin (H and E) stain, high power].

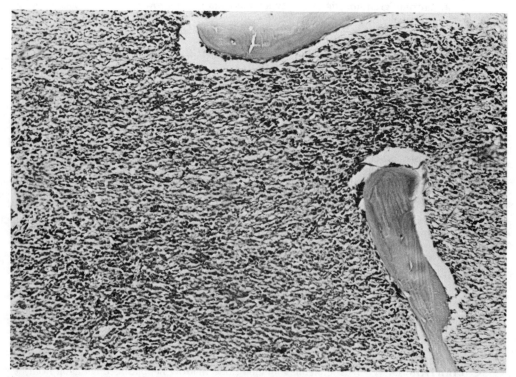

Figure 17-2. Marrow spaces replaced by leukemic blasts in acute granulocytic leukemia; no fat remains [hematoxylin and eosin (H and E) stain, high power].

lymphoid sites are called lymphomas. Lymphomas are divided customarily into Hodgkin's (disease) and nonHodgkin's lymphomas, and they often have leukemic phases. It is difficult to determine if leukemic cells have arisen from a marrow-based or a node-based neoplasm.

1. **Malignant Lymphomas.** Classification of neoplasms of the lymphoid system is based on the presumed cell of origin rather than solely on morphological features such as cell size.

   a. Malignant lymphomas are common neoplasms, comprising approximately 10 percent of all malignant tumors. Second only to acute leukemia as the most common form of cancer in children and young adults, lymphomas are also increasing in incidence in middle-aged and elderly adults. The lymphomas represent clonal expansions of lymphocytic elements blocked at particular stages of B- and T-cell differentiation. The cells of these tumors recapitulate the morphological and functional characteristics of the normal analogue.

   b. The **etiology** of human malignant lymphomas is unknown, but an increased incidence, up to 50 times that in normal individuals, is observed in patients with **congenital immunological defects** (e.g., ataxia, telangiectasia, and Wiskott-Aldrich syndrome). Patients with **acquired immunologic disorders** (e.g., Sjögren's syndrome, systemic lupus erythematosus, rheumatoid disease, and Hashimoto's disease) show an increased incidence of lymphomas, as do aging patients and those with altered immunological function induced by drug therapy (e.g., immunosuppression for transplantation). The common denominator is **alteration in immunoregulatory control mechanisms**. Certain viruses and chemicals have been implicated in the etiology of lymphomas. Epstein-Barr virus, probably not intrinsically oncogenic, is a potent polyclonal stimulator for B-cell proliferation. Certain chemicals, including the drug diphenylhydantoin, alter the surface membranes of certain lymphocytes, interfering with immunoregulatory control and promoting cellular proliferation in a manner favoring the development of lymphomas.

   c. **Pathophysiology.** Altered immunoregulatory control mechanisms predispose patients to significant risks of infectious disease.

      (1) Lymphomas of the **B-cell system** generally predispose patients to **bacterial disease** due to increased catabolism of immunoglobulins and suppression of all B-cell function.

      (2) Neoplasms of the **T-cell system** frequently predispose the patients to infections due to **viral, mycobacterial,** or **fungal elements**.

2. **Acute or chronic lymphocytic leukemia** may be of a non-T, non-B, T-cell, or B-cell type. Such lesions may present initially as marrow-based and peripheral blood disorders, but eventually almost all involve the lymph nodes, spleen, thymus, liver, and other solid organs.

   a. **Classification of T-Cell Neoplasms.**

      (1) **Acute lymphocytic leukemia** of the T-cell type represents approximately 30 percent of the acute lymphocytic leukemia population. The marrow shows sheets of cells with a high nuclear-cytoplasmic ratio, scant cytoplasm, and primitive nuclear chromatin. Nuclear convolutions are often prominent.

      (2) **Thymic lymphomas** are characteristically neoplasms of children and young adults. Patients typically present with a rapidly enlarging mediastinal mass (Fig. 17-3) manifested by respiratory embarrassment. Blood and bone marrow are uninvolved initially. Initially, the tumor is highly sensitive to radiation and corticosteroids. After a period of from 1 to several months, dissemination of the neoplasm occurs, producing progressive nodal, visceral, and marrow involvement and development of a leukemic phase. CNS involvement is common. The prognosis is poor (about 2 to 12 months survival).

      (3) **Skin-based T-cell lymphomas** are preceded by a prolonged symptomatic period in which the lymphoproliferative disorder appears rather indolent. Skin biopsies during the later stages of mycosis fungoides show extensive lymphocytic infiltration of the dermis and, to a lesser extent, the epidermis. In lymph node biopsies, nodal architecture is effaced by a diffuse lymphomatous process.

   b. **Classification of B-cell Neoplasms.**

      (1) **Chronic lymphocytic leukemia** is a heterogeneous group of diseases in which there is proliferation of small, usually B, lymphocytes. Cells of origin may be marrow-based or arise from nonfollicular center lymphocyte-plasma cell systems in nodes (as in well-differentiated lymphocytic lymphoma).

         (a) **Diagnosis.** Marrow may show diffuse or focal infiltrates of transformed lymphocytes. Peripheral blood is frequently involved.

         (b) **Clinical Data.** Chronic lymphocytic leukemia is a common form of leukemia, which affects older patients and has an indolent course. Splenomegaly and peripheral adenopathy are common. Rarely, patients die in an aggressive phase—equivalent to blast transformation in myeloid leukemia—in which large lymphoid cells are detected in nodes (Richter's syndrome).

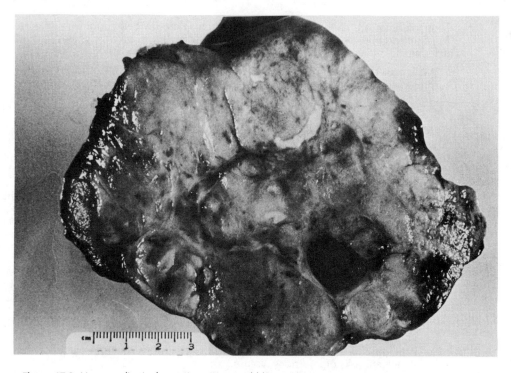

Figure 17-3. Huge mediastinal mass in a 14-year-old boy with respiratory distress. Thymic lymphoma.

(2) **Follicular center cell lymphomas**, lymphomas of effector cell precursors, comprise 30 percent of nonHodgkin's lymphomas and are the most common lymphomas in adults. Although these are generally rather indolent neoplasms, compatible with a long natural history, late-stage transformation into highly aggressive lymphomas commonly occurs. Follicular center cell lymphomas usually develop in superficial or retroperitoneal nodes (Fig. 17-4). Follicular center cell lymphomas have been divided into various cell types, representing the morphological variations of B cells during in vivo transformation: small and large cleaved follicular center cell lymphomas and small and large noncleaved or transformed follicular center cell lymphomas.

  (a) **Burkitt's lymphomas**, probably arising from small transformed follicular center cell lymphomas, are distinct clinical and pathological entities occurring most frequently in Africa.

    (i) **Clinical Data.** This primarily extralymphatic tumor, in its typical African form, arises in the jawbones, but it also has a predilection for abdominal viscera, ovaries, breasts, the epidural space, and meninges. Bone marrow is involved with peripheral blood manifestations. In its advanced forms, the disorder is rapidly fatal, but many patients are highly responsive to chemotherapeutic agents.

    (ii) **Histology.** The neoplastic cells are small, transformed lymphocytes, which are uniform in size and shape. Mitoses and macrophages are abundant, with the macrophages producing the nonspecific "starry sky" appearance.

  (b) **Multiple myeloma** is a plasma cell neoplasm primarily involving the bone marrow with minimal significant extension to extraosseous sites.

    (i) **Clinical Data and Pathophysiology.** Most patients are middle-aged to elderly and present with anemia, infection, and bone fractures. If the malignant clone retains the capacity to produce complete immunoglobulin molecules, the patient demonstrates the classic serum **immunoglobulin spike**, consisting of M protein-immunoglobulin molecules of a single light-chain type and a single heavy-chain class. The production of normal immunoglobulins is suppressed, as though the malignant plasma cells had replaced the normal B cells and their function, predisposing the patient to infection.

    (ii) **Diagnosis.** Massive replacement of marrow by homogeneous sheets of plasma cells is diagnostic of multiple myeloma.

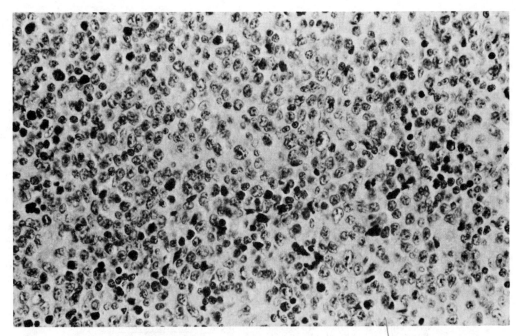

Figure 17-4. Malignant lymphoma of follicular center cells (B-cell neoplasm). The predominant cell is a cleaved lymphocyte. The pattern is diffuse [hematoxylin and eosin (H and E) stain, high power]. *starry sky appearance*

   (iii) Prognosis. Life expectancy in myeloma is usually a few years. Death may be caused by infection, the consequences of renal involvement and hypercalcemia, the development of amyloidosis, or occasionally the transformation to an aggressive B-cell lymphoma—the immunoblastic sarcoma of B cells.

  (c) Amyloidosis is characterized by the deposition in tissues of a highly organized glycoprotein material, which has a fibrillar appearance in the electron microscope (EM). This substance, deposited in smooth muscle, heart, tongue, nerves, kidney, carpal ligaments, skin, submandibular glands, and joints, is responsible for the uptake of Congo red stain and for polarized birefringence. Once formed, amyloid fibrils are not easily removed. The clinical picture is a composite of organ or tissue derangements resulting from the accumulation of amyloid. The amyloid fibrils of primary amyloidosis are frequently of immunoglobulin origin, consisting of portions of the light chains. Secondary amyloidosis is associated with myeloma, chronic infections, or rheumatoid arthritis.

  (d) Immunoblastic sarcomas of B cells are neoplastic proliferations of immunoblasts (transformed lymphocytes) often showing plasmacytic differentiation.

   (i) Clinical Data and Pathophysiology. These sarcomas usually are observed in patients with chronic abnormal immune disorders, such as Sjögren's syndrome, and congenital immune defects. They are also seen in recipients of immunosuppression. Most patients are unresponsive to therapy and have a very poor prognosis.

   (ii) Diagnosis is based on marrow or lymph node biopsy wherein plasmacytic immunoblasts are the predominant cells.

V. DISORDERS OF UNDETERMINED CELLULAR ORIGIN

 A. LEUKEMIC RETICULOENDOTHELIOSIS (hairy cell leukemia) is a proliferative disorder, most likely a malignant neoplasm, affecting primarily the spleen and marrow. A leukemic phase is common. The cell of origin is not known.

  1. Clinical Data. Leukemic reticuloendotheliosis affects adults who present with symptoms related to pancytopenia or splenomegaly. The clinical course is often prolonged for several years, even without therapy.

  2. Pathology. Marrow biopsies show focal or generalized effacement of architecture and infiltration by small cells with abundant **clear cytoplasms** and ovoid, folded nuclei. The peripheral blood usually contains numerous hairy cells with a distinctive appearance. The spleen is usually enlarged, shows effacement of white pulp, preservation of sinuses, and infiltration by hairy cells.

B. HODGKIN'S DISEASE

1. **Definition.** Hodgkin's disease is a neoplastic disease or diseases primarily affecting the lymph nodes, with later involvement of the liver, spleen, bone marrow, and lungs. Proliferating cells seem to be **mononuclear Reed-Sternberg** cells and possibly binucleate or multinucleated types of Reed-Sternberg cells. The cell of origin is probably lymphoid. Hodgkin's disease is a heterogeneous group of related lymphoid neoplasms, which together comprise approximately 45 percent of the malignant lymphomas. The distinctive features that delineate Hodgkin's disease from other malignant lymphomas include an aneuploid tumor cell line, Reed-Sternberg cells, and the invariable presence of a "host reaction," consisting of a variable admixture of lymphocytic elements, plasma cells, macrophages, eosinophils, and granulocytes. Hodgkin's disease is accompanied by early and profound systemic immunologic dysfunction. Cell-mediated immunologic responses are most severely depressed. Patients with Hodgkin's disease are therefore particularly susceptible to viral, mycobacterial, and fungal infections.

2. Hodgkin's disease is divided into four histopathological subtypes, each of which has particular clinicopathological correlations.

   a. **Nodular Sclerosis.**

      (1) **Clinical Data.** Comprising about 45 percent of all cases of Hodgkin's disease, it is most common in adolescents and young adults (Fig. 17-5). There is a strong association with initial involvement in the anterior mediastinum (thymus).

      (2) **Pathology.** Histologically, fibrous connective tissue bands demarcate involved tissues into nodules containing the tumor cells and accompanying cells of the immunologic reaction. Distinctive mononuclear Reed-Sternberg cell variants called **lacunar cells** are usually the most numerous tumor cells present in the nodules (Fig. 17-6). Nodular sclerosis is an indolent neoplasm, and results of current therapy are excellent.

   b. **Lymphocyte Predominance.**

      (1) **Clinical Data.** Generally presenting as early stage disease in middle-aged or elderly individuals, this type comprises about 10 percent of all cases of Hodgkin's disease and has the best prognosis.

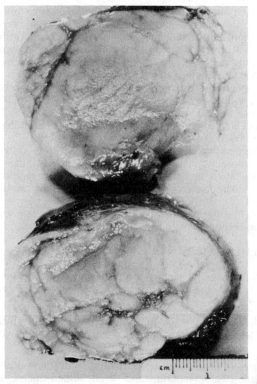

Figure 17-5. Axillary lymph node involved by Hodgkin's disease, nodular sclerosis variant. Note large size and nodular configuration.

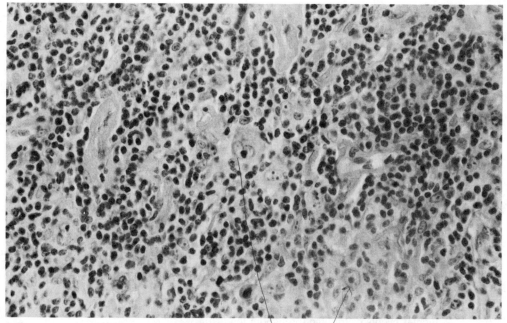

Figure 17-6. Hodgkin's disease showing mononuclear malignant cells (Reed-Sternberg variants) in center (high power).

[handwritten: Binucleate or multinucleated cell]

   (2) Pathology. The involved nodes demonstrate a rather small component of Reed-Sternberg cells dispersed in a lymphocytic and macrophagic immunologic reaction.
   c. Mixed Cellularity.
      (1) Clinical Data. Comprising about 40 percent of all cases, it is most common in middle-aged adults.
      (2) Pathology. Histologically, numerous Reed-Sternberg cells are distributed in an infiltrate in which eosinophils and plasma cells are most prominent and in which there are rather few lymphocytic elements.
   d. Lymphocyte Depletion.
      (1) Clinical Data. Comprising about 5 percent of cases, it is most common in elderly individuals who have disseminated disease and a rather poor prognosis.
      (2) Pathology. A very scanty immunologic reaction is present in the tumoral infiltrates.

VI. LYMPHADENOPATHIES OF NON-NEOPLASTIC CAUSES (WITH SPECIFIC CAUSATIVE AGENTS)

A. TOXOPLASMOSIS

   1. Clinical Data. Most patients are asymptomatic, but some have fever and sore throat. Posterior cervical nodes in young adults are typically involved.

   2. Pathology. The overall architecture of nodes is preserved, and follicles are usually prominent. Capsulitis with cellular proliferation in the capsule and in the subcapsular sinus is noted. The diagnostic feature of toxoplasmosis is the presence of macrophages in clusters both in the interfollicular areas and in the follicular centers. Rarely, toxoplasma cysts may be identified.

B. SYPHILIS

   1. Clinical Setting. Inguinal nodes usually are affected, but there may be generalized adenopathy in secondary syphilis.

   2. Pathology. Capsular inflammation and fibrosis are striking. The architecture of the nodes is preserved, and follicular centers are very active. Plasmacytosis is noted in the interfollicular areas and capsule. Spirochetes may be demonstrated by silver stain.

C. INFECTIOUS MONONUCLEOSIS. Variable distortion of the architecture is noted with obscuring of some follicular centers. The sinusoids of the nodes are generally preserved and often

are packed with cells. Generally there are large numbers of transformed lymphocytes in portions of all of the nodes, causing diagnostic confusion with malignant lymphomas.

VII. LYMPHADENITIS OF UNKNOWN CAUSES

A. DERMATOPATHIC LYMPHADENITIS is a fairly common disorder associated with a variety of chronic skin diseases. There is hyperplasia of the follicles and sinusoidal histiocytes. Ill-defined foci of histiocytes containing fat and melanin extend between the follicles.

B. ANGIOFOLLICULAR HYPERPLASIA (LYMPHOID HAMARTOMA) is a rare disorder associated with the production of solitary asymptomatic masses up to 7 cm in size and usually located in the mediastinum. Histopathologically, follicular centers contain centrally placed arterioles with a whorling of the follicular center cells, producing an appearance resembling Hassall's corpuscles or splenic follicles.

VIII. REACTIVE ADENITIS (Probably Due to Unknown Immunological Mechanisms)

A. SARCOIDOSIS

1. **Clinical Data.** This systemic granulomatous disease (probably heterogenous) is of unknown cause. In the United States young blacks are usually affected. Lungs, lymph nodes, and less commonly the liver, spleen, marrow, skin, eyes, and phalangeal bones are affected. Pulmonary dysfunction is common.

2. **Pathology.** There is typically a monotonous, recurrent pattern of small, noncaseating granulomas evenly distributed throughout the tissues.

B. IMMUNOBLASTIC ADENOPATHY (Angioimmunoblastic Lymphadenopathy)

1. **Clinical Data.** Immunoblastic lymphadenopathy affects adults of both sexes in middle and late life; the median age of onset is 60 years. In the typical advanced form, patients have fever, sweats, generalized lymphadenopathy, and hepatosplenomegaly; these symptoms are often associated with skin rash and sometimes with severe pruritus. Many patients have a polyclonal hypergammaglobulinemia and thrombocytopenia. Some patients have had recent exposure to drugs, and thus the condition is considered a hyperimmune allergic reaction. A few patients respond well to cytotoxic chemotherapy, but most do poorly.

2. **Pathology.** Although clinically distinct, the condition has often been confused with Hodgkin's disease. There are proliferations of arborizing small vessels. Immunoblasts, plasma cells, and often an amorphous, acidophilic, interstitial material are also present.

IX. DISEASES OF HISTIOCYTES (The Monocyte/Phagocyte System)

A. CLASSIFICATION OF THE HISTIOCYTIC DISORDERS

1. Neoplastic versus reactive: examples, eosinophilic granuloma; histiocytosis X, and Letterer-Siwe disease

2. Malignant neoplasms: examples, histiocytic medullary reticulosis and malignant histiocytosis

3. Lipid storage diseases

4. Reactive (agent known): example, tuberculosis

B. NEOPLASTIC VERSUS REACTIVE DISORDERS. Traditionally, diseases characterized by a proliferation of benign-appearing histiocytes containing Langerhans' granules are divided into three entities.

1. **Eosinophilic Granuloma.**
   a. **Clinical Data.** This disease may be monostotic or polyostotic or may present in the skin or lymph nodes. The lesion occurs in all age groups but is more common in the first decade of life. Bones most commonly involved are the skull, ribs, and femur. The prognosis is excellent, with good response to therapy (curettage and radiotherapy in most cases), and lesions often regress spontaneously.
   b. **Pathology.** Histologically, these lesions consist of accumulations of histiocytes with Langerhans' granules and eosinophils with varying amounts of giant cells and necrosis.

2. **Hand-Schüller-Christian disease** is composed of bone lesions, exophthalmos, and diabetes insipidus. The histologic appearance is very similar to that of eosinophilic granuloma.

    3. Letterer-Siwe Disease.
      a. Clinical Data. Letterer-Siwe disease is a systemic visceral disease from its onset. It occurs in infants less than 3 years old, is more common in males, and has an acute, usually fatal course. Skin rash and hepatosplenomegaly are usually present initially.
      b. Pathology. Lesions in bones, lymph nodes, skin, liver, lungs, and spleen show a diffuse growth of histiocytes. The lesions do not contain eosinophils or giant cells.

C. MALIGNANT HISTIOCYTOSES. Classification of these uncommon diseases is difficult since functional subpopulations of histiocytes have not been identified. The disorders listed below may represent the same disease.

    1. Histiocytic Medullary Reticulosis.
      a. Clinical Data. Signs and symptoms are fever, hepatosplenomegaly, lymphadenopathy, and wasting, followed by jaundice, purpura, and anemia.
      b. Pathology. There is a proliferation throughout hematopoietic and lymphoid tissues of erythrophagocytic histiocytes with nuclear atypia. Nodal lymphoid tissues characteristically show partial or complete filling of medullary and subcapsular sinusoids with masses of noncohesive neoplastic cells. The overall architecture is preserved, however, and only rare areas of infiltration of cortical or capsular tissue are found.

    2. Malignant Histiocytosis.
      a. Clinical Data. Malignant histiocytosis is an almost invariably fatal neoplasm that may occur at any age (the average age on onset is the fourth decade). In most series it shows a male to female predominance of approximately 2:1. Presenting features include fever, lymphadenopathy, hepatosplenomegaly, skin lesions, and pancytopenia. Clinically malignant histiocytosis is often confused with other hematopoietic or lymphoid malignancies.
      b. Pathology. Histologically lymph nodes show extensive accumulations of neoplastic histiocytes involving most portions of the individual nodes.

D. LIPID STORAGE DISEASES (LIPIDOSES). Genetic abnormalities in the catabolism of complex glycolipids, gangliosides, and globosides cause the lipid storage diseases. Reticuloendothelial disorders are rare hereditary causes of splenic enlargement and peripheral pancytopenia. Hereditary lipidoses are not caused by excessive production of the abnormally accumulated material. Enzymatic impairment of macrophage degradation of the membrane remnants of effete cells results in lysosomal accumulation of lipid. The metabolite accumulates in the central nervous system and in macrophages and produces a clinical disease according to the extent of displacement of normal tissue and the disruption of the tissue function.

    1. Gaucher's Disease. Deficiency of the enzyme **glucocerebrosidase**, with resultant accumulation of the sphingolipid glucocerebroside, causes Gaucher's disease. The disease is inherited as an autosomal recessive trait and is particularly prevalent among Ashkenazi Jews. Proliferation of histiocytes leads to hepatosplenomegaly and erosion of the cortices of long bones. Anemia and thrombocytopenia are mainly due to hypersplenism, with a possible element of decreased production due to cellular infiltration of the bone marrow. Diagnosis is made by identification of the Gaucher's cells in bone marrow or spleen aspirates (Fig. 17-7).

    2. Niemann-Pick disease is an autosomal recessive disease due to deficiency of the enzyme **sphingomyelinase.** As with other lipidoses, there is an increased prevalence among Ashkenazi Jews. Proliferation of "foamy histiocytes" containing sphingomyelin occurs in the liver, spleen, lymph nodes, and occasionally skin. A brown pigment, ceroid, also accumulates in these macrophages. Affected infants usually show hepatosplenomegaly and neurologic deterioration. No specific therapy is currently available.

    3. Tay-Sachs disease is an autosomal recessive disorder due to a defect of **hexosaminidase A**. Gangliosides accumulate in various organs, predominantly in the brain. Affected infants, mostly of Jewish ancestry, die before the age of three. They suffer from blindness and mental retardation.

X. DISORDERS OF THE SPLEEN

    A. HYPOFUNCTION. Congenital immunodeficiency states, radiation, chemotherapy, and steroids interfere with splenic function as does autoinfarction of the spleen as occurs in sickle cell anemia. Surgical removal of the spleen (e.g., in cases of trauma) also leads to asplenism or hypofunction. Infiltrative diseases (e.g., granulomas, neoplasms, and amyloidosis) can destroy sufficient splenic tissue as will cause hyposplenism. Most patients who suffer solely from

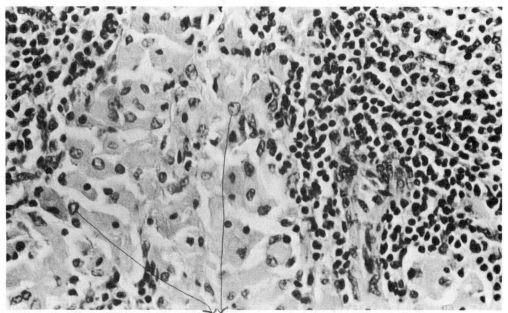

Figure 17-7. Gaucher's cells in the spleen. Large cells with clear cytoplasm are the diagnostic elements [hematoxylin and eosin (H and E) stain, high power].

hyposplenism or asplenia (especially after surgery) show an increased incidence of gram-positive bacterial infections (particularly pneumococcus) but apparently compensate well in regard to other splenic functions.

B. DISORDERS OF THE RED PULP. Diseases involving the splenic cords produce cord widening by accumulating abnormal blood cells (red cells and platelets) or by the infiltration of neoplastic and reactive cells.

    1. Congenital spherocytosis results in cord widening because the abnormal red cells cannot traverse the maze of the splenic cords. This stagnation and retention of red cells lead to their premature destruction.

    2. In **portal hypertension**, widened cords occur because of histiocytic proliferation and fibrosis, resulting in red cell stagnation.

    3. The **lipidoses** produce similar functional defects in the pulp by accumulations of histiocytes.

C. HYPERSPLENISM is any situation in which the spleen destroys excessive quantities of blood cells (red cells, white cells, or platelets). The spleen is usually enlarged and frequently palpable upon physical examination.

    1. Hypersplenism may result from **abnormal blood cells** and their increased sequestration by the spleen, **antibodies** produced by lymphocytes, which coat the blood elements and make them easy prey for splenic phagocytes, or **stagnation** and **hemoconcentration** of blood cells, leading to their increased vulnerability to splenic phagocytes.

    2. Causes of splenomegaly include hemolytic disorders, portal hypertension, infiltrative disorders and neoplasms—lymphatic, hematopoietic, or histiocytic.

    3. Consequences of Splenomegaly. In addition to the problems of the disease producing it, splenomegaly can lead to left upper quadrant pain, gastric discomfort, and, most serious and life threatening, spontaneous rupture of the spleen.

D. TUMORS AND CYSTS OF THE SPLEEN

    1. Primary tumors of the spleen are rare, although some patients with hematopoietic diseases may present with splenomegaly, and the diagnosis of a malignant lymphoma or leukemic reticuloendotheliosis may be made initially upon examination of the spleen.

2. The spleen is commonly involved in malignant lymphomas of all types, including Hodgkin's disease, and in all the leukemias (chronic and acute), including myeloproliferative disorders and histiocytic neoplasms.

3. Benign cysts of the spleen may represent parasitic *(Echinococcus)* diseases or mesothelial-lined (peritoneal inclusion) cysts. More commonly encountered, at least in the United States, are "false" cysts without recognizable lining cells, which represent encapsulated hematomas and probably are related always to trauma.

STUDY QUESTIONS

Directions: Each question below contains five suggested answers. Choose the **one best** response to each question.

1. Sickle cell disease (hemoglobin [Hb] SS) results in each of the following complications EXCEPT

(A) leg ulcers
(B) spleen infarction
(C) cholelithiasis
(D) pancreatitis
(E) osteomyelitis

2. Each of the following conditions can be confused histologically with malignant lymphoma EXCEPT

(A) toxoplasmotic lymphadenitis
(B) syphilitic lymphadenitis
(C) herpesvirus lymphadenitis
(D) infectious mononucleosis lymphadenopathy
(E) dermatopathic lymphadenopathy

reduction of productive capacity of bone marrow due to space occupying lesions → bone marrow depression

3. Myelophthisic anemia can occur in patients with each of the following conditions EXCEPT

(A) miliary tuberculosis
(B) carcinomatosis
(C) osteopetrosis
(D) multiple myeloma
(E) uremia

not due to space occupying lesion but bone marrow depression due to toxin production.

4. All of the following associations with human acute leukemia are valid EXCEPT

(A) viruses
(B) irradiation
(C) antibiotics
(D) antineoplastic drugs
(E) benzene compounds

5. For 2 weeks a 36-year-old man has complained of purpura and bleeding of the gums. On examination, he is pale and his temperature is 39° C. This clinical picture is compatible with

(A) chronic lymphocytic leukemia
(B) acute lymphocytic leukemia
(C) chronic myelogenous leukemia
(D) acute myelogenous leukemia
(E) infectious mononucleosis

6. Iron deficiency anemia in males most often is caused by which of the following disorders?

(A) Severe liver disease
(B) Cardiomyopathy
(C) Peptic ulcer
(D) Pancreatitis
(E) Renal failure

7. A 14-year-old boy who has difficulty breathing is brought to the emergency room. Examination discloses moderate respiratory distress, fever to 39° C, and skin pallor. His white blood count is 100,000 with 95 percent lymphoblasts. To evaluate his respiratory distress, a chest x-ray is taken, which most likely shows

(A) right lower lobe pneumonia
(B) bilateral pleural effusion
(C) cardiomegaly
(D) a mediastinal mass
(E) diffuse pulmonary fibrosis

Blast transformation to acute — leukemia

8. Blast crisis may occur during the course of each of the following disorders EXCEPT

(A) polycythemia vera
(B) chronic myelogenous leukemia
(C) chronic lymphocytic leukemia
(D) Hodgkin's disease
(E) myelofibrosis

9. Nonimmune hemolytic anemia can be recognized in patients with

(A) systemic lupus erythematosus
(B) malarial infection
(C) chronic lymphocytic leukemia
(D) Hodgkin's disease
(E) Rh incompatibility

10. Which of the following indicators of hemolytic anemia is always diagnostic?

(A) Red blood cell antibodies
(B) Red blood cell destruction
(C) Red blood cell enzyme deficiency
(D) Hemolysis
(E) Abnormal hemoglobin

11. Which of the following statements concerning sickle cell anemia is true?

(A) It occurs in 20 percent of the black population of the United States
(B) It produces splenomegaly
(C) It results from decreased hemoglobin synthesis
(D) It is accompanied by iron deficiency
(E) It protects against malaria

12. A 42-year-old man presented with acute leg thrombophlebitis. After symptomatic therapy and the administration of warfarin for several months, he was well for 1 year, when another episode of thrombophlebitis occurred, complicated by pulmonary embolism. Appropriate therapy is administered for the acute problems, but the diagnostic approach includes

(A) a complete blood count, bone marrow biopsy, and liver-spleen scan
(B) a complete blood count, measurement of fibrin split products and prothrombin time
(C) a complete blood count, clotting factor assay, and abdominal tomography
(D) a clotting factor assay, intravenous pyelogram, and bone marrow biopsy
(E) a clotting factor assay, measurement of prothrombin time, and a venogram

Directions: The question below contains four suggested answers of which **one or more** is correct. Choose the answer

A   if **1, 2, and 3** are correct
B   if **1 and 3** are correct
C   if **2 and 4** are correct
D   if **4** is correct
E   if **1, 2, 3, and 4** are correct

13. The similarities between thalassemia major and thalassemia minor include which of the following?

(1) Severity of anemia
(2) Incidence of infection
(3) Life span
(4) Familial occurrence

ANSWERS AND EXPLANATIONS

1. The answer is D. [*II A 3 a (3) (a)*] Leg ulcers and spleen infarction result from small vessel occlusion by sickled red cells. Cholelithiasis results from hemolysis and excessive bilirubin; this problem also occurs in patients with other congenital hemolytic disorders. Sickle cell patients are prone to develop a variety of infections—osteomyelitis, especially that caused by unusual organisms (*Salmonella*), is a very serious one.

2. The answer is E. (*VII A*) The histiocytic reaction in toxoplasmosis infection can be confused with Hodgkin's disease as can the extensive capsular and nodal fibrosis of syphilitic lymphadenitis. Viral infections of lymph nodes may efface normal architecture, and reactive lymphocytes can appear abnormal. However, the lack of one-cell lymphocyte population proliferation, as would be seen in a lymphoma, is a useful diagnostic feature. Dermatophatic lymph node enlargement reflects changes that are seen in nodes draining excoriated skin lesions; such nodes show follicular hyperplasia and melanin in sinus histiocytes. The latter feature is useful in the diagnosis. No evidence suggesting malignancy is seen.

3. The answer is E. [*II A 3 b (3)*] Myelophthisis is reduction of the productive capacity of the bone marrow through the presence of space-occupying lesions. Granulomata replace marrow in tuberculosis. Metastatic carcinoma and myeloma produce mass lesions, replacing and destroying marrow. Osteopetrosis involves excessive bone formation with little or ineffective resorption; hence, marrow spaces are overgrown by bone. The anemia of uremia, however, is not related to space-occupying lesions but to a toxic effect, resulting in marrow depression.

4. The answer is A. (*IV B 2*) Although viruses have been shown to be associated with leukemia in animals, this association has not been proved in man. Irradiation has been linked with the subsequent development of leukemia, probably as a result of marrow stem cell damage leading to chromosomal aberrations and consequent malignancy. Certain antibiotics and benzene compounds, which share specific chemical configurations, have also been associated with leukemia development. Finally, chemotherapeutic agents, by causing marrow damage, have been implicated.

5. The answer is D. (*IV B 6 b*) The short history of the symptoms and the signs of anemia, infection, and thrombocytopenia indicate acute myelogenous leukemia. The duration of symptoms excludes both chronic lymphocytic leukemia and chronic myelogenous leukemia. Acute lymphocytic leukemia rarely, if ever, is present beyond the pediatric age. Purpura, evidence of anemia, and thrombocytopenia are unlikely to occur in mononucleosis.

6. The answer is C. [*II A b (1)*] Peptic ulcer leads to chronic blood (therefore, iron) loss. Although severe liver disease may produce upper gastrointestinal bleeding (varices), the bleeding is usually acute, not chronic. The anemia of renal failure is due to toxic damage to the marrow; the iron stores are normal. Cardiomyopathy and pancreatitis are not normally associated with anemia.

7. The answer is D. [*IV C 2 a (2)*] The patient has T-cell acute lymphoblastic leukemia with a thymic mass. Although he might have an associated infection, it is not the cause of his respiratory distress. Pleural effusion can occur but would rarely be present at the time of the initial diagnosis. Neither cardiomegaly nor diffuse pulmonary fibrosis are relevant to this case.

8. The answer is D. (*II B 1*) Polycythemia vera and myelofibrosis are chronic conditions in which dysplastic marrow elements occur. Each carries a risk of acute leukemia, although the risk in polycythemia vera is lower than that in myelofibrosis. Both chronic myelogenous and chronic lymphocytic leukemia can undergo blast transformation to acute leukemia; however, this occurs more commonly in the myeloid type.

9. The answer is B. [*II A 3 a (3) (b)*] Of the distractors, only malarial infection is a nonimmune disorder. Autoantibodies, which lyse red cells, can be demonstrated in lupus erythematosus and in chronic lymphocytic leukemia. In Rh incompatibility, nonhost antibodies lyse red cells.

10. The answer is B. [*II A 3 a (3) (b)*] Although red blood cell antibodies, red blood cell enzyme deficiency, hemolysis, and abnormal hemoglobin at times can each be indicative of hemolytic anemia, only red cell destruction is always diagnostic.

11. The answer is E. [*II A 3 a (3) (a)*] Sickle cell anemia occurs in only 1 percent to 2 percent of the United States black population, although sickle cell trait may occur in up to 10 percent. The spleen is tiny due to autoinfarction. The anemia results from production of abnormal hemoglobin and the subsequent hemolysis of the red blood cells containing the hemoglobin; therefore, it cannot be the result of decreased hemoglobin synthesis. Since the hemolyzed cell products release iron back into the reticuloendothelial system, there is excess, rather than deficient, iron. In parts of the world where malaria is endemic, individuals with sickle cell anemia fare better.

12. The answer is C. (*III A*) It is necessary to assess deficiencies or excesses in clotting factors that could lead to increased coagulability; therefore, polycythemia (either primary or secondary) with associated vascular stasis must be ruled out by a blood count. To rule out an underlying malignant tumor that can produce hypercoagulability (especially pancreatic cancer), abdominal tomography is very helpful. By taking a complete blood count, assessing the clotting factor, and taking an abdominal tomograph, the three most important underlying reasons for the patient's clinical problem have been evaluated.

13. The answer is D (4). [*II A 3 a (3) (a) (iii)*] Of the choices, the only similarity between thalassemia major and thalassemia minor is that both conditions are determined genetically. Whereas anemia is marked in thalassemia major, it may be mild or nonexistent in thalassemia minor. Infection is a common complication only in thalassemia major; most patients with this disease die in young adulthood or before, but, in contrast, thalassemia minor is compatible with a normal life span.

18
Head and Neck

I. INTRODUCTION. This chapter will review the lesions that commonly affect the mucous membranes of the mouth as well as those that affect the nasopharynx, larynx, jaw, and salivary glands.

II. MOUTH

A. CONGENITAL ABNORMALITIES. These malformations may be hereditary.

1. Cleft lip occurs usually in the upper lip and is due to the failure of union of the globular processes with the maxilla.

2. Cleft palate is caused by premature closure of the coronal or lambdoid sutures and may involve the soft, the hard, or both palates. It usually is associated with cleft lip, and in such cases the nasal cavities communicate with the oral area, interfering with feeding.

3. Fordyce's disease, a benign asymptomatic condition, is characterized by the presence of painless yellow-to-white granules in the mucosa of the cheeks, lips, and gingivae. The plaques consist of displaced ectopic sebaceous glands.

B. INFLAMMATIONS. Inflammation of the oral mucosa is called **stomatitis**, and the term **gingivostomatitis** is used when the inflammation also involves the gingiva. These conditions are produced usually by ill-fitting dentures or poor dental hygiene.

1. Herpetic gingivostomatitis is a disease caused by herpes simplex and is characterized by the development of vesicular lesions that fuse and rupture, forming small ulcers (Fig. 18-1).
  a. These lesions occur most frequently in infants and children, who commonly present with soreness of the oral cavity, malaise, and fever.
  b. The disease resolves within 7 to 12 days.

2. Moniliasis is caused by *Candida albicans* and occurs predominantly in children with neglected oral hygiene and in adults who have debilitating diseases or who are receiving immunosuppressive therapy. The lesions appear as white elevated patches, which are scattered over the oral mucosa, tongue, palate, and pharynx. Confluence of these lesions may lead to the formation of extensive membranes consisting of a mixture of necrotic epithelia, fungal organisms, and acute inflammatory cells. If the disease advances, systemic involvement of organs may occur.

3. Aphthous stomatitis is a painful condition characterized by yellow-white ulcers of different sizes, the etiology of which remains unknown.
  a. Histologically, the epithelium is preserved, but there is fibrinous exudate in varying amounts beneath it.
  b. The duration of the ulcers varies from 7 to 10 days, but chronic conditions lasting years may occur.

4. Syphilis in any stage can involve the oral mucosa. The primary stage is characterized by chancres, the second stage by patches in the oral mucosa and macules on the tongue, and the third stage by gummas in the hard or soft palate and glossitis (inflammation of the tongue). Histologically, there is marked lymphoplasmocytic infiltration more prominently around the small- and medium-sized vessels.

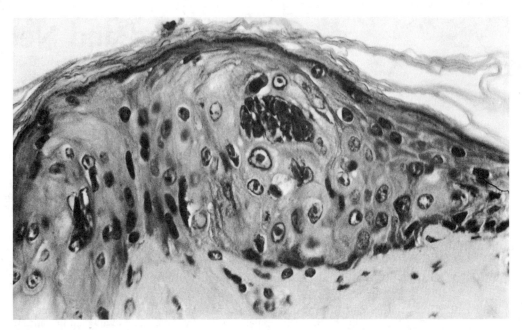

Figure 18-1. High-power view of herpes stomatitis. Notice the multinuclear inclusion cell characteristic of herpes infection.

C. BENIGN TUMORS AND TUMOR-LIKE CONDITIONS

1. **Gingival hyperplasia** occurs predominantly in patients receiving Dilantin therapy. The gingiva appears as a pink lobulated mass due to the proliferation of collagenous tissue with new blood vessel formation. This abnormality usually disappears after the drug is discontinued.

2. A **ranula** is a unilateral cyst on the floor of the mouth near the frenulum linguae. It varies in size and is believed to be a retention cyst that results from mechanical interference with secretions of the sublingual glands, or it is a remnant of a branchial cleft cyst.

3. A **mucocele** is a benign cyst that occurs predominantly on the lips and is characterized by pools of mucus and inflammatory cells within the minor salivary glands.

4. **Epulis** is a tumor-like mass located in the gingiva and is characterized by the presence of sessile or pedunculated masses of rubbery consistency, red-blue or pink in color. It is situated on the outer surface of the gum and involves the mandible more often than the maxilla. Histologically, it consists of a fibrous stroma in which numerous multinucleated giant cells are seen mixed with chronic inflammatory cells.

5. **Fibroma** occurs predominantly on the inner surface of the cheeks and lips. Usually it follows irritation from dentures or other trauma to the area. It is an exophytic type of soft tissue proliferation with chronic inflammatory cells covered by squamous mucosa that may be either thickened or atrophic.

6. **Granular cell myoblastoma** is one of the most common benign tumors occurring in the tongue. Histologically, it is identical to those seen in soft tissues. Hyperplasia of the squamous mucosa overlying the lesion may simulate cancer.

D. LEUKOPLAKIA is regarded by some as a precancerous condition occurring in the mucous membranes. The lesion is more common in males than in females. Chronic irritation and trauma to the area are believed to be the local etiological factors.

1. **Clinical Data.** The lesion consists of one or several white patches not less than 5 mm in diameter with raised, ill-defined borders.

2. **Histologically**, there is hyperkeratosis, parakeratosis, thickening of the stratified squamous

mucosa, and varying degrees of cellular atypia, especially in the basal layer. Inflammation may be present in the underlying connective tissue.

E. SQUAMOUS CELL CARCINOMA OF THE MOUTH

1. **Incidence.** Cancer of the mouth is an important clinical problem, constituting about 5 to 10 percent of all malignant tumors. The lips, larynx, and tongue are the sites most often involved. The most common malignant lesion of the oral mucous membranes is **squamous cell carcinoma**.

2. **Etiology.**
   a. Cancer of the tongue and larynx occurs often in smokers, especially in those who smoke and drink heavily.
   b. There is a high incidence in tobacco chewers of buccal mucosa tumors, especially at the site in the mouth where tobacco is held.
   c. Carcinoma of the lips affects pipe smokers and individuals chronically exposed to sunlight.

3. **Clinical Data.** The lesion starts as a small indurated plaque, nodule, or ulcer, which may increase in size and project as a large cauliflower-like mass, interfering with speech and chewing and destroying the adjacent tissues.

4. **Histology.**
   a. Carcinoma in situ is considered a precursor of invasive cancer and may be found at the margins of an obvious cancer. It is characterized by immaturity and disorganization of the squamous epithelium, with pleomorphism and atypia of individual cells. Mitoses are present. The lesion is limited by an intact basement membrane.
   b. Infiltrating carcinoma is usually well differentiated, exhibits abundant keratin formation, and invades adjacent tissues (Fig. 18-2).

5. **Prognosis** depends on several factors such as degree of differentiation, size of the primary tumor, depth of invasion, and metastatic spread. Multiplicity is commonly associated with a poor prognosis.

6. These tumors frequently **metastasize** by lymphatics to the neck lymph nodes.

7. **Treatment** usually depends on the site and size of the tumor and the surgical accessibility. If surgical resection is possible, a radical lymph node dissection should be performed, followed by radiation of the involved area.

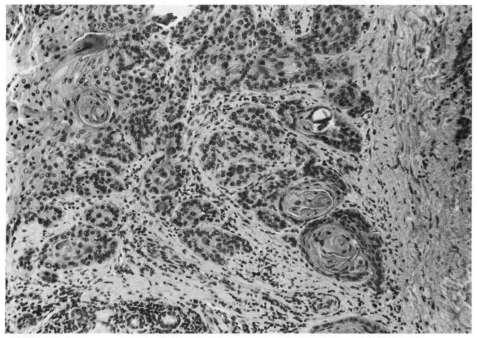

Figure 18-2. Low-power view of an invasive well-differentiated squamous cell carcinoma of the larynx. Notice the keratin formation.

III. NASOPHARYNX. The pharynx is encircled by aggregations of lymphoid tissue forming the tonsillar ring of Waldeyer (the nasopharyngeal, tubal, palatine, and lingual tonsils). These lymphoid aggregates are covered by either pseudostratified columnar epithelium or stratified squamous epithelium.

A. INFLAMMATIONS

1. **Tonsillitis** is the acute or chronic inflammation of the tonsils, which appear enlarged and red. Histologically, the crypts of squamous epithelia contain numerous polymorphonuclear leukocytes and desquamated epithelial cells. The causative agents are most commonly *Streptococcus hemolyticus* and pneumococcus, but tonsillitis may result from viruses and other organisms.

2. **Pharyngitis.** Infections of the oropharynx are commonly caused by viruses or bacteria, such as streptococci and less frequently staphylococci. There is intense infiltration by inflammatory cells, edema, and hyperplasia of tissues. With antibiotics, the process resolves in a few days.

B. BENIGN TUMORS

1. **Nasal polyp** is a nonspecific proliferation of edematous stroma and nasal mucosa found in patients with clinical histories of allergies. It is a very common condition.

2. **Angiofibroma** is an infrequent tumor that predominantly affects males between the ages of 12 and 25 years.
   a. **Clinical Data.** The characteristic symptoms are nasal obstruction, epistaxis, and nasal discharge.
   b. **Grossly**, the lesion is a firm tumor of rubbery consistency, gray or purple-red in color, and usually with a broad attachment to the wall of the nasopharynx. The surface may become ulcerated.
   c. **Microscopically**, the tumor is composed of vascular fibrous connective tissue with intermingled spindle-shaped cells and chronic inflammatory cells, such as lymphocytes and plasma cells. The vessels are of small- to medium-capillary size. The vascularity is so pronounced that the tumor may be confused with a hemangioma.
   d. **Treatment.** Removal of the lesion is a difficult and dangerous procedure because of potential severe hemorrhage, which may be difficult to control. An endocrine pathogenesis has been suspected. As an androgen-dependent tumor, it may respond to hormonal manipulation. Angiofibroma has a tendency to spontaneous remission.

C. LYMPHOEPITHELIOMA

1. **Clinical Data.** This malignant tumor occurs in young adults, often of Oriental lineage. It can appear in any site of the upper respiratory tract but most frequently is found in the lateral wall around the ostium of the eustachian tube. The patient usually presents with nasal obstruction, bleeding, middle ear disease, cranial nerve palsies, and enlarged lymph nodes in the neck.

2. **Pathology.** There is an admixture of lymphoid elements with malignant epithelial cells identical to those of a poorly differentiated squamous cell carcinoma. The lymphoid cells are not considered neoplastic.

3. **Prognosis.** This tumor grows rapidly and has an early tendency to metastasize. However, only the epithelial component is present in the metastases.

4. **Treatment.** The treatment of choice is radiotherapy as surgical control of this cancer is virtually impossible.

IV. LARYNX

A. INFLAMMATION of the larynx, or **laryngitis**, occurs usually as part of any inflammatory process in the respiratory tract. Special attention should be paid when it occurs in children because significant edema may cause laryngeal obstruction with difficulties in breathing. Hoarseness is the most common symptom of laryngeal disease.

B. TUMORS

1. **Polyps** are sessile or pedunculated nodules that occur predominantly in the vocal cords. Laryngeal polyps are most common in adult males and generally cause hoarseness.
   a. **Pathology.** A laryngeal polyp is composed of a proliferative stroma covered by benign squamous epithelium. The stroma may be very vascular and exhibit varying degrees of chronic inflammation.

   b. Treatment. These benign lesions are best treated with surgical excision.
   2. **Papillomatosis** is probably of viral origin.
      a. Clinical Data. The lesion can occur at any age, including childhood. It is a true neoplasm composed of friable nodules or excrescences located on the true vocal cords.
      b. Histology. There is a central core of fibrous tissue covered by squamous epithelium. This tumor is believed to predispose to carcinoma, although malignant transformation is rare in children.

C. CARCINOMA

   1. The most common epithelial tumor of the larynx is **squamous cell carcinoma**, similar to that arising in the oral cavity. It occurs in situ or as an invasive form. Prognosis is directly related to the extent (i.e., stage) of the tumor (Fig. 18-3).
   2. **Verrucous carcinoma** has a gross appearance of a large fungating papillary growth. Histologically, it is a very well-differentiated tumor and may be difficult to diagnose. Resection is the treatment of choice. Radiotherapy should not be used because it may alter the biological behavior of the lesion to that of a highly aggressive neoplasm.

V. JAW

   A. OSTEOMYELITIS. Inflammation of the bone can occur in an acute or chronic form. The chronic variety is usually secondary to a dental or periodontal infection. The radiological and pathological features are identical to those seen in any other bone.

   B. CYSTS of the maxilla and mandible may arise as a result of a developmental defect (odontogenic) or secondarily to inflammation of the dental pulp (nonodontogenic).

   1. **Odontogenic Cysts.**
      a. A **radicular cyst**, arising in epithelial dental granulomas, is the result of inflammation

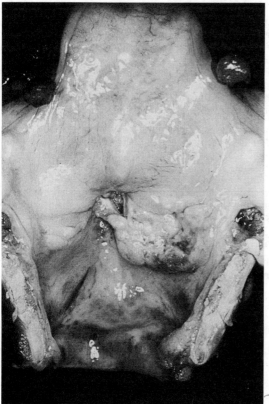

Figure 18-3. Invasive carcinoma of the larynx in the vocal cord. The tumor protrudes into the lumen of the larynx.

and necrosis of the dental pulp. This cyst is attached to the roots of the teeth and may become very large. As a rule, it is lined by squamous epithelium and, rarely, by columnar epithelium. It is the most common cyst of the jaws.

    b. A **follicular cyst** (dentigerous cyst) occurs commonly in the maxilla, where it is derived from misplaced tooth epithelial buds. The cyst is lined by stratified squamous epithelium and contains serous or mucoid material. Secondary infection may occur. The treatment of choice is curettage of the lesion, and recurrences are unusual.

    c. A **primordial cyst** usually has no special relationship with teeth, although it may appear in the area of a missing tooth. It is lined by stratified squamous epithelium, and the lumen is filled with keratinocytes.

    d. An **eruption cyst** is a small dentigerous cyst that occurs on teeth that have already erupted, and it is responsible for swelling of the gingiva. Microscopically, the cyst is lined by stratified squamous epithelium.

2. Nonodontogenic Cysts.

    a. A **nasopalatine cyst** is found in the midline of the maxilla behind the central incisors and superior to the incisive papilla. The cyst wall contains numerous mucous glands, nerves, and vessels. The epithelial lining may be squamous, transitional, or cylindrical.

    b. A **globulomaxillary cyst** is located beneath the maxillary lateral incisor and cuspid and is only symptomatic if infected. It is lined by stratified squamous cuboidal epithelium.

    c. A **nasolabial cyst** may develop from epithelial remnants at the site of fusion of the facial processes. It is situated on the alveolar process near the base of a nostril. The lining of the cyst is similar to those of the previously described cysts.

C. TUMORS

1. Adamantinoma (ameloblastoma) is a true neoplasm resembling the morphology of a developing tooth. This lesion occurs most commonly in the mandible.

    a. Clinical Data. There is a slight predilection for women between the fourth and fifth decades of life, and the lesion presents as a painless swelling, which may ulcerate and cause limitation of function in later stages.

    b. Radiologically, the lesion appears as a unilocular or multilocular radiolucency with well-defined margins. An embedded tooth may be present.

    c. Pathology. An adamantinoma is composed of epithelial strands of varying size, which resemble the enamel of a tooth. The peripheral layer of cells shows centrally placed nuclei with pink cytoplasms facing the surrounding stroma. Toward the center of the epithelial strands, the cells undergo hydropic degeneration, giving rise to cyst formation. The older the lesion is, the more cystic development there is. The origin of this lesion has not been definitely established.

    d. Prognosis. This tumor is very radioresistant and is locally aggressive and destroys bone and adjacent structures by expanding. The usual therapy is curettage or resection of the lesion, but there is often recurrence. Metastases to lungs and lymph nodes have been described, but it is not clear whether or not they represent other types of tumors.

2. An odontoma is a hamartoma arising from tissues involved in tooth formation.

    a. Clinical Data. It is often diagnosed in the second decade of life, predominantly in women. A lesion presents as an asymptomatic mass in the premolar-molar area of the mandible. Expansion into the jaws is very unusual.

    b. X-ray shows a radiolucent lesion with varying degrees of radiodensity.

    c. Pathology. The lesion is composed of varying proportions of dentin, enamel, cementum, and pulp tissue. When the tissues exist in random arrangement, the lesion is called **complex odontoma**. If the tissues follow normal formation patterns, the lesion is called **compound odontoma**.

    d. Treatment is simple curettage, and recurrences are rare.

3. A cementoma is a tumor in which the soft tissues have been partly or entirely replaced by cementum-like structures. They can be single or multiple and occur predominantly in women.

    a. Clinical Data. It appears almost always around the root of a premolar or molar and sometimes is fused to the tooth. The mandible is often more affected than the maxilla.

    b. Radiologically, a central radiopaque mass, surrounded by a uniform radiolucent shell, is present.

    c. Pathology. Histologically, irregular osteoid formation and large hyperchromatic osteoblasts are seen within a background of proliferative fibrovascular tissue.

4. Other Tumors. The jaw may be affected by benign and malignant tumors similar to those occurring in the long bones. Of these, the most common are osteoid osteomas, giant cell tumors, fibrous dysplasia, the tumors of Paget's disease, ossifying fibromas, and osteosarcomas. Secondary involvement of the mandible is common from squamous cell carcinomas of the buccal and oral mucosae. Other primary tumors, such as those of the breast and lungs, can also metastasize to the mandible and simulate primary neoplasms.

VI. SALIVARY GLANDS

A. NON-NEOPLASTIC DISEASES usually manifest themselves clinically as salivary gland enlargement.

1. **Sialadenosis** is asymptomatic enlargement of salivary glands unrelated to inflammation, salivary stones, or tumors. It occurs most frequently in the parotid glands (chipmunk facies). The diagnosis can be suggested by the history of the patient and confirmed by chemical analysis of the saliva or by needle biopsy of the parotid glands. A number of associated conditions may lead to sialadenosis.
   a. Nutritional deficiencies, especially protein malnutrition as is seen in prisoners of war and alcoholics.
   b. Ingestion of drugs containing iodides, lead, or mercury.
   c. Hormonal imbalances, especially those that occur in hypothyroidism, diabetes mellitus, and pregnancy.

2. **Sialolithiasis.**
   a. **Sites.** Stones are found in the large ducts of the major glands, with 80 percent occurring in the submandibular, less than 20 percent in the parotid, and about 1 to 2 percent in the sublingual glands.
   b. **Etiology.** The cause is unknown, but sialolithiasis probably reflects subtle abnormalities of salivary secretion, local electrolyte imbalance, and local dehydration, leading to precipitation of insoluble calcium salts.
   c. **Clinical Data.** Most stones occur in adults. Salivation produces acute pain, and there is swelling of the gland after ingestion of spicy or tart food.
   d. **Diagnosis.** If the patient history and physical examination are typical (e.g., pain on salivation and a palpable mass), the diagnosis is obvious. If stones are small or multiple, x-ray and sialography (the introduction of a radiopaque medium into major salivary ducts) are useful.
   e. **Therapy.** In many cases, manual removal of the stones under local anesthesia is curative. If, however, this proves difficult (because of the location of the stone or stones), surgical excision of the entire submandibular gland or parotid lobectomy is curative. The treated patient should watch carefully dietary intake and maintain adequate hydration to prevent a recurrence.

3. **Parotitis.**
   a. **Acute.**
      (1) Acute suppurative parotitis is seen in very young or elderly patients. Predisposing factors are debilitation and dehydration. Injection of virulent bacteria directly into the parotid duct of normal subjects will not produce the disease. About 50 percent of patients with acute parotitis have major systemic infections, and 25 percent have malignancies and usually are undergoing chemotherapy.
      (2) The organism that is cultured most frequently is *Staphylococcus aureus*.
      (3) **Treatment** consists of appropriate antibiotic therapy pursuant to culture results. Occasionally surgical drainage is required.
      (4) The approximate 20 percent mortality rate is a reflection of the seriousness of the underlying infections or tumors, rather than of the parotitis per se.
   b. **Chronic.**
      (1) Chronic recurrent parotitis can occur in the presence or absence of stones. It is characterized by recurring pain and infection, decreased secretion, and increased sodium concentration in resting saliva. Sialography demonstrates parotid duct irregularities due to stenosis and dilatation.
      (2) Submaxillary gland inflammation, in contrast to that of the parotid, is invariably due to stones.
   c. **Mikulicz's Disease, Mikulicz's Syndrome, and Sjögren's Syndrome.**
      (1) Many conditions have been included in the wastebasket diagnosis of **Mikulicz's disease**: lymphoma, tuberculosis, sarcoidosis, and salivary gland enlargement due to nutritional deficiencies. Mikulicz described 1 patient with bilateral lacrimal, submandibular, and parotid gland swelling that histologically resembled severe chronic inflammation with atrophy of these glands. It is now believed that this patient had Sjögren's syndrome.

    (2) **Mikulicz's syndrome** defines bilateral swelling of the lacrimal, submandibular, and parotid glands due to known causes such as sarcoidosis and tuberculosis. It is advisable to define the specific lesion rather than to employ the eponym.

    (3) **Sjögren's syndrome** is a **systemic condition**, presenting both inflammatory and neoplastic characteristics.

       (a) **Clinical Data.** Women, frequently postmenopausal, are afflicted more commonly than men in a ratio of 9:1. There may or may not be swelling of salivary and lacrimal glands, and it may be unilateral. The triad of dry mouth, dry eyes (due to a marked decrease in the secretion of the salivary and lacrimal glands), and arthritis is classic, although these symptoms may not always appear in one patient. The combination of xerostomia and xerophthalmia is often referred to as the "sicca syndrome." Although rheumatoid arthritis is seen in more than half of the patients, other collagen diseases, such as systemic lupus erythematosus, polyarteritis, scleroderma, and polymyositis, may also be found. Abnormal immunoglobulins (antibodies to normal salivary duct epithelium) in the serum of patients with Sjögren's syndrome have been demonstrated by immunofluorescent techniques. Although Sjögren's syndrome is a benign disease in the majority of cases, recent evidence suggests that some patients may have a predisposition to lymphoma.

       (b) **Pathology.** The histologic findings in salivary glands of patients with Mikulicz's syndrome or Sjögren's syndrome are similar. These similarities also extend to an ipsilateral isolated salivary gland mass termed **lymphoepithelial lesion of Godwin**. In each syndrome, there is atrophy of acinar tissue with fibrosis of inter- and intralobular tissue and lymphoplasmocytic infiltration. The diagnosis is confirmed by the presence of **epimyoepithelial islands**, the result of altered (metaplastic) ducts that become suspended in lymphoid tissue. They are most valuable in distinguishing the lesion from lymphoma, a diagnosis that had been made frequently in error because of marked lymphoid infiltration of the salivary glands. The distinctive epimyoepithelial islands found in Sjögren's syndrome are not present in diseases of the minor salivary glands, in which only atrophy and lymphocytic infiltration are seen.

       (c) The **diagnosis** is obvious clinically in classical cases of Sjögren's syndrome. Although needle biopsy of the parotid gland is often valuable, characteristic microscopic changes are present throughout the salivary and lacrimal system and are reflected in the minor salivary glands as well. A biopsy of these glands taken from beneath the mucosal surface of the lip can be performed as an office procedure under local anesthesia, without risking injury to the facial nerve. The simplicity and reliability of this method have made it increasingly popular.

B. NEOPLASMS. Most tumors (approximately 80 percent) of the salivary glands occur in the parotid gland; the next most common site is the submandibular gland. Excluding the major salivary glands, the palate is the most frequently affected site of salivary gland tumors.

    Most present as painless swellings. The presence of pain, functional disturbances (e.g., seventh nerve weakness), or ulceration (in minor glands) should alert one to the presence of a malignant lesion.

    The diversity of the neoplasms that can arise in salivary tissue is not exceeded in any other part of the body. Almost all salivary tissue tumors are now believed to be epithelial, either acinar or ductal cell in origin.

  1. Benign Tumors.

    a. Benign Mixed Tumor [BMT] (Pleomorphic Adenoma).

      (1) **Clinical Data.** A mixed tumor appears as an asymptomatic, slowly enlarging mass. Although it can reach an enormous size in the parotid, it does not invade the facial nerve or infiltrate the skin. This type of tumor comprises 80 to 85 percent of all salivary gland tumors. A BMT is usually found in the superficial lobe of the parotid; occasionally, it may lie on or near the seventh nerve.

      (2) **Grossly**, a BMT is well-circumscribed and, less often, encapsulated. Often, small outpouchings or satellite nodules are noted; hence, if the tumor has just been enucleated or shelled out, there is a high rate of recurrence because satellites remain (Fig. 18-4).

      (3) **Microscopically**, the cartilaginous material in a BMT has been identified as mucins of epithelial origin (Fig. 18-5). It is suggested that myoepithelial cells undergoing metaplastic change have the capacity to act as facultative chondrocytes, elaborating a matrix of mesenchymal components similar to hyaline cartilage.

      (4) **Prognosis.** A BMT may be seeded in the operative site if the tumor is incised. The

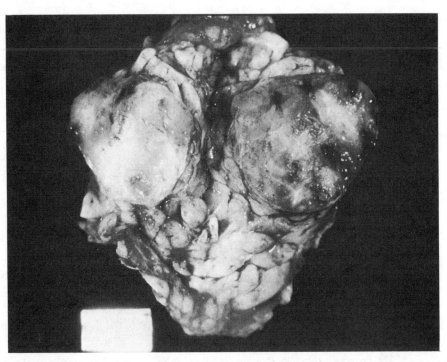

Figure 18-4. Circumscribed nodule in parotid gland with the cartilaginous appearance characteristic of a benign mixed tumor (BMT).

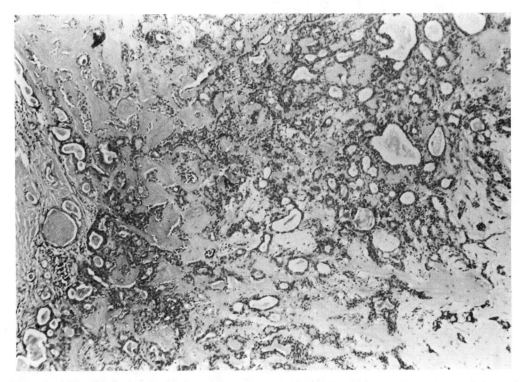

Figure 18-5. Benign mixed tumor (BMT) with fibrous and myxoid stroma and epithelial structures [tubules and glands] (low power).

patient may eventually present with multiple nodules in the scar, which may grow locally and expand. This is a recurrent BMT, not a malignancy.

b. Papillary Cystadenoma Lymphomatosum (Warthin's Tumor).

(1) **Clinical Data.** This neoplasm constitutes about 10 percent of benign salivary tumors. Warthin's tumor is found almost exclusively in the parotid gland, frequently in the tail, and occasionally separate from the main body of the gland. About 10 percent are bilateral. There is a 8:1 to 10:1 male predominance in the occurrence of this tumor.

(2) **Pathology.** Grossly, the lesion is soft, almost fluctuant, brown in color, and shows cystic areas. Its histologic appearance is that of salivary epithelium in lymphoid stroma.

(3) **Diagnosis.** Warthin's tumor, alone among salivary neoplasms, concentrates technetium 99m, which makes its identification possible preoperatively.

(4) **Prognosis.** The tumor is frequently multicentric in origin, accounting for its tendency to recur after local excision. There is no known malignant transformation.

2. Malignant Tumors.

a. Mucoepidermoid Carcinoma.

(1) **Clinical Data.** These are the most common, constituting about one-third of malignant salivary tumors. Sixty to seventy percent occur in the parotid. A greater proportion (15 to 20 percent) are found in the minor salivary glands than are found in the submaxillary glands (10 percent). The tumors often may be seen in the hard and soft palate.

(2) **Pathology.** Circumscribed but nonencapsulated, the tumor contains mucus-secreting and epidermoid cells and an intermediate type of basal or nonmucus-secreting cell. Low-grade, well-differentiated tumors, intermediate-grade lesions, or high-grade aggressive cancers are seen.

(3) **Prognosis** depends directly on the grade of the tumor. The majority of patients have an excellent prognosis; the 5-year survival has approached 90 percent. However, in approximately 10 percent of patients, the tumor takes a highly malignant course. Two-thirds of the patients with high-grade tumors develop regional node metastases, and one-third have distant metastases over a 5-year period. Death is often due to uncontrolled local and distant metastases. The low-grade tumors have a clinical course that approaches that of BMTs.

b. Malignant Mixed Tumor (MMT).

(1) **Clinical Data.** Comprising about 10 to 15 percent of salivary gland cancers, this neoplasm, which occurs twice as frequently in women as in men, most often involves the parotid gland, less so the submaxillary glands, and rarely the minor salivary glands. Patients usually have a typical clinical history: an untreated salivary gland tumor has been present for many years, with recent rapid enlargement. The average age of patients with MMT is 10 to 20 years greater than that of those with BMT. Pain and facial nerve paralysis are often seen.

(2) **Pathology.** The finding of a BMT associated with an obvious carcinoma supports the diagnosis of a MMT. Recurrences and metastases from an MMT do not show the pleomorphic spectrum of a BMT. A MMT consists of carcinomas of the single-cell type, such as epidermoid, adeno-, and spindle cell carcinomas. One of these carcinomas appears to become malignant, overgrowing and infiltrating the benign tumor.

(3) **Prognosis.** Extensive tumors, or those previously treated, have a poor prognosis. There is a high rate of local recurrence, frequent nodal metastases, and widespread bone and visceral metastases.

c. Cylindroma (Adenocystic Carcinoma).

(1) **Clinical Data.** Cylindromas occur in all salivary glands but are found in relatively greater proportion in the submaxillary and minor salivary glands. They are the most frequently encountered neoplasms of minor salivary glands, accounting for 16 to 25 percent of all tumors of these glands. Local pain is a prominent feature in one-half of the cases of cylindroma. Facial paralysis is an ominous sign.

(2) **Pathology.** The term cylindroma portrays the structural pattern of the tumors—the enclosure of mucin or hyaline cylinders within epithelial islands. Often the small, darkly stained cells appear as anastomosing cords lying in a mucoid or hyaline stroma. The neoplasm is nonencapsulated.

The most striking characteristic is the tumor's affinity for **nerves**, with growth into and within the **perineural spaces**. The tumor may extend along nerves to the base of the brain. Hence, at line of resection, the nerves should be carefully examined. In patients in whom a solid histologic pattern of a larger cell type with areas of necrosis is found, the clinical course is more rapid and fulminant.

(3) Prognosis. The lesion is deceptively slow growing but has a relentless clinical course. Because the tumor may infiltrate insidiously at margins and resection is often inadequate, recurrence is common and the **ultimate prognosis** (i.e., 10- to 15-year survival) **is poor**. While the cure rate for 5 years is approximately 75 percent, it drops to 15 to 20 percent when patients are followed for 10 to 20 years.

In the late stage, metastases to lungs, bones, and viscera are common. Silent-lung metastases are not unusual and should not deter the surgeon from trying to control local disease. Radiotherapy is a useful adjunct in controlling a local, persistent, or recurrent malignant tumor.

d. Acinic Cell Carcinoma.

(1) Clinical Data. Most acinic cell carcinomas arise in the parotid gland. Only 5 percent arise from the submaxillary gland, and rarely have these tumors been reported in minor salivary glands. Seventy percent of acinic cell tumors are found in women. Clinically, an acinic cell carcinoma mimics a mixed tumor.

(2) Pathologically, this grossly circumscribed but microscopically invasive tumor resembles the cellular lining of the acini of the parotid gland; it is composed of basophilic cells with granular cytoplasms. Cyst formation is common.

(3) Prognosis. It is a low-grade carcinoma, recurring locally and rarely producing distant metastases. Regional nodes are involved infrequently. The 5-year cure rate is 90 percent; however, the cure rate drops off if longer follow-up periods are evaluated.

e. Other Malignant Tumors. Rare examples of carcinomas, which are not easily classifiable into the above groups, do occur.

(1) Squamous cell carcinomas, originating primarily in salivary tissue, have been recorded, but it is unknown whether these are part of high-grade mucoepidermoid tumors or are carcinomas arising in a BMT in which the latter is not identified or has been destroyed by the malignancy.

(2) Malignant lymphomas may appear initially as intraparotid masses since nodes occur in the parotid gland.

(3) Metastatic tumors of the intraparotid nodes may mimic primary salivary gland cancers. Usually these are melanomas of head or eye origin or squamous cell carcinomas from the head and neck.

3. Summary of Tumors.

a. A benign tumor is usually a painless lump that gradually increases in size. Recurrence is common after inadequate resection.

b. A malignant tumor has a **variable** course depending on the histologic type. The tumor may be painful as a result of rapid growth, may produce nerve palsy through invasion of nerves, and may spread to the base of the brain. It may extend to the skin or bones. The tumor may grow to the floor of the mouth, into the tongue or pharynx; dysphagia may result, and aspiration may occur. Some patients die from the local disabling effects of the tumor, or it may invade the jugular vein or carotid artery, leading to exsanguination.

4. Treatment of Tumors. Surgery is the primary therapy for all salivary gland tumors.

a. Benign neoplasms are best treated by lobectomy when in the parotid gland, total excision when in the submandibular or sublingual gland, and wide excision when in the minor salivary glands.

b. Therapy of **malignant** neoplasms is determined by the grade, type, and extent of the lesion. High-grade, aggressive tumors may require radical excision, including sacrifice of the seventh nerve, and radical neck dissection. Wide excision usually suffices in low-grade, slowly growing cancers. Shell-out procedures are to be condemned. Radiation therapy postoperatively may be of secondary value to control microscopic residues or may be used for palliation in unresectable local disease. The value of adjuvant chemotherapy requires additional study.

STUDY QUESTIONS

Directions: Each question below contains five suggested answers. Choose the **one best** response to each question.

1. The preferred surgical treatment for a pleomorphic adenoma [benign mixed tumor (BMT)] of the parotid gland is

(A) superficial parotidectomy
(B) superficial parotidectomy with lymph node dissection
(C) radical parotidectomy
(D) radical parotidectomy with neck dissection
(E) simple enucleation of the tumor

2. The condition in which there is painless development of small yellow granules in the posterior region of the oral muscosa is called

(A) Addison's disease
(B) Albright's syndrome
(C) Fordyce's disease
(D) Warthin's tumor
(E) Vincent's disease

3. The odontogenic tumor of the jaw with morphologic features resemblinng those of a developing tooth but with invasive, highly destructive growth is called

(A) odontogenic fibroma
(B) dentinoma
(C) cementoma
(D) ameloblastoma
(E) odontogenic fibrosarcoma

Directions: Each question below contains four suggested answers of which **one or more** is correct. Choose the answer

A if **1, 2, and 3** are correct
B if **1 and 3** are correct
C if **2 and 4** are correct
D if **4** is correct
E if **1, 2, 3, and 4** are correct

4. True statements concerning sialolithiasis include

(1) it occurs most often in the parotid gland
(2) it presents clinically with painless swelling
(3) it is treated successfully with antibiotics
(4) it occurs most often in the submandibular gland

5. Characteristics that typically are associated with a benign mixed tumor (BMT) of the salivary glands include

(1) it most commonly occurs in the parotids
(2) it is a slow-growing, asymptomatic mass
(3) it does not invade the skin or nerves
(4) it is the most common salivary gland tumor

6. Characteristics of angiofibroma of the nasopharynx include

(1) frequent occurrence in young males
(2) common incidence in cigarette smokers
(3) a tendency to regress spontaneously
(4) capability of undergoing malignant transformation

7. Cylindroma is a tumor of the salivary glands that is characterized by

(1) frequent involvement of the minor salivary glands
(2) frequent nerve invasion in the area of the tumor
(3) hyaline cylinders found among the nests of epithelial cells
(4) short survival rates for affected patients

8. Lymphoepithelioma is a malignant neoplasm occurring in the nasopharynx. The tumor typically

(1) has both lymphoid and epithelial elements
(2) occurs most often in young oriental men
(3) responds to external radiation therapy
(4) undergoes spontaneous regression when untreated

9. Characteristics of Mikulicz's syndrome include

(1) swelling of lacrimal and salivary glands
(2) metastasis to regional lymph nodes
(3) association with granulomatous diseases
(4) pulmonary infiltration

10. Which of the following cysts of the mandible and maxilla may be classified as odontogenic cysts?

(1) Dentigerous
(2) Radicular
(3) Primordial
(4) Eruption

ANSWERS AND EXPLANATIONS

1. The answer is A. *(VI B 1 a)* Because pleomorphic adenoma is a benign tumor, radical parotidectomy with or without neck dissection is unnecessary. Pleomorphic adenoma is usually found in the superficial lobe of the parotid gland and may at times be located very close to the seventh nerve. Most of these benign mixed tumors (BMTs) are well-circumscribed; however, satellite nodules or small fingers may project from the main tumor mass. Therefore, it is not sufficient simply to enucleate or shell out the main tumor since there is a high rate of recurrence from the remaining tumor tissue.

2. The answer is C. *(II A 3)* Fordyce's disease is characterized by the presence of painless, yellow or white granules in the mucosa of the cheeks, lips, and gingivae. These granules are actually ectopic sebaceous glands. The disease is a purely benign asymptomatic condition.

3. The answer is D. *(V C 1)* The ameloblastoma, also called the adamantinoma, is a true odontogenic neoplasm with several morphologic features that resemble the features of a developing tooth. This tumor is locally highly invasive and destructive. Whether true metastases of this tumor occur is still controversial; however, a great deal of local bone destruction occurs as the ameloblastoma expands as it grows.

4. The answer is D (4). *(VI A 2)* Sialolithiasis (stone formation within the salivary gland ducts) occurs most often in the submandibular salivary gland. Nearly 80 percent of cases involve this gland, about 18 to 20 percent of cases occur in the parotid gland, and only 1 to 2 percent occur in the sublingual glands. In most cases, surgical removal of the stone is curative. The stones produce acute pain and swelling of the affected gland.

5. The answer is E (all). *(VI B 1)* Benign mixed tumors of the salivary glands are also called pleomorphic adenomas. The most common location for these tumors is the parotid salivary gland. They usually occur in patients between the ages of 20 and 40 years. The histology of pleomorphic adenomas is dominated by epithelial and myoepithelial cells in a matrix of myxomatous tissue, which sometimes contains islands of cartilage and bone.

6. The answer is B (1, 3). *(III B 2)* Angiofibroma of the nasopharynx is an uncommon benign tumor that occurs in young males between the ages of 12 and 25 years. This lesion is composed of vascular fibrous connective tissue intermingled with spindle cells and chronic inflammatory cells. It is extremely vascular and may present with frequent epistaxis. Angiofibroma is postulated to have a hormonal dependency, and it commonly regresses spontaneously.

7. The answer is A (1, 2, 3). *(VI B 2 c)* A cylindroma (adenocystic carcinoma) can be found in any salivary gland but occurs frequently in the minor salivary glands. The most striking characteristic of the tumor is its propensity for nerve invasion and subsequent growth in the perineural spaces. The tumor is slow-growing but relentless; the 5-year survival rate is nearly 75 percent, but the 10- to 15-year survival rate is only 15 to 20 percent. The name cylindroma refers to the histopathologic finding of mucin or hyaline cylinders within islands of neoplastic epithelial cells.

8. The answer is A (1, 2, 3). *(III C)* Lymphoepithelioma is a highly malignant tumor of the upper respiratory tract; it occurs in young adults, particularly those of an oriental lineage. The tumor is composed of malignant epithelial cells as well as lymphoid cells, which probably represents an immune response to the malignant epithelial component. Radiotherapy is the treatment of choice since the epithelial component grows rapidly and will metastasize.

9. The answer is B (1, 3). *(VI A 3 c)* Characteristics of Mikulicz's syndrome include lacrimal and salivary gland enlargement due to a variety of conditions, including Sjögren's syndrome, sarcoidosis, leukemia, lymphoma, and tuberculosis. Mikulicz's original case report, which led to the name of the syndrome, probably was a description of a patient with Sjögren's syndrome.

10. The answer is E (all). *(V B 1)* Odontogenic cysts are believed to result from a defect in tooth formation or in the organization of the epithelial cells involved in tooth formation. Dentigerous, radicular, primordial, and eruption cysts are all considered to be odontogenic. The other major group of jaw cysts are termed nonodontogenic and usually occur secondary to epithelial cell inclusions in fusion sites during embryonic jaw development.

19
Bones and Joints

I. BONES

A. BONE HISTOLOGY

1. Bone tissue consists of the **cortex**, a dense outer layer that is covered by connective tissue called the periosteum, and an inner network of thin trabeculae called the medulla within the marrow cavity. The inner surface of the cortex and the outer surface of the medulla are lined by the endosteum. The cortex is essential for mechanical functions, and also it is less sensitive to metabolic disorders than the medulla.

2. Three types of cells compose bone.
   a. **Osteoblasts** are mononuclear cells with basophilic cytoplasm due to abundant endoplasmic reticulum. The cytoplasm of the cells have blurred borders; however, narrow spaces do exist between them. Osteoblasts are actively engaged in synthesizing collagen and ground substance and in mineral transport for the calcification of the organic matrix. The origin of osteoblasts is unknown and remains controversial.
   b. **Osteocytes** are osteoblasts that become embedded and incorporated into an osteoid matrix. They communicate with the overlying osteoblasts by canaliculi through which cell processes extend and are able to either form or resorb bone.
   c. **Osteoclasts** are large, usually multinucleated (5 to 10 nuclei) cells that in the presence of parathyroid hormone cause bone resorption by first releasing phosphorus and calcium from the bone and then digesting the bone matrix, creating Howship's lacunar spaces (pits) along bone surfaces.

3. **Bone development** occurs by means of two phenomena.
   a. Long bones develop by endochondral ossification. There is replacement of the cartilaginous surface by bone, and the cartilage is left serving as the epiphyseal plate and articular surface.
   b. Flat bones develop by intramembranous ossification. The mesenchymal cells differentiate directly into bone. There is no cartilaginous phase.

4. **Hormones.** Three major hormones control calcium and phosphate metabolism: parathyroid hormone (PTH), calcitonin, and the metabolites of vitamin D, 25-hydroxyvitamin D_3 and 1,25-dihydroxyvitamin D_3 [1,25-$(OH)_2D_3$].

B. CONGENITAL BONE DISORDERS

1. **Osteogenesis imperfecta** is a hereditary disorder of connective tissue that is clinically manifested by a predisposition toward multiple bone fractures.
   a. In **osteogenesis imperfecta congenita** the fetus develops multiple fractures and thus is born with crippling deformities. Few patients are capable of reproduction; hence the genetic pattern remains uncertain.
   b. **Osteogenesis Imperfecta Tarda.** Usually transmitted as an autosomal dominant trait, this disorder appears after the perinatal period with bowing of the extremities, blue sclerae, and other manifestations of collagen synthesis defects. Fractures usually heal normally. The bones show marked osteopenia with porous cortex because osteoblasts do not synthesize as much bone matrix as is standard. The disease is less severe after puberty.

2. **Osteopetrosis** is hereditary and is characterized by an extreme reduction in the size of the medullary cavities and an increased density and widening of all cortical bones except the membranous bones such as the cranium. The ends of the long bones appear club-shaped, and there are alternating zones of radiolucency and radiopacity, depending on the pro-

gression of the disease. A large number of osteoclasts are present but are incapable of resorbing bone because they cannot release acid phosphatase.

  a. The **benign** form is autosomal dominant and affects males and females who may have multiple fractures. Diagnosis of the disease often is not made until the second or third decade of life. Osteomyelitis is a common complication.

  b. The **malignant** form is recessive and may cause slow growth, mental retardation, and deafness. Affected children usually die before the second decade of life because of anemia and secondary infections.

C. METABOLIC BONE DISEASES: DISORDERS OF REMODELING (FORMATION AND RESORPTION). There is a decrease in the amount of osseous tissue per unit of bone volume. The entire skeleton may show low density with conspicuous sparsity and thinning of the spongy trabeculae of the affected bone, resulting from an imbalance between resorption and formation in the remodeling sequence.

  1. Osteopenia is characterized by a decrease in bone mass.

  a. **Senile.** With increase in age, there is a continuous loss of bone both at the trabecular and cortical layers, which become thinner by internal resorption.

  b. **Steroid-Induced.** Corticosteroid therapy, with its catabolic effect, may affect trabecular bone, producing a decrease in bone formation. Steroids also decrease intestinal absorption and renal resorption of calcium so that less calcium goes to the bone.

  2. Osteoporosis is characterized by bone rarefaction. It has been suggested that the term **osteoporosis** be reserved for those cases where **osteopenia** causes clinical symptoms.

  a. **Postmenopausal** osteoporosis is most common in women, especially after the fifth decade of life. In this form of osteopenia, there is decreased bone volume due not only to a disorder in remodeling but also to a decreased amount of bone deposited by osteoblasts. No effective treatment has been found for this condition, which may cause compression of vertebral bodies and fractures.

  b. **Immobilization Osteoporosis.** Bed confinement for periods longer than 6 months can result in a loss of 30 percent of initial bone volume. The lack of exercise probably leads to an increase in bone resorption and a decrease in bone formation.

D. HORMONAL BONE DISORDERS

  1. Primary Hyperparathyroidism. PTH stimulates the active phase of the remodeling sequence. When the blood levels of PTH are elevated due to parathyroid hyperplasia or adenoma, bone is affected. PTH also affects the renal tubules by increasing the excretion of phosphorus in the urine and elevating calcium levels in the blood serum.

  a. **Clinical Data.**

   (1) The clinical symptoms are similar to those of hypercalcemia. Primary hyperparathyroidism predominantly affects women 30 to 50 years of age who present with bone pain, which is more severe in the lower extremities. Renal symptomatology, such as polyuria and polydipsia, with unexplained renal stones may be an early complaint. In advanced cases, hypotonia, uncoordination, loss of appetite, and constipation may be present. Pathologic fractures and bone deformities may be seen.

   (2) Serum levels of calcium are elevated higher than 11.5 mg/100 ml, and phosphorus levels are reduced to less than 2 mg/100 ml.

  b. **Histologically**, there is an increased number of osteoclasts, which resorb the walls of the haversian canals of cortical bone and the surfaces of spongy trabeculae, and it is replaced with fibrous tissue. Occasionally, proliferation of osteoclasts that contain hemosiderin pigment is very prominent within the fibrous stroma. The lesions are called **brown tumors** and can occur in any bone but are most common in the jaws.

  c. **Treatment** consists of removal of the parathyroid lesion.

  2. Secondary Hyperparathyroidism.

  a. The most common causes are renal failure, hypercorticism, vitamin D deficiency, and pseudohypoparathyroidism. In circumstances where hypocalcemia or hyperphosphatemia occur, there is an increase in the secretion of PTH by the parathyroid gland in order to compensate for these abnormalities.

  b. The histologic appearance is the same as that in primary hyperparathyroidism but with more severe marrow fibrosis.

  3. Hypoparathyroidism is produced commonly by the accidental surgical removal of the parathyroid glands, although idiopathic hypoparathyroidism can occur.

  a. **Clinical Data.** The signs and symptoms are dominated by hypocalcemia, with soft tissue calcification and ossification, abnormal dentition, and otosclerosis.

b. Histologically, bone shows a markedly decreased turnover rate with active osteoblasts and a lack of osteoclasts.

c. Treatment is the administration of synthetic PTH or vitamin D.

E. NUTRITIONAL BONE DISORDERS

1. Vitamin D Deficiency [Rickets (Osteomalacia)].

a. **Clinical Data.** If vitamin D deficiency occurs before epiphyseal closure, bone deformities and pain will result. In children symptoms may include a **rachitic rosary** (swelling at the osteochondral junctions of the ribs), bowing of the legs, fractures, and pelvic disorders. The diagnosis of osteomalacia in adults can be made only on bone biopsy because bone growth has already been completed.

b. **Histologically**, there is an increase in uncalcified osteoid cartilage and a decrease in calcified bone.

c. **Treatment.** The disease responds to the administration of vitamin D.

2. Vitamin C Deficiency.

a. **Clinical Data.** This condition occurs predominantly in children, but it is rarely seen in the Western Hemisphere. The symptoms are due to increased capillary fragility, which results in hemorrhages in the gums, skin, and periosteum.

b. **Histologically**, the trabecular bone mass is decreased, and osteoblasts are abnormal.

3. Vitamin A Disorders.

a. **Hypervitaminosis A.** There is abundant mineralization of the periosteum and abnormal bone formation. In children with this condition, there is premature epiphyseal closure, resulting in permanent skeletal deformities.

b. **Vitamin A Deficiency.** In this condition remodeling ceases, and osteoclastic activity disappears. The bones are short and thick, with predominance of new cancellous periosteum.

F. INFECTIOUS BONE DISEASES

1. Osteomyelitis is inflammation of the medullary and cortical portions of bone, including the periosteum. As bone is altered or destroyed by inflammation, repair and remodeling take place with new bone formation. Occasionally, inflammation may persist in regions of relative avascularity where it is impossible to achieve high tissue levels of antibiotics.

a. The **pathogenesis** is a result of
   (1) Most commonly, the hematogenous spread of bacteria from a distant focus of sepsis
   (2) Invasion of bone from adjacent septic arthritis or soft tissue abscesses
   (3) Penetrating trauma
   (4) Complication of fractures
   (5) Postoperative complications
   (6) A natural part of certain diseases such as sickle-cell disease

b. **Clinical Data.** Fever, local pain, marked leukocytosis, and an elevated sedimentation rate often occur. X-rays are normal until bone resorption takes place or the medullary cavity shows increased density.

c. **Types.**
   (1) **Pyogenic osteomyelitis** most commonly affects children and young adults and involves the femur, tibia, humerus, and radius. Often no source of infection is obvious, but the usual causative organism is *Staphylococcus aureus.*
   (2) **Chronic Osteomyelitis.** When the acute process is not properly treated, a chronic condition may develop and cause flare-ups of osteomyelitis at intervals of months or years.
   (3) **Tuberculous osteomyelitis** affects both children and adults and occurs by hematogenous spread of tuberculous organisms to bone; however, the primary focus of the disease may be difficult to find. Spinal involvement **(Pott's disease)** produces destruction and collapse of vertebral bodies. Hips, knees, ankles, and hands are also often affected. Progressive destruction with little ossification is the rule, and there may be marked epiphyseal involvement.

d. The **pathology** of osteomyelitis is variable, depending upon the causative organism (fungi but usually bacteria), host factor, and therapy. Suppurative inflammation is initiated in the marrow cavities, haversian canals, or subperiosteal spaces. Repair is a feature that follows the initial acute phase. In osteomyelitis, fibrosis, granulation tissue formation, and lymphocytes, plasma cells, and macrophages are seen. The structural integrity of the bone depends upon the degree of new bone formation and bone remodeling.

e. **Treatment** consists of the administration of antibiotics and surgical débridement.

G. IDIOPATHIC BONE DISORDERS

1. **Paget's disease of the bone (osteitis deformans)** affects 3 to 4 percent of the population over 40 years of age, most commonly men.
   a. **Clinical Data.**
      (1) The initial symptoms may be bone pain, fractures, and deformities. The disease is usually, but not always, polyostotic, with a predilection for the skull, pelvis, tibia, and femur. Deafness is common when the skull is affected. Height distortion may occur due to vertebral compression. Serum alkaline phosphatase is markedly elevated.
      (2) X-ray findings of bone lysis and reformation are characteristic.
      (3) Occasionally, Paget's disease of the bone may be associated with a malignant neoplasm, such as an osteosarcoma.
   b. **Histology.**
      (1) There is a high turnover of bone characterized by the presence of numerous osteoclasts and osteoblasts, an increased calcification rate, and accumulation of woven bones. This turnover leads to the "mosaic" pattern, so termed because a cement-type material forms narrow boundaries between the original bone and the actively remodeling foci.
      (2) There is marked medullary fibrosis, and numerous osteoclasts appear abnormal because of the increase in the number of nuclei. Lytic and formative phases rapidly succeed one another, leading to local increase in bone mass and disorganization of the normal trabecular pattern.
   c. **Treatment** consists of administration of calcitonin or one of the diphosphonates, which decreases the resorption and, therefore, the high turnover rate.

2. **Avascular necrosis** affects predominantly the femoral head in men. It is often associated with alcoholism, corticosteroid therapy, hyperuricemia, Gaucher's disease, systemic lupus erythematosus, and trauma.
   The reparative foci are seen radiologically to replace necrotic bone.

3. **Legg-Calvé-Perthes disease** is a childhood disorder of the head of the femur similar to avascular necrosis of adulthood. The typical age of onset is 5 to 9 years, and the earliest manifestation is an intermittent limp and pain.

H. NEOPLASTIC BONE LESIONS (see Table 19-1)

1. **Cystic Lesions.**
   a. **Solitary Bone Cyst.**
      (1) **Clinical Data.** This benign lesion of unknown etiology occurs predominantly in the distal end of the long bones (humerus and femur) of young males. The most common symptoms are pain of the affected areas, swelling of the soft tissues, and, occasionally, fractures.
         A cyst with a smooth thin cortex is seen in x-rays in close proximity to the epiphysis.
      (2) **Pathology.** Grossly, the cyst has ridges dividing the cavity, giving it a multiloculated appearance. The cavity is filled with clear or bloody fluid. Specific microscopic features are lacking, but strands of fibrous tissue with occasional osteoid and granular tissue formation may be present.
      (3) **Treatment.** The lesion is successfully treated by curettage followed by insertion of bone chips. Recurrences are very rare.

Table 19-1. Bone Tumors

	Cystic	Chondroblastic	Osteoblastic	Other
Benign	Solitary bone cyst Aneurysmal bone cyst	Chondroma Osteochondroma Chondroblastoma Chondromyxoid fibroma	Osteoma Osteoid osteoma Osteoblastoma	Fibrous dysplasia
Malignant		Chondrosarcoma	Osteosarcoma	Giant cell tumor Plasma cell myeloma Ewing's sarcoma Malignant lymphoma Metastatic tumors

b. Aneurysmal Bone Cyst.
  (1) Clinical Data.
    (a) This tumor is seen most frequently in females in the second and third decades of life. It occurs in the metaphysis of the long bones and in the vertebrae. Swelling, pain, and tenderness of the affected area are the most common symptoms.
    (b) In x-rays, there is seen a circumscribed zone of rarefaction with extension into the soft tissues.
  (2) Pathology.
    (a) The lesion varies in size from a few to 20 cm. The bone is greatly distorted and has an irregular outline. On cut surface it has a spongy appearance with cystic spaces of various sizes containing blood in different stages of organization.
    (b) Microscopically, the essential feature is the presence of cavernous spaces, the walls of which lack normal endothelial linings. Solid areas of fibrous tissue contain osteoid and mature bone, and giant cells may be present. The histologic differential diagnosis of this tumor includes giant cell tumor of the bone and telangiectatic osteosarcoma.
  (3) Treatment. The most successful treatment is removal of the entire lesion or as much of it as is possible, followed by insertion of bone chips. Recurrences may appear in up to 21 percent of the cases.

2. Benign Lesions.
  a. Fibrous Dysplasia.
    (1) Clinical Data.
      (a) These poorly understood lesions are usually monostotic, although 20 percent are polyostotic. When polyostotic, the lesion is part of Albright's syndrome, evidenced by precocious puberty and cutaneous pigmentation.
      (b) Symptomatology varies from vaginal bleeding and endocrinologic symptoms in the infant to bone pain in the elderly. Repeated fractures may lead to bone deformities.
      (c) Although any bone can be affected, the ribs, femur, tibia, and maxilla are those most commonly involved.
      (d) X-rays usually demonstrate well-defined zones of rarefaction surrounded by narrow rims of sclerotic bone.
    (2) Pathology. Histologically, the major feature is the proliferation of fibroblasts, which produce a dense collagenous matrix. There is no evidence that the woven immature bone ever grows into trabecular lamellar bone. In some areas of the lesion poorly oriented trabeculae of semicalcified bone are present. Fibrosis with osteoid, giant cells, macrophages, and islands of cartilage is seen.
    (3) Treatment. A monostotic lesion is treated by either curettage or local resection. The treatment of a polyostotic lesion should be conservative because the lesion commonly stops growing after puberty.
  b. Chondroma (Endochondroma).
    (1) Clinical Data.
      (a) This benign cartilaginous lesion, which can be solitary or multiple, occurs frequently between the second and fifth decades of life. It is usually asymptomatic and affects the small bones of the hands and feet.
      (b) X-rays show a localized, radiolucent, cystic defect with distortion of the bony contour. Central areas of calcification may be present.
    (2) Pathology.
      (a) This neoplasm is thought to originate from heterotopic cartilaginous cell nests in the medullary cavities of bones. It appears grossly as a confluent mass of bluish hyaline cartilage with a lobular configuration.
      (b) Histologically, the cartilage is moderately cellular with occasional binucleated cells. Mitoses are absent.
    (3) Treatment is curettage of the lesion.
    (4) Syndromes.
      (a) Ollier's disease (enchondromatosis) is a rare nonhereditary disorder in which multiple chondromas are present in the metaphysis and diaphysis of various bones. There is a relatively high incidence of malignant transformation and development of chondrosarcomas.
      (b) Maffucci's syndrome is a congenital disease characterized by dyschondroplasia and multiple hemangiomas in the skin and viscera. Patients have a relatively high risk of developing chondrosarcomas.

c. **Osteochondroma.**
  (1) **Clinical Data.** This is the most common benign tumor of bone affecting patients under the age of 21 years. The symptoms are usually pain and compression of adjacent structures by large tumor masses. The lesions may be single or multiple, involving predominantly the metaphysis of long bones.
  (2) **Pathology.**
    (a) This tumor appears as stalked protuberances with a lobulated surface jutting from the affected bone. The periosteum of the adjacent bone covers the lesion, which may range in size from 1 to several cm.
    (b) Microscopically, the cartilaginous cells appear lined-up, mimicking the orientation of cartilaginous cells in a normal epiphysis. There are no mitoses present.
  (3) **Treatment.** Resection of the lesion is usually curative.
d. **Chondroblastoma.**
  (1) **Clinical Data.**
    (a) This is a rare cartilaginous tumor that predominantly affects males in their second decade of life, who present with local pain, stiffness, and limitation of motion. The lesion almost always involves the epiphyseal portion of the long bones.
    (b) X-rays show a central area of bone destruction delineated from the surrounding normal bone by a thin margin of increased bone density.
  (2) **Pathology.**
    (a) Grossly, the tumor is round or oval in shape, with areas of cystic degeneration and hemorrhage.
    (b) Microscopically, there is proliferation of chondroblasts intermixed with varying amounts of fibrous stroma and chondroid material. Multinucleated giant cells and calcifications are present. Mitoses are virtually absent.
  (3) **Treatment and Prognosis.** A conservative approach such as curettage or local excision is advocated as the best modality of treatment. Although chondroblastomas are considered to be benign, there are cases in which metastases to the lungs have occurred.
e. **Chondromyxoid Fibroma.**
  (1) **Clinical Data.** This tumor primarily affects males in the first and second decades of life. Pain is the most common symptom. The lesion appears in x-rays as a sharply outlined mass with a rim of sclerotic bone. The tumor is most commonly located in the metaphysis of long bones, but it occasionally can involve the epiphysis.
  (2) **Pathology.**
    (a) Grossly, the tumor is a well-circumscribed solid mass with a cartilaginous appearance. The cortex of the bone is expanded by the tumor, which is limited by the periosteum.
    (b) Histologically, there is a variety of fibrous, myxomatous, and chondroid elements together with multinucleated giant cells and macrophages that contain hemosiderin pigment. When the tumor forms lobules, there is a condensation of nuclei beneath the rim of the compressed adjacent tissue.
  (3) **Treatment and Prognosis.** Cure can be obtained by complete excision of the lesion, including a rim of normal bone. The incidence of local recurrence is about 20 percent.
f. **Osteoma.**
  (1) **Clinical Data.** An osteoma is a benign tumor mass that almost exclusively involves the skull and facial bones; the frontal sinus is the most common location. Males are affected more often than females, and the lesion can occur at any age. The lesion is asymptomatic unless it interferes with the paranasal sinus drainage.
  (2) **Pathology.** The tumor is composed of normal dense and mature bone originating from the periosteum. There is little evidence of osteoblastic activity. Although osteoma is predominantly a solitary lesion, multiple osteomas can occur in association with intestinal polyposis and soft tissue tumors (e.g., Gardner's syndrome).
g. **Osteoid Osteoma.**
  (1) **Clinical Data.**
    (a) This lesion is common in young persons, mostly males, who present with increasing pain that tends to be more severe at night and is relieved by aspirin.
    (b) X-rays show the lesion itself as a **nidus**, a central radiolucent area surrounded by dense sclerotic bone.
  (2) **Pathology.**
    (a) Grossly, an osteoid osteoma appears as a small round or oval mass in which a central red-brown, friable area of nidus is recognized. Frequently the nidus becomes dislodged from the surrounding sclerotic bone.

      (b) Histologically, the nidus appears as a maze of irregular bone trabeculae, fibrous tissue, and vessels. The center of the nidus is rich in osteoblasts, calcification, and multinucleated giant cells.

    (3) Treatment. It is necessary to excise the entire nidus together with a rim of sclerotic bone to avoid recurrences of the lesion or persistence of the symptoms.

  h. Osteoblastoma.

    (1) Clinical Data.

      (a) This is a lesion that affects predominantly the vertebrae and long bones of young males in the first 3 decades of life. Symptoms are rarely present.

      (b) X-rays demonstrate a well-circumscribed lesion surrounded by a zone of sclerotic bone and thickened periosteum. Some tumors may appear as obstructive and expansile masses.

    (2) Pathology. The lesions vary in size from a few to several cm. Histologically, there is a proliferation of osteoblasts and increased osteoid production. Osteoclasts and multinucleated giant cells may be very numerous, especially in areas where there is blood extravasation.

    (3) The **treatment** of choice is removal of the entire lesion by curettage.

3. Malignant Tumors.

  a. Osteosarcoma (Osteogenic Sarcoma).

    (1) Incidence. An osteosarcoma is a highly malignant bone tumor characterized by the production of osteoid and bone. It is the most common primary tumor next to multiple myeloma, accounting for approximately 16 percent of all bone malignancies. The disease predominantly affects young males between 10 and 20 years of age.

    (2) The **etiology** of the tumor remains unknown; however, two factors that predispose to its development are radiation and preexisting conditions such as Paget's disease. The suspected roles of trauma and viral disease are not clearly established.

    (3) Clinical Data.

      (a) In general, the presenting symptoms are pain and swelling of the affected region; however, in cases of large tumor masses, there might be limitation of motion of the nearby joints. Patients with rapidly growing tumors may experience weight loss and secondary anemia.

      (b) Most osteosarcomas arise in the metaphyseal end of long bones (predominantly the femur, humerus, and tibia), but they can involve any bone, including the small bones of the hands, feet, and face.

      (c) Radiologically, there is evidence of bone destruction with penetration of the cortex, subperiosteal elevation (Cadman's triangle), and infiltration of adjacent soft tissues.

    (4) Pathology.

      (a) On gross examination the tumor appears as a large necrotic and hemorrhagic mass. The lesion usually ends in the epiphyseal cartilage and rarely extends into the nearby joint space (Fig. 19-1).

      (b) Three types of osteosarcomas have been differentiated according to their predominant histologic patterns: **osteoblastic, fibroblastic,** and **chondroblastic.** The hallmark of the tumor is the presence of a malignant stroma that contains osteoid and bone (Fig. 19-2). The stroma shows bizarre pleomorphic cells with hyperchromatic, irregular nuclei and abundant mitoses. Malignant cartilage may be present either in small foci or as a large proportion of the tumor. Multinucleated giant cells are seen, usually near zones of necrosis and calcification.

    (5) Treatment and Prognosis. Surgical amputation of the affected limb is the best treatment in order to avoid early dissemination of the tumor. Good results and longer survival are obtained with adjunct chemotherapy. Radiation therapy has proven ineffective.

      (a) Osteosarcoma is a highly malignant tumor with a 5-year survival rate of 5 to 20 percent; the lower percentage generally prevails.

      (b) Death usually occurs by hematogenous dissemination of the disease to the lungs and liver and to other bones.

  b. Chondrosarcoma.

    (1) Incidence. A chondrosarcoma is a malignant cartilaginous tumor, the **incidence** of which comprises between 7 and 15 percent of all bony neoplasms. It occurs in patients between 30 and 60 years of age and is found more often in men than in women in a ratio of 3:1.

    (2) Etiology. The tumor may arise de novo (primary chondrosarcoma) or originate from a preexisting benign cartilaginous lesion (secondary chondrosarcoma).

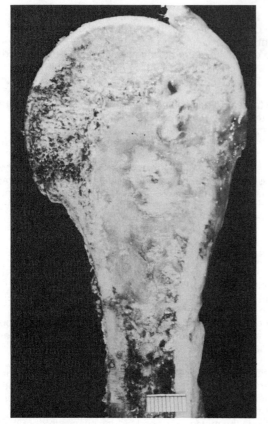

Figure 19-1. Section of a femoral head with osteosarcoma. The necrosis and hemorrhage involve the medullary cavity and extend into the cortical bone.

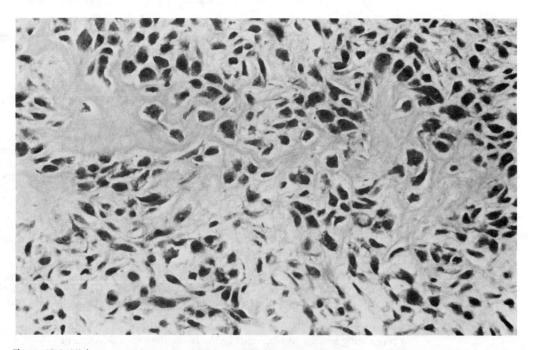

Figure 19-2. High-power microscopic view of an osteosarcoma showing malignant stroma and osteoid formation.

(3) Clinical Data.

    (a) Local swelling and pain are the most common symptoms. A history of a mass that has been present for months or years can be obtained in many cases.

    (b) In x-rays, the affected areas show cortical bone destruction with occasional medullary involvement and mottled densities produced by calcification and ossification.

    (c) The most common locations of this tumor are the spine, pelvic bones, and upper ends of the femur and humerus.

(4) Pathology.

    (a) A chondrosarcoma appears as a lobulated white-gray mass that contains mucoid material and foci of calcification (Fig. 19-3).

    (b) Histologically, there are islands of immature or poorly developed cartilage, which contain anaplastic cells with more than one nuclei present within the lacunar space. Mitoses are common.

(5) Treatment and Prognosis.

    (a) Total resection of the tumor is the treatment of choice, but it may be difficult to accomplish depending upon the location of the tumor.

    (b) The neoplasm is slow growing and can remain locally aggressive for years, with a high tendency to recur and implant in soft tissues. Hematogenous dissemination to the lungs, liver, and kidneys takes place over the years with eventual death of the patient. The 10-year survival rate for this tumor ranges from 50 to 60 percent.

c. Giant Cell Tumor (Osteoclastoma).

(1) Incidence. This is an uncommon malignant tumor characterized by the presence of multinucleated giant cells or osteoclasts. It occurs predominantly in women beyond the age of 19 years and peaks in the third decade of life.

(2) Etiology. The etiology of this tumor is unknown, but it is believed that it originates from the mesenchymal cells of connective tissue.

(3) Clinical Data.

    (a) Patients present with pain, tenderness, functional disability, and large bulky masses.

    (b) The lesion is almost always localized in the distal portion of the long bones (femur or humerus), but occasionally it involves the skull, pelvis, or small bones of the hands and feet. Half of the cases, however, occur in the area of the knee.

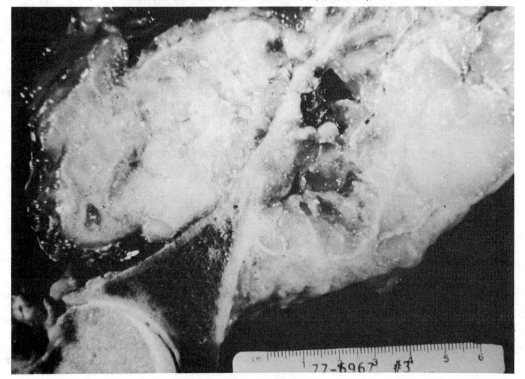

Figure 19-3. Chondrosarcoma of the ischium with characteristic white-grey lobulated appearance.

      (c) X-rays show an expanding zone of radiolucency with no reactive sclerosis in the surrounding margins.

   (4) Pathology.

      (a) The characteristic gross appearance shows multiple hemorrhagic cystic cavities that destroy the adjacent bone and are enclosed by a thin shell of new bone formation.

      (b) Histologically, there is a vascularized stroma composed of spindle cells, which contains multinucleated giant cells mixed with areas of hemorrhage, inflammation, and hemosiderin deposits. Mitoses are present.

   (5) Treatment and Prognosis.

      (a) Adequate removal of the lesion by complete resection or curettage is the treatment of choice.

      (b) The behavior of giant cell tumors is not predictable on a histologic basis because well-differentiated benign-appearing tumors have been known to metastasize. In general, approximately one-third of the tumors will behave in a benign fashion, one-third will recur, and the remaining one-third will be frankly malignant.

      (c) Metastatic spread can occur to any organ, but the lungs are most commonly involved.

d. Multiple Myeloma (Plasma Cell Myeloma).

   (1) Incidence.

      (a) Multiple myeloma, the most common primary bone tumor, is characterized by the proliferation of plasma cells in the marrow cavity.

      (b) The disease is common in the sixth to eighth decades of life and affects men more often than women in a ratio of 3:2.

      (c) Myeloma is a multicentric disease, involving several sites at the time of diagnosis.

   (2) Etiology. The origin of this tumor remains unknown, but observations suggest that chronic inflammation may play an important role.

   (3) Clinical Data.

      (a) Patients present with pain in areas such as the back, thorax, and head, where occasionally a tumor mass may be palpated. Frequently there is associated weight loss, fever, and anemia.

      (b) A range of immunoglobulins can be detected by serum electrophoresis. These immunoglobulins are biochemically normal but are produced in abnormal levels. The majority is of the immunoglobulin G (IgG) or immunoglobulin M (IgM) type. Myeloma protein is present in the blood serum of up to 90 percent of the patients.

      (c) Abnormal protein (Bence Jones protein) is found in the urine.

      (d) Multiple destructive or punched-out lesions are seen radiologically.

   (4) Pathology. Histologically, the tumor is composed of masses of mature plasma cells with varying degrees of atypia and anaplasia. Binucleated forms and mitoses can be present (Fig. 19-4).

   (5) Treatment and Prognosis.

      (a) The course of the disease varies according to the degree of differentiation and extension of the lesion. Death usually occurs due to associated infection, anemia, or renal failure. In general, there is a 10 percent 5-year survival rate.

      (b) Chemotherapy (Alkeran) has proven to be successful in some cases. Radiation therapy is used to relieve pain.

e. Ewing's Sarcoma.

   (1) Incidence. Ewing's sarcoma is a rare primary malignant tumor, accounting for fewer than 2 percent of all bone malignancies. The disease is found most commonly in young males between the ages of 10 and 30 years.

   (2) Etiology. The etiology remains unknown, but the disease is believed to originate from undifferentiated mesenchymal cells of the medullary cavity.

   (3) Clinical Data.

      (a) Pain is the most common symptom, but there also may be a palpable mass, tenderness, and compromised function of the involved area.

      (b) The tumor originates predominantly in the medullary cavities of the long bones, although any bone can be involved.

      (c) A destructive lesion is seen radiologically. As the tumor breaks through the cortex, it gradually elevates the periosteum, producing multiple layers of subperiosteal, reactive, new bone, which give the characteristic "onion skin" appearance of the lesion.

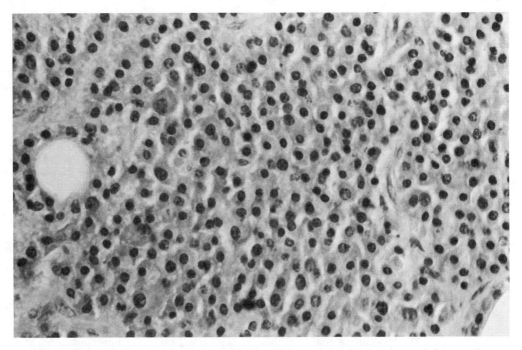

Figure 19-4. High-power microscopic view of a multiple myeloma showing sheets of plasma cells.

    (4) Pathology.
        (a) The affected bone characteristically shows destruction of the medullary cavity by hemorrhage and necrosis, which can permeate the cortex and extend into adjacent soft tissues. Grossly, the extent of the lesion is greater than is appreciated on x-rays.
        (b) Microscopically, the tumor is composed of undifferentiated small round cells arranged in sheets or cords. The cells are slightly larger than lymphocytes and have prominent nuclei with scanty cytoplasms. The tumor has a rich vascular background, and fibrous tissue is seen.
    (5) Treatment and Prognosis. The treatment consists of amputation of the affected limb, if possible. New chemotherapeutic agents have been used with relative success. However, the disease is highly aggressive and malignant, with 5-year survival rates that range from 0 to 12 percent. Metastases occur through hematogenous dissemination and can involve any organ.
  f. Lymphoma. Primary malignant lymphoma of the bone is quite rare and generally arises in the diaphyseal area of the long bones. The histology is similar to that of the diffuse histiocytic lymphomas of the lymph nodes.
  g. Metastatic tumors to bones are the most common form of malignancy in adult bones. The tumors that frequently metastasize are carcinomas of the prostate, breast, thyroid, and renal cell. Other metastatic tumors include those of the lungs, stomach, and bowel.

II. JOINTS. A joint consists of two molded bone ends connected through the joint capsule, which is formed by dense fibroconnective tissue. The bone and cartilaginous surfaces are covered by a thin membrane, or synovium, which can produce a clear (synovial) fluid that acts as a lubricant.
    Joints serve as attachment points of the skeletal muscles.
    All of the elements that form joints are of mesenchymal derivation.

  A. INFLAMMATORY PROCESSES

    1. Infectious Arthritis.
      a. Incidence. Arthritis is the inflammation of a joint. In general, the bacterial forms of the disease are more common in individuals between the ages of 20 and 40 years because this group is most susceptible to the diseases that predispose to arthritis. Children are prone to arthritis in one joint (monoarticular).
      b. Etiology. Gonococcus, *Staphylococcus, Streptococcus,* and pneumococcus are the most common organisms involved in the development of the disease, which is acquired through

hematogenous spread from a primary septic focus such as pneumonia, otitis media, and endocarditis or any site of gonorrheal infection.

c. Clinical Data.
  (1) Affected patients present with acute pain, swelling, tenderness, and redness of the involved joint, with associated systemic symptoms such as fever and malaise. There may be limitation of joint motion.
  (2) Any joint may be involved, but the most frequently affected are those of the knee, hip, ankle, and wrist. Infectious arthritis can be either monoarticular or polyarticular (involving several joints), although the former is more common.
  (3) Radiologically, the early phase of the disease shows prominent accumulation of fluid. In the later stages, there is evidence of destruction of the articular surfaces.

d. Pathology. Pathologic findings depend largely on the nature of the causative organism and the stage of the disease process.
  (1) In the early stages, there is congestion and edema of the synovial membranes, with collection of fluid in the joint space.
  (2) As the process progresses there is an intense purulent inflammatory exudate with areas of necrosis in the synovium and articular cartilage.
  (3) If the disease is controlled in an early phase, there is resolution of the process without sequelae; if not, fibrosis and calcification of the joint occur, resulting in ankylosis.

e. Treatment. Antibiotics are the treatment of choice.

2. Tuberculous Arthritis.
  a. Incidence. This type of arthritis occurs predominantly in children as a complication of pulmonary or miliary tuberculosis.
  b. Clinical Data.
    (1) The clinical manifestations are the same as those of infectious arthritis, but they present late in the course of the disease when joint destruction has already occurred.
    (2) The spine is the most common location.
  c. Pathology.
    (1) Tuberculous arthritis is characterized by the presence of confluent tubercles and necrotizing granulation tissue. The joint space may be filled with thick purulent material, and acid-fast bacilli may be identified in cultures.
    (2) Destruction and obliteration of the joint space is common. Erosion of articular cartilage and bone leads to ankylosis.
  d. Treatment. Antituberculous drugs should be administered.

3. Rheumatoid Arthritis.
  a. Incidence. Rheumatoid arthritis is an inflammatory disease of the joints that affects approximately 4 percent of the American population. It is more common in women than in men by a ratio of 3:1, and it usually starts during the fourth or fifth decade of life.
  b. Etiology. The etiology is unknown, but two sources are suspected—infection and an autoimmune response.
  c. Clinical Data.
    (1) Rheumatoid arthritis is a systemic disease in which a variety of organs may be involved, and the initial symptoms, such as fatigue, fever, and malaise, may not be related to joint involvement.
    (2) When joints are affected, there is morning stiffness, pain on movement, hypersensitivity to pressure, joint swelling, redness, and warmth. In later stages there is permanent ankylosis.
    (3) The disease usually involves the interphalangeal joints of the fingers and the metacarpophalangeal joints of the hands and the feet in a bilaterally symmetrical fashion. Eventually any joint may be involved.
    (4) In the terminal stage of the disease, the joints may be contracted into various deforming and incapacitating positions. The hands are distorted as a result of ulnar deviation of the fingers and dislocation of the interphalangeal joints. The wrists become fixed, and there is ankylosis of the elbows in flexion.
    (5) The patients present with hypergammaglobulinemia, and their blood serum contains an antibody against IgG known as **rheumatoid factor**. This factor is an IgM that will cross-react with immunoglobulins of other species. The serum titers depend upon the severity of the disease.
    (6) Since the disease process may involve other mesodermal surfaces, the patients may develop pericarditis, pleuritis, and cardiac problems.
    (7) Typically, x-rays show erosion of the juxta-articular surfaces.
  d. Pathology.
    (1) The inflammatory process causes diffuse thickening and hyperplasia of the synovium. Eventually the synovium is replaced by a vascularized mass, called the **pannus**,

composed of lymphocytes and plasma cells surrounding areas of necrosis with palisading fibroblasts.

    (2) The pannus and inflammatory component wear away the articular surfaces and erode the bone, leading to hemorrhage and granulation tissue formation, which diminishes the synovial spaces.

    (3) Fibrosis is the end result of the disease.

  e. Treatment and Prognosis. Steroids and aspirin are used in the treatment of rheumatoid arthritis, but recurrences and exacerbation of the disease are common. Approximately 15 percent of these patients will develop systemic amyloidosis.

B. DEGENERATIVE AND METABOLIC DISEASES

  1. Osteoarthritis.

    a. Incidence. Osteoarthritis is the most common degenerative, noninflammatory disease affecting the movable joints. It afflicts approximately one-fifth of the American population. It is a progressive disease of the fifth decade of life and beyond.

    b. Etiology. Of the factors involved in the development of osteoarthritis, aging (wear and tear) is probably the most important. Other factors include

      (1) Obesity

      (2) Previous injury to the joint (particularly infections and traumas)

      (3) Excessive use of the part involved (through athletics)

      (4) Synovial diseases

    c. Clinical Data.

      (1) The disease has an insidious beginning with decreased mobility of the affected joint. With progression of the disease, there might be pain, crepitation, and effusion, but there is no clinical evidence of inflammation.

      (2) Nodules occasionally can be noted at the base of the terminal phalanges of the fingers (Heberden's nodes).

      (3) The joints most frequently involved include the hips, knees, the distal joints of the fingers, and the vertebral joints. Osteoarthritis may be monoarticular or polyarticular.

      (4) Radiologically, there is evidence of erosion of articular surfaces and the underlying bone, with a decrease in size of the articular spaces.

    d. Pathology.

      (1) The initial changes are in the articular cartilage. There is gradual loss of the amount of cartilage, and articulation takes place over a smaller surface area than is normal. Therefore these articular surfaces erode and appear chipped, pitted, and shredded. Macroscopic pieces of cartilage (joint mice) may flake into the joint space.

      (2) Perichondrial soft tissues proliferate, which may give rise to cartilaginous formation and ossification. This produces "lipping" of the bone ends, which is responsible for the loss of joint motion and deformities.

      (3) Histologically, the synovial tissues are thickened, but there is little evidence of inflammation.

    e. Treatment. There is no adequate treatment for this chronic disease, but supportive measures, such as aspirin and occasionally steroids, are indicated.

  2. Gout.

    a. Incidence. Gout is rare and accounts for 2 to 5 percent of articular diseases. The majority of patients are middle-aged or elderly men.

    b. Etiology. Gout has its origin in an inborn error in the metabolism of purines, the result of which is an abnormally high production of uric acid. The disease is familial and is inherited as a recessive trait.

    c. Clinical Data.

      (1) Gout begins as an acute attack of arthritis in the metatarsophalangeal joint of a great toe, which becomes tender and swollen. Occasionally other joints are the sites of first attack, such as those elsewhere in the feet, in the fingers, and the knees. The attacks usually occur first at night and may last several days.

      (2) There are elevated serum levels of uric acid (more than 6 mg/100 ml).

    d. Pathology.

      (1) Histologically, there is evidence of deposits of urates, called tophi, anywhere in and around the joints. The tophi appear as a collection of filamentous urate crystals when fixed in absolute alcohol. Many of the individual agglomerations of urates have roundish contours and are surrounded by foreign body giant cells.

      (2) Deposition of urates can also occur in the kidney.

    e. Treatment should include a balanced, purine-free diet and the administration of colchicine to reduce swelling and pain. Probenecid is effective in the prevention and amelioration of chronic deforming gout.

C. **MALIGNANT NEOPLASMS: SYNOVIAL SARCOMA** may affect patients of all ages, but it is most frequently found in early adult life. In most series the tumor has a slight preponderance in males.

1. **Clinical Data.** Synovial sarcoma commonly occurs in the lower limbs, specifically in the region of the knee. The tumor may develop, however, in any site where there are tendons, joints, or bursae. The sarcoma may be small or large, is often well circumscribed and painless, and usually is slow in enlarging.

2. **Histologically,** the tumor does not arise from synovial membranes but is classified as being of synovial origin because it is **biphasic,** having a spindle-cell fibrosarcoma-like element and a pseudoglandular (epithelioid) one, resembling normal synovial membrane. Calcification is often noted, radiologically and microscopically.

3. The **prognosis** is generally poor. Nodal metastases occur in up to 30 percent of cases, and bloodborne spread, especially to the lungs, is common.

4. Wide excision, including amputation, is the **treatment** of choice. Surgical intervention usually is performed late in the course of the disease and often is inadequate because the tumor appears encapsulated. The incidence of local recurrence is high, reflecting this failure.

5. A recently recognized and probably related lesion is the **epithelioid sarcoma,** which arises in distal portions of the extremities, frequently producing multiple nodules along the length of the tendon.

   a. **Histologically,** this lesion shows granulomatous features with large histiocytic or epithelioid cells surrounding zones of necrosis. This latter feature has led to misdiagnosis of the lesion as a rheumatoid nodule.

   b. The natural history is one of multiple recurrences and eventual distant metastasis, although the course may extend over many years.

STUDY QUESTIONS

Directions: Each question below contains five suggested answers. Choose the **one best** response to each question.

1. Synovial sarcoma is most likely to occur in which of the following sites?

(A) Head and neck
(B) Knees
(C) Hands
(D) Spine
(E) Shoulders

2. A 40-year-old woman who complains of a low-grade fever, malaise, and stiffness in her joints each morning most likely has which of the following diseases?

(A) Metastatic carcinoma
(B) Osteoarthritis
(C) Rheumatoid arthritis
(D) Gout
(E) Villonodular synovitis

3. What is the most common degenerative disease affecting the joints?

(A) Rheumatoid arthritis
(B) Osteoarthritis
(C) Gouty arthritis
(D) Villonodular synovitis
(E) Migratory polyarthritis

4. A 12-year-old boy complains of leg pain and swelling, and an x-ray of the affected limb shows the classic sign of Codman's triangle. What is the most likely diagnosis?

(A) Chondrosarcoma
(B) Osteomyelitis
(C) Osteosarcoma
(D) Multiple myeloma
(E) Aneurysmal bone cyst

5. Which of the following bone disorders tends to occur in the femoral epiphyses of young women?   or humerus

(A) Chondroblasoma
(B) Unicameral bone cyst
(C) Giant cell tumor
(D) Fibrous dysplasia
(E) Osteosarcoma

6. Osteomalacia is characterized by which of the following mechanisms?

(A) Pronounced mineralization of the periosteum
(B) Increased deposition of uncalcified osteoid
(C) Abnormal osteoblastic activity
(D) Increased capillary fragility
(E) Abnormal crystalline structure of the bone

Directions: Each question below contains four suggested answers of which **one or more** is correct. Choose the answer

A	if **1, 2, and 3** are correct
B	if **1 and 3** are correct
C	if **2 and 4** are correct
D	if **4** is correct
E	if **1, 2, 3, and 4** are correct

7. A decrease in bone mineral mass can be seen in which of the following groups?

(1) Elderly patients of both sexes
(2) Postmenopausal women
(3) Individuals on chronic steroid therapy
(4) Patients with hypoparathyroidism

8. True statements concerning multiple myeloma include

(1) it may affect several bones simultaneously
(2) it causes abnormal protein electrophoresis
(3) it occurs commonly in the elderly
(4) it is not a true bone neoplasm

ANSWERS AND EXPLANATIONS

1. The answer is B. *(III C 1)* Approximately 75 percent of synovial sarcomas develop in the lower extremities, particularly in the area of the knee. Synovial sarcoma is a malignant neoplasm of the synovial membrane and can occur in the joint synovium, tendon, sheaths, or bursae. The tumor generally carries a poor prognosis, with less than 25 percent of patients surviving 5 years.

2. The answer is C. *(II A 3)* Rheumatoid arthritis is a systemic inflammatory disease of the joints, producing symptoms such as fever, malaise, anemia, and leukocytosis along with joint stiffness and soft tissue swelling around the affected joints. Other complications may occur, including pericarditis, pleuritis, and cardiovascular conditions.

3. The answer is B. *(II B 1)* Osteoarthritis is the most common form of arthritis. Unlike rheumatoid arthritis, which affects the synovial membranes, osteoarthritis destroys articular cartilage. Osteoarthritis may be monoarticular or polyarticular, but typically it affects the large joints of the spine and extremities.

4. The answer is C. *(I H 3)* When an osteogenic sarcoma (osteosarcoma) penetrates the bone cortex, it elevates the periosteum. This periosteal elevation usually produces an acute angle with the underlying remaining cortical bone, which is known as Codman's triangle. As a significant radiographic sign, Codman's triangle aids in the diagnosis of osteogenic sarcoma.

5. The answer is C. *(I H 3 c)* Giant cell tumor or osteoclastoma is a rare bone tumor that is characterized by the presence of multinucleated giant cells, which some authors believe are osteoclasts. This tumor occurs most frequently in women between the ages of 20 and 30 years. The lesion is usually found in the distal portion of long bones, such as the femur or humerus.

6. The answer is B. *(I E 1)* Osteomalacia (rickets) is caused by vitamin D deficiency, the effect of which is an increase in uncalcified osteoid and cartilage and a decrease in the amount of calcified bone. The disease responds to administration of vitamin D.

7. The answer is A (1, 2, 3). *(I C)* Osteopenia is characterized by decreased bone mineral mass, which occurs with increasing age. The catabolic effects of steroid therapy can decrease trabecular bone formation and alter calcium metabolism. Osteoporosis is characterized by bone rarefaction and occurs often in postmenopausal women. Hyperparathyroidism, not hypoparathyroidism, produces progressive calcium waste and demineralization of bone.

8. The answer is E (all). *(I H 3 d)* Multiple myeloma is a malignant tumor of the plasma cells growing in the marrow cavity of the bone. It is thus not a true primary tumor of the bone. The tumor produces excessive amounts of immunoglobulins, hence the abnormal protein electrophoresis. Multiple myeloma is most frequently seen in patients between the sixth and eighth decades of life.

20
The Skin

I. GENERAL PATHOLOGY (Fig. 20-1)

A. EPIDERMIS

1. **Hyperkeratosis** is thickening of the stratum corneum, as occurs in the common wart.

2. **Acanthosis** is thickening of the stratum pinosum (prickle-cell layer), which results from chronic external irritation, as in the formation of a callus.

3. **Parakeratosis** is the retention of the keratocyte nuclei in the stratum corneum, as occurs in psoriasis vulgaris. The condition appears under conditions of rapid keratin formation when there is not time for normal resorption of the keratinocyte nuclei.

4. **Spongiosis** is intercellular edema of the epidermis, as is seen in acute inflammatory disorders such as contact dermatitis from poison ivy.

B. DERMIS

1. With **age** there is a decrease in elastic tissue and mucopolysaccharide content, resulting in a thinner dermis. The subcutaneous fat also atrophies.

2. With **chronic light exposure** the dermis undergoes elastotic degeneration of collagen, which gives the clinical appearance of severe wrinkling.

3. Extreme **stretching** of skin leads to the rupture and loss of elastic tissue, as seen during pregnancy in the striae gravidarum.

4. In **wound repair** a scar is formed when new collagen fibrils are deposited parallel to the surface of the skin. In keloidal wound repair, seen predominately in blacks, there is a neoplastic proliferation of collagen.

5. **Hair.**
   a. **Male pattern alopecia** (balding) is a common abnormality seen in 80 percent of Caucasian males in approximately the sixth decade of life. It is induced by androgens; the active moiety is thought to be 5-dihydroxytestosterone. This irreversible process is not found in males castrated before puberty, and it may be induced in a castrate by the administration of androgens.
   b. Excessive hair loss may be **secondary** to other conditions.
      (1) Extreme **stress**, for example, after a myocardial infarction
      (2) Administration of a **toxic drug**, for example, chemotherapy for a neoplasm

II. LESIONS

A. TYPES

1. A **macule** is a circumscribed flat area of skin distinguishable by color (e.g., a freckle).

2. A **papule** is a solid elevated skin lesion occupying a relatively large surface area (e.g., seborrheic keratosis).

3. A **nodule** is a palpable, solid, round or ellipsoidal lesion in the deep skin or subcutaneous tissues; it is situated deeper than a papule (e.g., a nodule of rheumatoid arthritis).

4. A **wheal** is a rounded or flat-topped elevation of skin. It is short-lived and results from edema of the upper dermis (e.g., a mosquito bite).

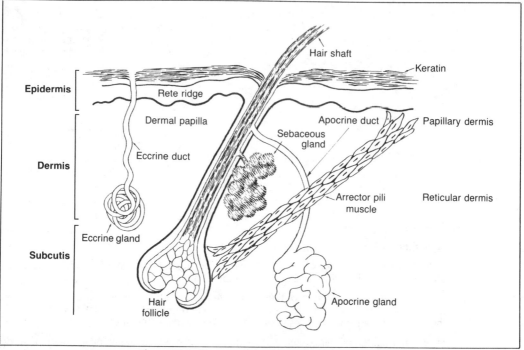

Figure 20-1. Diagram of the skin and its adnexa.

5. A **vesicle** is an elevated lesion that contains fluid. When it is larger than 0.5 cm it is referred to as a **bulla** or **blister** (e.g., the blister of a second-degree burn).

B. DISTRIBUTION

1. When lesions are **localized** they can be bilateral and symmetrical and occur in sun-exposed areas, intertriginous areas, and areas of trauma and dermatomal pattern.

2. **Generalized** lesions are widespread throughout the skin.

3. **Universal** lesions involve the entire integument: the skin, hair, and nails.

III. SKIN DISORDERS

A. COMMON SKIN DISEASES

1. **Acne vulgaris** Is distributed equally between the sexes and predominates between the ages of 14 and 19 years.

   a. **Clinical Data.** The disease is an inflammatory reaction of the pilosebaceous apparatus. It predominately affects the face, neck, and upper trunk areas, which are rich in sebaceous follicles. The initial lesions are comedones, commonly called black heads and white heads. The complicated lesions include papules, pustules, nodules, and cysts, which result ultimately in scars.

   A genetic component is apparent. Diet, inadequate cleansing, stress, and weather all have been implicated in the exacerbation of acne. Approximately 60 to 70 percent of females present with a flare-up of the disease before menstruation.

   b. **Pathology.** The current pathogenic concept is that in adolescence two important changes occur: Sebaceous glands become hyperplastic, and the shedding of keratin from the outer follicle becomes sluggish. A keratinous plug forms in the outer hair follicle and sebaceous material accumulates below it. As the proximal follicle accumulates debris, it becomes distended and eventually ruptures into the surrounding dermis. The follicular contents stimulate an intense acute inflammatory reaction. The anaerobic bacterium *Corynebacterium acnes* is involved in the development of the complicated acne lesions; however, its role is not clear.

   c. **Treatment.** Acne is treated, often successfully, with tetracyclines.

2. **Acne rosacea** is a disease of the pilosebaceous apparatus, which occurs in middle age (30 to 50 years). The patient has facial erythema, follicular papules, and pustules. In one form, known as rhinophyma, which is seen predominately in men, there is diffuse sebaceous hyperplasia of the nasal skin, leading to a bulbous nose.

3. **Miliaria** (heat rash) is a disease of the eccrine (sweat) apparatus. It occurs following excessive sweating in parts of the body covered by clothing. In certain cases, such as diaper rash, urine is the irritant. There are two major types: **miliaria crystallina** and **miliaria rubra**.
   a. **Pathology.** In miliaria crystallina there are vesicles, within or beneath the horny layer, caused by a ruptured sweat duct. In miliaria rubra spongiotic vesicles are found in the stratum malpighii. A chronic inflammatory infiltrate is seen around and within the vesicles as well as in the adjacent dermis. Both types result from poral occlusion caused by a horn plug swollen through excessive hydration.
   b. **Treatment.** The best treatment is removal of the cause of the plugging and reduction of the stimulus that produces the excessive perspiration.

4. **Psoriasis** is a disease affecting 1 to 2 percent of individuals of European lineage. Men in the third decade of life are affected more often than women.
   a. **Clinical Data.** Scaley plaques appear, predominately on the surfaces of extensor areas such as the elbows and knees. The disease is thought to be genetically determined and probably represents an autosomal dominant trait with incomplete penetration.
   b. **Pathology.** The psoriatic lesion is an elevated whitish plaque and is associated with rapidly dividing epidermal cells. Normally epidermal cells take 28 days to ascend from the basal layer to the skin surface; in the psoriatic patient they take 3 to 4 days, and two to three layers of dividing cells are often present in the epidermis. Typically the epidermis is thin over the dermal papillae, and there is a parakeratotic scale. The dermis is so richly vascularized that bleeding easily occurs (Auspitz sign).
   A regular feature of psoriasis is the outward migration of polymorphonuclear neutrophil leukocytes into the epidermis. A serine protease, released by the outer epidermal keratinocytes of the psoriatic plaque, cleaves complement, which then serves as the chemotactic agent for polymorphonuclear neutrophil leukocytes. Why and how this serum protease is activated is not clear.

5. **Seborrheic dermatitis** is an erythematous lesion of unknown etiology. The most common and mildest form of the disease is known as **dandruff**. Generalized seborrheic dermatitis in infants is often referred to as Leiner's disease.
   a. **Clinical Data.** The disease may be generalized or may affect focal areas such as the scalp, eyebrows, face, and ears. The lesions appear as sharply demarcated brown-red areas covered with fine yellowish scales. Oozing may be present, but no vesiculation is found.
   b. **Pathology.** The histologic picture is not diagnostic. The horny layer shows focal areas of parakeratosis, occasionally containing a few pyknotic leukocytes. Moderate epidermal acanthosis, with elongation of the rete ridges, and spongiosis appear. The dermis has a mild chronic inflammatory infiltrate.

6. **Contact dermatitis** is caused by contact of the skin with an agent that acts either as a specific allergic sensitizer or as a primary irritant. The disease may be acute, subacute, or chronic. In the acute and subacute forms, diffuse erythema, edema, oozing, and crusting predominate. In the chronic form, erythema, scaling, and lichenification prevail.
   a. **Acute contact dermatitis,** particularly if a specific allergic sensitizer is the cause, is characterized by the presence of vesicles or bullae, separated from one another by thin fibrous septa. The vesicles and bullae contain lymphocytes, eosinophils, neutrophils, and disintegrated epidermal cells. The epidermis shows extensive edema. The upper dermis shows vascular dilatation, edema, and inflammation.
   b. **Subacute contact dermatitis** is characterized by spongiosis and the presence of small vesicles. There are abundant chronic inflammatory cells. Moderate epidermal acanthosis with varying degrees of parakeratosis appears.
   c. **Chronic Contact Dermatitis.** There is slight intercellular edema of the epidermis with acanthosis and elongation of the rete ridges. The dermis contains varying amounts of chronic inflammatory cells.

B. DISORDERS OF KERATIN PRODUCTION

1. **Cutaneous horn** is a large, horn-like, gray-brown projection of keratin, which can arise on almost any papillary lesion including carcinoma. Histologically, the horn is composed of a thickened stratum corneum with focal areas of parakeratosis.

2. Warts.

    a. Verruca vulgaris (common wart) is a circumscribed, firm, elevated growth. The fingers are the most common sites of verruca vulgaris, but the lesion may occur anywhere on the skin and, in rare instances, on the oral mucosa.

        (1) Etiology. The lesion is caused by a virus commonly found in the nuclei of the vacuolated cells present in the granular layer and stratum malpighii.

        (2) Pathology. Verruca vulgaris shows acanthosis, papillomatosis, and hyperkeratosis with areas of parakeratosis, but the basal layer of the epidermis is intact. The dermis is unremarkable. Intracytoplasmic inclusions are seen in approximately 25 percent of cases.

        (3) Treatment. Excision and cryosurgery of the lesion are the treatments of choice. The lesion, however, can resolve spontaneously.

    b. Verruca plana is a slightly raised, smooth wart. It occurs usually in multiples and is seen chiefly in children.

    c. Verruca plantaris, also known as a plantar wart, is located on the soles of the feet.

3. Condyloma acuminatum is a lesion consisting of soft verrucous nodules that often fuse and form large cauliflower-like masses around the anal and genital regions. It is of viral origin and may be transmitted sexually, although many of these lesions do arise without sexual contact.

    a. Pathology. There is marked acanthosis of the epidermis, and vacuolated epithelial cells with clear cytoplasms and hyperchromatic nuclei are present. The surface of the condyloma is papillomatous, wavy, and covered by a slightly thickened parakeratotic layer. The dermis may contain some chronic inflammatory cells.

    b. Treatment is resection of the lesion.

4. Seborrheic keratosis, also called verruca senilis or basal cell papilloma, is a lesion that arises on the trunk, face, and arms of elderly people. It is often seen in large numbers, but single lesions may occur.

    a. Clinical Data. Presenting as brownish, slightly raised, circumscribed, and verrucous, the lesion varies in size from a few mm to several cm.

    b. Histologically, there is hyperkeratosis, acanthosis, and papillomatosis. Melanin may be present in different amounts in the epidermis. Interspersed among the epithelial cells are cystic inclusions of horny material. The border of the tumor is sharply demarcated, and the dermis is unremarkable, although chronic inflammatory cells may be present.

    c. Treatment. This lesion is not malignant, and surgical resection is sufficient.

5. Actinic (solar) keratosis is a common lesion that occurs on the face, the dorsum of the hands, and the forearms of individuals in or past middle life. Prolonged exposure to sunlight is the essential predisposing factor. Usually the lesion measures less than 1 cm in diameter.

    a. Pathology. The presentation is that of a dry scale, firmly adherent to an erythematous base. Histologically, there is hyperkeratosis, acanthosis, and papillomatosis. The epidermal cells are arranged in a disorderly fashion and have hyperchromatic nuclei. Mitoses are commonly found. The upper portion of the dermis shows solar degeneration of the collagen (solar elastosis) and dense chronic inflammatory lymphocytic infiltration.

    b. Treatment. Although this process is not considered malignant per se, it is regarded by most pathologists as precancerous because of its progression to squamous cell carcinoma. The treatment should consist of wide excision.

6. Ichthyosis (fish skin) is an inherited, lifelong disease caused by overproduction of keratin and decreased keratin desquamation or by a molecular defect, which is not known. It appears that the keratin itself is faulty since the keratin layer does not shed normally. Affected patients have increased water loss.

C. BULLOUS DISEASES

1. General Considerations. This group of diseases is characterized by the presence of blisters, vesicles, or bullae. The lesions can be formed by the destruction of either individual cells or intracellular connections. In trauma, which results in a rip of keratinocytes within the epidermis itself, fluid accumulation forms a balloon structure referred to as a blister. A blister may also result from suction, which separates the epidermis from its dermal junction.

2. Bullous Pemphigoid.

    a. This disease occurs in elderly people (80 percent of the patients are older than 60 years of age) who may look sick because of their multiple bullae but who usually do not feel ill. The blisters do not rupture easily.

    b. The lesion starts as an erythema, which then evolves into a tense bulla. The roof of the bulla is the entire epidermis. Immunofluorescent studies show that there are deposits of immunoglobulin G (IgG) in the basement membrane.

3. **Pemphigus.** In this disease the split in the skin occurs within the epidermis. The roof of the blister is quite thin and ruptures easily. In time, the patient develops large weeping wounds over the body. These wounds encourage fluid loss and infection.

4. **Pemphigus vulgaris** occurs mainly in individuals 40 to 60 years of age, 60 percent of whom are Jewish. A mouth lesion is the presenting sign in 50 percent of the patients. There appears to be an immunologic etiology in that the patient has circulating antibodies to his or her epidermis.

5. **Dermatitis Herpetiformis.**
   a. This is a chronic, recurrent, pruritic disease in which groups of papules and vesicles appear symmetrically. The extensor surfaces of the extremities, the shoulders, and the buttocks are commonly affected. The oral mucosa is not affected.
   b. The typical **histologic** feature is the presence of neutrophils and eosinophils at the tips of the papillae and the subepidermal vesicles or bullae (Fig. 20-2).
   c. When the disease occurs during pregnancy, it is known as **herpes gestationis**, and it usually disappears after termination of the pregnancy.
   d. As a rule the eruption responds well to sulfapyridine and the sulfones.

6. **Erythema Multiforme** (Stevens-Johnson Syndrome).
   a. This acute, self-limited dermatosis, with a tendency to recur, is believed to be produced by an allergic sensitivity reaction. The lesions may be multiple and widespread or focally localized, and they present as macules, papules, vesicles, or bullae. They commonly produce the so-called iris lesion, a papule with peripheral extension and central cleaving.
   b. **Histologically**, there are no specific features. Severe cases may start abruptly with high fever, prostration, and extensive bullous eruption of the skin and mucous membranes. When bullae form, they are localized in the subepidermis and contain fibrin as well as eosinophils, lymphocytes, and polymorphonuclear cells. The dermis contains an inflammatory infiltrate, the severity of which varies as do its clinical manifestations.

7. **Herpes simplex** is a viral infection that characteristically leads to necrosis of the epidermal cells, resulting in blister formation.
   a. **Herpes labialis** appears often on the edges of the lips or nostrils. It commonly is referred to as a cold sore. A burning sensation and hyperesthesia occur. The vesicles may develop

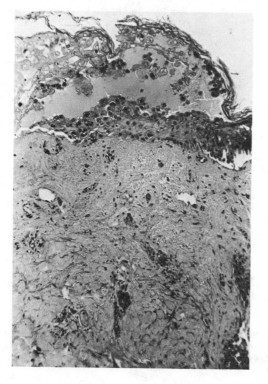

Figure 20-2. Low-power magnification of dermatitis herpetiformis. Notice the epidermal vesicle formation filled with fibrin, neutrophils, and degenerating epidermal cells.

in association with trauma, sun exposure, menstruation, and stress. Healing may take place spontaneously within 1 to 2 weeks, although the condition may become chronic with common recurrences.

   b. Herpes genitalis presents in the same way, but the sores are on the genitals.

   c. When there is accompanying fever (fever blisters), the condition is referred to as **herpes febrilis**.

8. Impetigo.

   a. This is an infectious disease of childhood, caused by staphylococcal or streptococcal infections of the outer epidermis. It begins with the development of erythematous macules and progresses to thin-walled, pus-filled vesicles.

   b. The bullae develop secondary to the bacteria-induced inflammatory reaction apparently because of cell lysis and necrosis.

   c. When impetigo is produced by streptococcus, it may be the source of other infections such as glomerulonephritis.

9. Epidermolysis Bullosa.

   a. This congenital disease may be inherited as an autosomal-recessive condition. It is rare, occurring in 1 of 300,000 births.

   b. Affected patients lack anchoring fibrils and have blisters over areas common to trauma, such as the abdomen, knees, elbows, hands, and feet. The bullae heal readily, but often the resultant scarring is immobilizing.

D. INFLAMMATIONS

1. Bacterial.

   a. Hidradenitis suppurativa is a chronic infection caused by *Staphyloccocus* and *Streptococcus*. The lesion begins as a red, subcutaneous nodule in the axillary or anogenital regions. Eventually the nodules coalesce to form cordlike, elevated bands, and there is suppuration and tenderness with eventual drainage of the purulent material. The bacteria enter via the hair follicles and spread to the apocrine sweat glands. Diffuse scarring is the end result of the disease.

   b. Leprosy is a slowly developing disease caused by *Mycobacterium leprae*. Although it manifests itself first in the skin, the bacterium also may be found in parenchymal organs. Typically, the patient has hypoesthesias and hypopigmented papules over the skin of the face, ears, cheeks, chin, neck, and trunk. The several forms of the disease are defined in part by host resistance to the infecting organism.

   (1) In the **lepromatous** form, host defense is inadequate, and bacterial multiplication is uncontrolled.

   (2) In the **tuberculoid** form, there is strong resistance to the infection.

   c. Tuberculosis (Lupus Vulgaris).

   (1) Clinical Data. The lesions are found most commonly on the face and consist of well-demarcated, red-brown patches. Superficial ulceration occurs occasionally.

   (2) Histologically, tubercules composed of epithelioid and giant cells are present. Caseation and other forms of necrosis are almost always absent. The upper portion of the dermis may show extensive inflammation, but occasionally the infiltrate can extend into the subcutis, destroying the cutaneous appendages. The acid-fast bacilli may be difficult to demonstrate by special staining methods.

2. Fungal.

   a. Moniliasis (Candidiasis).

   (1) Clinical Data. *Candida albicans* is not only a cutaneous pathogen that may affect mucosal surfaces, but in certain instances it can also cause systemic problems. In the skin, the primary lesion of moniliasis is a subcorneal pustule. When in the mucocutaneous areas, the lesions appear as confluent white patches with surrounding erythematous borders and inflammation of adjacent tissues.

   (2) Pathology. The organism is present in the stratum corneum, but occasionally it can infiltrate adjacent tissues. It consists of branching mycelia (2 μ to 4 μ in diameter) and ovoid spores.

   (3) Once the causative organism is determined, the diagnosis can be made.

   b. Tinea (dermatophytosis) is the most important type of superficial fungal infection. The designation varies according to the area of the body that is affected. The diagnosis is based on demonstration of the fungi histologically.

   (1) Tinea of the **feet** and **hands** is caused by *Trichophyton rubrum*. The lesion presents with maceration between and underneath the toes, erythematous scaling, and vesicular eruption on the soles and the palms.

(2) Tinea cruris, common in males, is caused by *Trichophyton rubrum* and produces erythematous areas on the scrotum and inner surfaces of the thighs.

(3) Tinea capitis occurs predominately in children and affects the hair, which tends to break off, and the scalp. It is caused by *Microsporum audouini*.

(4) Tinea barbae is characterized by inflammation of the bearded regions of the face and neck and is produced by *Trichophyton mentagrophytes*.

(5) Tinea versicolor is caused by *Malassezia furfur*. It is noninflammatory and affects predominately the trunk, where there are areas of brown discoloration with fine brawny scales.

   c. Other fungal diseases such as sporotrichosis, mycetoma, coccidioidomycosis, and nocardiosis may affect the skin and be the entrance for systemic infections. The diagnosis is made when the causative agent is determined.

E. NONMALIGNANT PIGMENTED LESIONS

1. **Freckles** are benign, circumscribed areas of hyperpigmentation. They vary from light to dark brown and usually become darker after sun exposure. Histologically, the increased pigmentation is in the basal layer of the epidermis.

2. **Nevocellular nevus** (the common mole) is a benign neoplasm composed of nevus cells and melanocytes. The lesion may appear flat, papillomatous, or pedunculated, and it may show marked hyperpigmentation and hairs. Three types are recognized.

   a. Intradermal Nevus. The upper dermis shows nests and cords of nevus cells, some of which contain varying amounts of melanin. In the lower dermis the nevus cells are scattered and embedded in collagenous tissue. Occasionally these cells fuse and form multinucleated giant cells; this occurs more commonly with mature nevi. The epidermis may show changes, such as papillomatosis and hyperkeratosis (Fig. 20-3), or it may appear normal.

   b. Junction Nevus. The nevus cells, which contain melanin, are arranged in nests in the lower epidermis. They can occur in the upper dermis but to a minimal extent and always in conjunction with the epidermis. The dermis is unremarkable.

   c. Compound nevus is a lesion that possesses features of the two just discussed. Although nevus cells are present in both the dermis and epidermis, they may predominate in the dermis. When the lower third of the dermis is involved and the pilar units are surrounded, the lesion is probably congenital.

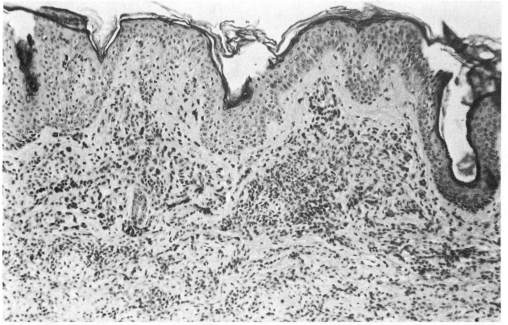

Figure 20-3. High-power view of an intradermal nevus. Nevus cells lie in the dermis in nests and cords. The epidermis here is unremarkable.

3. **Blue Nevus.**
    a. This is a small, round or oval, well-circumscribed, soft nodule and is blue to black in color. It commonly occurs on the buttocks, face, and arms, but it can be seen anywhere on the body.
    b. **Histologically,** the lesion involves the entire dermis, where fibroblastic pigmented cells are present. In addition, there are melanophages grouped in irregular bundles extending into the subcutaneous layer. The epidermis is normal.

F. **TUMORS OF THE DERMIS**

1. **Granuloma Pyogenicum.**
    a. **Clinical Data.** This is predominately a single lesion that is composed of a dull-red, soft, raised nodule. The surface may be smooth but often shows superficial ulceration and crusting. Bleeding occurs easily when the lesion is traumatized. As a rule, the epidermis has an inward growth at the base of the lesion, causing slight pedunculation.
    b. **Histologically,** the lesion is circumscribed and is covered by a flattened epidermis. The dermis contains numerous newly formed capillaries with prominent endothelial cells. The stroma is edematous and is usually free of inflammatory infiltration.
    c. **Treatment** is resection of the lesion.

2. **Keloid** (see Chapter 21, IV E).

3. **Dermatofibroma.**
    a. **Clinical Data.** This lesion is an indolent nodule that occurs predominately on the extremities of adults. It is usually small, a few mm in diameter, and varies in color from red to yellow.
    b. **Histologically,** the dermal collagen appears as irregularly arranged intertwining and anastomosing bands mixed with scattered small capillaries. It forms nodules that merge gradually with the surrounding normal collagen. Occasionally, multinucleated giant cells and foamy macrophages are present. The overlying epidermis may frequently show marked acanthosis, predominately in the center of the lesion (Fig. 20-4).
    c. **Treatment** is resection of the lesion.

4. **Dermatofibrosarcoma Protuberans.**
    a. **Clinical Data.** This is a slow-growing tumor that originates in the dermis. Originally it presents as an indurate plaque from which red or blue multiple nodules arise.

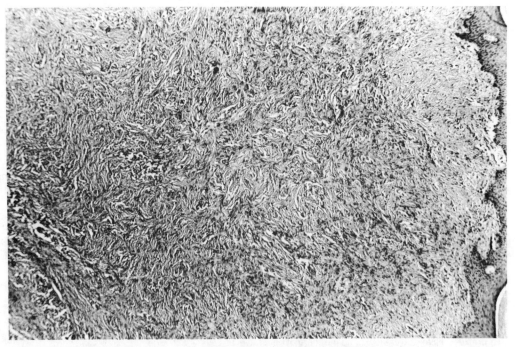

Figure 20-4. Low-power magnification of a dermatofibroma. There is an increased amount of dermal collagen arranged in an irregular fashion.

    b. Histologically, the tumor is composed of fibroblasts arranged in irregular strands and whorls. The fibroblasts may be atypical to varying degrees, and mitoses may be present. The tumor cells penetrate the subcutaneous fat and occasionally may infiltrate the fascia and underlying muscle. The epidermis may show atrophy or ulceration, but it does not show acanthosis. Metastasis to other organs are very rare.

    c. Treatment. Complete surgical excision of the lesion is necessary to avoid recurrences.

5. Kaposi's Sarcoma.

    a. This is a disease with a marked preponderance in men, but approximately 4 percent of the cases are found in children. Cases have been reported in all countries, but it predominates in the black population in certain parts of Africa. The etiology of this tumor is not clear, but it is believed that affected individuals have a deranged immune status. The basic cell of origin is an immature pluripotential vascular cell.

    b. Clinical Data. Kaposi's sarcoma is characterized by one or more blue-to-red skin nodules or by a maculopapular eruption. The lesion is most commonly located on the lower extremities, but it can occur on any body surface. In approximately 15 percent of the cases there is visceral involvement affecting the liver, lungs, gastrointestinal tract, and lymph nodes. In rare instances, the visceral lesion precedes the skin manifestations.

    Recently there has been an increase of Kaposi's sarcoma in homosexual males. When the disease occurs in this clinical setting, it presents with prominent visceral involvement and carries a dismal prognosis.

    c. Microscopically, there is a proliferation of capillaries, prominent endothelial cells, and the vascular spaces sometimes show free anastomoses. The capillaries may be inconspicuous because they are intermingled with a stroma that is composed of spindle-shaped fibroblasts. The stroma contains varying amounts of hemosiderin, extravascular red blood cells, and inflammatory cells, mainly lymphocytes.

    d. Prognosis. The disease is ordinarily slow, unrelenting, and progressive, causing death after varying intervals. Death may result from hemorrhage or infection. Kaposi's sarcoma tends to coexist with lymphoma, leukemia, and other malignancies.

6. Mycosis Fungoides Cutaneous Lymphoma.

    a. Mycosis fungoides is a cutaneous lymphoproliferative disorder that pursues an indolent but progressive course, frequently spanning many years. Prolonged localization of this lymphoma in the skin suggests that it arises from immunocompetent T cells specialized to provide cutaneous immunity.

    b. Clinical Data. The disease may present as a diffuse, generalized erythema or as elevated plaques consisting of irregularly shaped, raised, brown-red lesions, which often undergo ulceration.

    c. Histologically, skin biopsies show extensive lymphocytic infiltration of the dermis and, to a lesser extent, of the epidermis. The neoplastic cells are intermediate to large in size, and their nuclei have a characteristic cerebriform folding pattern. An almost pathognomonic finding is the presence in the epidermis of **Pautrier microabscesses** (small groups of mononuclear cells surrounded by halo-like clear spaces). When dissemination occurs to the lymph nodes they show involvement of the T-zone areas by foci of neoplastic cells.

    d. Prognosis. In the cutaneous tumor stage, ulceration of the lesion may precede sepsis and death, but the natural history is eventual dissemination to the involvement of the lymph nodes, viscera, and bone marrow. The mortality is approximately 70 percent within 6 years.

7. Sézary syndrome is characterized by generalized pruritic erythroderma, peripheral lymphadenopathy, and the presence of Sézary cells in the peripheral blood. The course of the disease is similar to that of a malignant lymphoma.

G. TUMORS OF THE EPIDERMIS. Carcinomas may metastasize to the skin either directly from underlying tumors or via lymphatics or the bloodstream. Cutaneous metastases from primary sites, such as the kidneys, breasts, and lungs, are not uncommon.

    1. An **inclusion cyst** is a benign cystic lesion in the epidermis.

        a. Clinical Data. This slow-growing, elevated, firm, intracutaneous, or subcutaneous "tumor" can occur at any site on the body.

        b. Histologically, the cyst, lined by epidermis with all layers present, is filled with keratin, often arranged in laminated layers. Rupture of the cyst is common, and its contents excite a florid, foreign-body giant cell reaction in the surrounding tissues.

        c. Treatment is surgical excision of the lesion.

    2. Basal Cell Carcinoma. Derived from the basal cells of the epidermis, this tumor occurs predominately on the hair-bearing surfaces of the adult. The face and scalp areas are the regions most commonly affected; mucous membranes, the palms, and the soles are never involved. The tumor grows by direct extension and infiltration of adjacent structures, but it very rarely metastasizes.

    a. Clinical Data. This lesion can arise without apparent reason, but prolonged sun exposure or large doses of x-radiation are important predisposing factors. Basal cell carcinoma can occur as single or multiple lesions, which measure a few cm in diameter and have raised, rolled borders with a central area of depression that may be ulcerated.

    b. Histologically, the tumor is composed of characteristic basal cells, that is, cells with large oval or elongated nuclei and little cytoplasms. The nuclei are very uniform and show no anaplasia.

        (1) The basal cells form masses of various sizes and shapes and infiltrate the dermis. Some of the masses may show contact with the epidermis. The periphery of these masses often shows an arrangement of palisade cells; the nuclei of the cells inside are disorganized. Occasionally pigmentation, calcification, or mucinoid degeneration are present (Fig. 20-5).

        (2) The connective tissue adjacent to the tumor shows proliferative changes, with an increased number of young fibroblasts. Chronic inflammatory cells may be seen.

        (3) Since the basal cell has a pluripotential capacity, it can differentiate toward squamous epithelium, hair, or adnexal structures, accounting for the different patterns of basal cell carcinomas.

    c. The best **treatment** is complete excision of the lesion.

   3. Squamous cell carcinoma can occur anywhere on the skin as well as in the mucous membranes.

    a. Clinical Data. This lesion commonly arises on sun-damaged skin, but it can also arise in association with ulcers, scars, and foci of chronic osteomyelitis. Men are affected more often than women in a ratio of 2:1. The lesion consists of a shallow ulcer surrounded by a wide, elevated, and indurate border. The ulcer may be covered by a crust with a red granular base. Occasionally, a raised, verrucous lesion occurs without evidence of ulceration.

    b. Histologically, the tumor is composed of irregular masses of epidermal cells, which proliferate and invade the dermis. The squamous cells may show different degrees of anaplasia, as well as pleomorphism with prominent hyperchromatic nuclei. There is absence of intercellular bridges. Individual cells may undergo keratinization and pearl formation, and mitoses are present. The dermis surrounding the invasive tumor shows prominent chronic inflammatory reaction.

    c. The **prognosis** depends largely on the site of the lesion. Carcinomas that arise in mucous membranes have a high rate of metastasis, if not properly treated, and the regional lymph

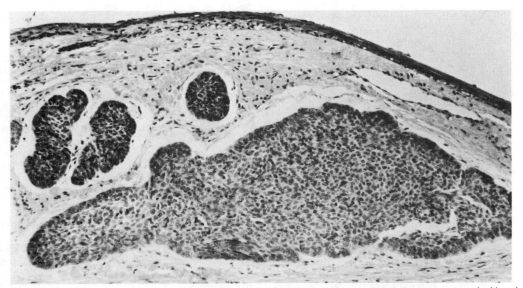

Figure 20-5. High-power view of a basal cell carcinoma. Masses of varying sizes and shapes composed of basal cells are present. The periphery of the masses shows a palisade arrangement.

nodes are the first sites to be invaded. Tumors that originate in sun-exposed areas have a low propensity toward metastasis.

    d. Treatment is surgical excision of the tumor.

4. **Malignant melanoma** is the most malignant of the cutaneous neoplasms. It arises from melanocytic cells of the epidermis in a preexisting nevus or de novo from the melanocytes. Malignant melanoma is rare before puberty, but fatal cases have been reported in children.

    a. Clinical Data. This lesion presents as a gradually enlarging pigmented nodule surrounded by erythema. The nodule may show crusting, bleeding, or ulceration.

    b. Histologically, the tumor originates at the epidermal-dermal junction, where there is irregular activity with streaming of atypical and malignant nevus cells down toward the dermis. The tumor cells may vary in size and shape, but most have large nuclei with prominent nucleoli and abundant granular eosinophilic cytoplasms. Multinucleated, bizarre giant cells are present, and mitoses are common. The amount of melanin and inflammatory infiltrate varies greatly with each case (Fig. 20-6).

    c. There are three types of malignant melanoma: **superficial spreading**, **nodular**, and **lentigo maligna**. The superficial spreading and nodular types are the most common, occurring on any part of the body but most often on the legs, shoulders, and upper back. Lentigo maligna occurs in the sun-damaged skin of older people. Both of these types may rest in a superficial location for many years before invading. Nodular melanoma is the most aggressive variant; in part because it is usually diagnosed after it has deeply invaded. In rare instances, malignant melanoma occurs in areas such as the oral cavity, the upper respiratory and gastrointestinal tracts, and the vagina.

    d. Prognosis depends on the type of melanoma, the level of invasion, and the presence or absence of metastasis. The superficial spreading and lentigo maligna melanomas usually have a better prognosis than the nodular type.

       Of the five levels of invasion, the prognosis is best for the first three.

      (1) At **level 1** tumor cells are limited to the epidermis.

      (2) At **level 2** tumor cells extend into the papillary dermis.

      (3) At **level 3** tumor cells fill the papillary dermis.

      (4) At **level 4** tumor cells invade the reticular dermis.

      (5) At **level 5** the tumor extends through the skin into the subcutis.

      (6) It is believed that those tumors measuring less than 0.76 mm **(Breslow's level)** in thickness have an excellent prognosis with low metastatic rates.

    e. Metastases. The melanomas that metastasize tend to spread in early stages to adjacent skin and regional lymph nodes. In later stages, hematogenous spread with diffuse visceral involvement occurs.

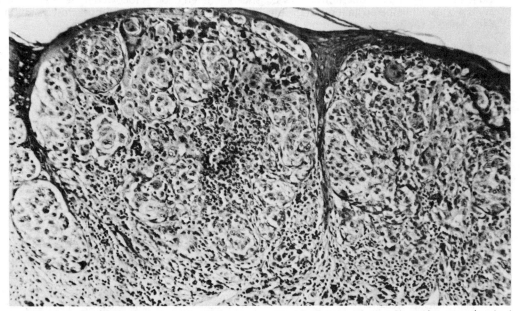

Figure 20-6. High magnification of a malignant melanoma. The nests of tumor cells infiltrate the upper dermis. A moderate lymphocytic response is also present.

STUDY QUESTIONS

Directions: The question below contains five suggested answers. Choose the **one best** response.

1. What is the primary predisposing factor for actinic keratosis?

(A) Autoimmune disease
(B) Chemical exposure
(C) Sunlight exposure
(D) Cigarette smoking
(E) Inheritance

Directions: Each question below contains four suggested answers of which **one or more** is correct. Choose the answer

A   if **1, 2, and 3** are correct
B   if **1 and 3** are correct
C   if **2 and 4** are correct
D   if **4** is correct
E   if **1, 2, 3, and 4** are correct

2. Characteristics of psoriasis include

(1) dermatosis of extensor surfaces
(2) rapidly dividing epidermal cells
(3) outward migration of polymorphonuclear leukocytes
(4) Auspitz sign

3. Malignant pigmented skin lesions include which of the following?

(1) Superficial spreading melanoma
(2) Nodular melanoma
(3) Lentigo maligna
(4) Mycosis fungoides

Directions: The group of questions below consists of lettered choices followed by several numbered items. For each numbered item select the **one** lettered choice with which it is **most** closely associated. Each lettered choice may be used once, more than once, or not at all.

Questions 4–8

The most important superficial fungal infections of the skin are termed dermatophytoses or tinea. Match the tineal infections described below with the causative fungi.

(A) *Trichophyton rubrum*
(B) *Microsporum audouini*
(C) *Trichophyton mentagrophytes*
(D) *Malassezia furfur*
(E) *Candida albicans*

4. Tinea cruris—the erythematous lesion found on the scrotum and inner thigh surfaces

5. Tinea capitis—the fungal infection of the scalp, which affects the hair follicles and causes the hair shafts to break off

6. Tinea barbae—fungal infection of the bearded facial skin in men

7. Tinea versicolor—affects the trunk area, where it produces brown discoloration with a very fine scale

8. Tinea pedis—the fungal infection of the feet, producing erythema and erosion beween the toes

ANSWERS AND EXPLANATIONS

1. The answer is C. *(III B 5)* Actinic keratosis is also called solar keratosis because prolonged exposure to sunlight is the essential predisposing factor. The lesions usually develop on the face, on the dorsum of the hand, and on other skin surfaces chronically exposed to the sun. Although actinic keratosis is not considered to be malignant per se, the lesions are precancerous because of frequent progression to squamous cell carcinoma. Treatment is wide margin surgical excision.

2. The answer is E (all). *(III A 4)* Psoriasis is a relatively common dermatosis, reportedly affecting 0.5 to 1.5 percent of the population. It produces erythematous plaques covered by fine, silvery scales, which typically involve the extensor surfaces (i.e., elbows, knees, back, and scalp). Migration of polymorphonuclear leukocytes into the parakeratotic epidermis produces Munro microabscesses. The dermis becomes so highly vascularized that bleeding occurs easily with minor trauma such as scratching (Auspitz sign).

3. The answer is A (1, 2, 3). *(III F 6; III G 4)* The primary types of malignant melanoma, a highly malignant neoplasm of the melanocytic cells of the skin, include superficial spreading melanoma, nodular melanoma, and lentigo maligna. Most melanomas produce melanin and are thus darkly pigmented with variable amounts of ulceration, crusting, bleeding, and surrounding erythema. Mycosis fungoides is an indolent but malignant lymphoma of the T lymphocytes of the skin. It produces a diffuse, generalized erythema or elevated plaques consisting of raised, red-brown lesions, which can undergo ulceration. Mycosis fungoides does not, however, produce additional pigment.

4–8. The answers are: 4-A, 5-B, 6-C, 7-D, 8-A. *(III D 2)* Tinea cruris, which is caused by the fungus *Trichophyton rubrum,* is an erythematous lesion found on the scrotum and inner surfaces of the thigh. *Trichophyton rubrum* is also the cause of tinea pedis, the fungal infection of the feet, which produces erythema and erosion between the toes. Tinea capitis is a fungal infection of the scalp caused by *Microsporum audouini.* It affects the hair follicles and causes the hair shafts to break off. The infection of the bearded facial skin in men is termed tinea barbae and is caused by *Trichophyton mentagrophytes. Malassezia furfur* produces tinea versicolor, which affects the trunk area where it produces brown discoloration with a very fine scale.

21
Soft Tissues

I. INTRODUCTION

A. DEFINITION AND CLASSIFICATION OF SOFT TISSUE LESIONS

1. Soft tissues are found between the dermis and the skeleton, including those of nonvisceral origin. Thus, soft tissues are muscles, connective tissues, blood vessels, nerves, and fat.

2. Lesions involving soft tissues can be divided into four main groups.
   a. Pseudotumors (reactive or reparative processes)
   b. Benign neoplasms
   c. Malignant neoplasms
   d. Locally aggressive lesions

B. CLINICAL PRESENTATION OF SOFT TISSUE LESIONS

1. Most soft tissue lesions produce a noticeable lump, which is frequently painless and often enlarging over a variable period of time. In some instances, trauma may be related to the production of the lump (as in fasciitis—see II D). True neoplasms probably are not induced by trauma, but trauma may draw a patient's attention to a lesion.

2. A **solitary lump** may represent anything, such as an epidermal inclusion cyst (sebaceous cyst), a skin adnexal tumor, or a metastasis from a carcinoma elsewhere, but the present discussion will be limited to those lesions the origin of which is considered mesenchymal (i.e., classic "soft-tissue tumors").

II. PSEUDOTUMORS (REACTIVE OR REPARATIVE PROCESSES)

A. GENERAL CONSIDERATIONS

1. Pseudotumors may be related temporally to a specific traumatic event, frequently are discovered soon after onset, and often are tender or painful.

2. These lesions may vary in size but are commonly under 2 cm. Simple surgical excision is curative.

3. Among a, b, d, and e, below, any two or more can coexist, and variable amounts of inflammatory cells, hemorrhage, and hemosiderin may be found in any individual lesion. Any of these lesions also may include the relatively newly described **myofibroblasts**, with their properties of contraction (myo-) and collagen production (fibroblast). Such cells participate in normal wound healing as well as in the exaggerated or abnormal processes of repair and regeneration described below.

4. **Classification.** Pseudotumors can be classified into seven groups, which are listed here in descending order of importance.
   a. Hematoma
   b. Fat necrosis
   c. Pseudosarcomatous (nodular) fasciitis
   d. Foreign-body granuloma
   e. Xanthogranuloma
   f. Proliferative myositis
   g. Myositis ossificans

B. HEMATOMA

1. This lesion results when extravasation of blood into the soft tissues following vascular disruption (usually post-traumatic) leads to the development of a mass of blood cells, serum, and proteins in a confined space. An inflammatory response proceeds in and around the hematoma, with the presence of granulation tissue and "organization" of the hematoma leading to eventual resorption and disappearance of the mass.

2. The reparative process includes the proliferation of many mesenchymal elements. Microscopically, one sees proliferating capillaries lined by plump endothelial cells, fibroblasts, and histiocytes, as well as red blood cells and leukocytes. Sometimes, the reparative process shows such marked cellularity as to suggest a sarcoma.

C. FAT NECROSIS

1. A post-traumatic reaction of adipose tissue, either idiopathic or iatrogenic (at an injection site), this lesion demonstrates a disruption of fat cells with release of fat and fatty esters and a histiocytic response. A localized liquefaction of fat then occurs, forming a cystic or solid lump that enlarges slowly and may imitate a neoplasm.

2. Ingestion of the liquid fat by phagocytes, inflammatory cells, and later fibrosis and calcification are noted. The histiocytes in fat necrosis tend to be mononuclear with finely granular to bubbly cytoplasm.

D. PSEUDOSARCOMATOUS (NODULAR) FASCIITIS

1. Clinical Data.
    a. The lesion appears in the subcutaneous (rarely deeper) tissues as a nodule that is usually tender and discovered soon after onset. Approximately 30 to 50 percent of affected patients remember an episode of trauma to the area involved.
    b. Although it can occur at any age, fasciitis is chiefly a lesion of young adults. There is no predilection for either sex.
    c. The favored site is the upper body, particularly the forearm and trunk, and fasciitis is relatively rare in the lower extremities.
    d. The lesion is usually small, seldom attaining a size of more than 3 cm.

2. Histology.
    a. The lesion is composed of highly cellular, well-vascularized tissue, proliferating spindle cells with numerous mitotic figures and foci of myxoid change, and scattered inflammatory and red blood cells. Typically, the lesion is nonencapsulated and interdigitates with surrounding tissues.
    b. The gross and microscopic infiltrative patterns together with the mitoses and dense cellularity can produce diagnostic confusion with malignant mesenchymal tumors; the recognition of fasciitis in this case must be based on its vascularity, inflammatory cell component, and resemblance to exuberant granulation tissue.

E. FOREIGN-BODY GRANULOMA

1. This poorly circumscribed mass is comprised of an array of inflammatory cells and many histiocytes (macrophages), predominantly multinucleated forms.

2. Foreign material (e.g., hair shafts, keratin, cholesterol, wood, cotton, suture material, and metallic fragments) may be identified readily in the lesion, either in the giant cells or around them. Occasionally, the foreign material may be demonstrated only by examining the tissue under polarized light.

F. XANTHOGRANULOMA

1. Some authors consider xanthogranuloma to be a benign neoplasm; others believe it is a reactive pseudotumor. This lesion is distinguished from fat necrosis by the presence of lipid-filled histiocytes (foam cells) dominating in the microscopic field. Xanthogranulomas also contain fibroblasts, giant cells, and capillaries.

2. This lesion is located most frequently in the retroperitoneum, but it may be found in the kidneys, lungs, mediastinum, and mesentery. It may grow to a large size, and when it occurs in the retroperitoneum, the lump may be confused clinically with retroperitoneal fibrosis or sarcoma.

G. PROLIFERATIVE MYOSITIS. This lesion represents fasciitis of skeletal muscle. The regenerating

and degenerating striated muscle cells may assume bizarre configurations and lead to an erroneous diagnosis of skeletal muscle malignancy (rhabdomyosarcoma).

H. MYOSITIS OSSIFICANS, probably the result of direct trauma to striated muscle, consists of a mass of bone, cartilage, or both in muscle, interdigitating with muscle fibers at the periphery. The more cellular areas tend to be placed centrally, while maturation of bone in various degrees is noted near the periphery. Such lesions probably represent an exaggerated reparative response in the organization of a hematoma involving striated muscle.

III. NEOPLASMS OF SOFT TISSUE—GENERAL CONSIDERATIONS

A. THE QUESTION OF ENCAPSULATION. On physical examination or at surgery, soft-tissue lesions may demonstrate encapsulation, circumscription (without a true capsule), or infiltration into surrounding tissues. Benign tumors are usually encapsulated; malignant ones are not. Gross impression may be misleading because some sarcomas show "encapsulation," but microscopic examination of malignant tumors usually shows definite invasion outside the gross confines of the lesion. On the other hand, some soft-tissue lumps that are reactive and non-neoplastic, so-called pseudosarcomas, may show gross and microscopic interdigitation with surrounding tissues. Hence, the presence or absence of a capsule cannot be taken as prima facie evidence of benignity or malignancy.

B. Neoplasms can be divided into benign, malignant, and locally-aggressive lesions. A summary of soft tissue tumors is given in Table 21-1.

Table 21-1. Soft Tissue Tumors

Presumed Origin (or Cells Resembled)	Benign Neoplasms	Locally Malignant Neoplasms	Aggressive Forms
Fat cells	Lipomas Lipoblastomas Hibernomas	Liposarcomas	Well-differentiated myxoid liposarcomas
Smooth muscles	Leiomyomas	Leiomyosarcomas	
Blood vessels	Hemangiomas	Angiosarcomas	
Fibrocytes	Keloids (dermal)	Fibrosarcomas	Fibromatosis (desmoid tumors)
Histiocytes	Fibrous histiocytomas (fibrous xanthomas, giant cell tumors of the tendon sheath, and sclerosing hemangiomas)	Malignant fibrous histiocytomas	Dermatofibrosarcoma protuberans
Striated muscles	Rhabdomyomas	Rhabdomyosarcomas (embryonal, sarcoma botryoides, alveolar, and pleomorphic)	
Nerves	Neural sheath tumors [schwannomas] (neurofibromas, neurilemomas, and granular cell tumors)	Malignant schwannomas	
? Synovial cells		Synovial sarcomas (? epithelioid sarcomas)	

IV. BENIGN NEOPLASMS

A. GENERAL CONSIDERATIONS

1. Benign tumors are frequently encapsulated, slowly growing masses, which may attain very large sizes.

2. They never metastasize, and the prognosis is usually excellent.

3. **Classification.** Benign tumors can be divided into seven types.
   a. Lipoma
   b. Fibrous histiocytomas
   c. Hemangioma
   d. Keloid (dermal)
   e. Neural sheath tumors
   f. Leiomyoma
   g. Rhabdomyoma

B. LIPOMA

1. A lipoma is the most common soft tissue tumor. It resembles adipose tissue but is encapsulated and lacks the lobulations of normal fat. Frequently found on the extremities or the back, it may be small or reach considerable size.

2. Degeneration of a lipoma into a liposarcoma has never been documented adequately.

3. A rare variant of lipoma is **lipoblastoma**, a lobulated, encapsulated, soft tumor, which occurs almost exclusively in infants and children. Despite infiltration into surrounding tissues, it has a benign clinical course with a low recurrence rate after surgical excision.

4. Another rare variant is the **hibernoma**, which derives its name from its morphologic resemblance to the brown fat of hibernating animals. It presumably arises from the multivacuolated fat that may occur in the back, hips, but especially the neck of both adults and infants.

C. FIBROUS HISTIOCYTOMA

1. This term is used to describe an entire group of lesions composed of cells that have light-microscopic and ultrastructural features of both histiocytes and fibroblasts.
   a. The histiocytes range from mononuclear forms to foam cells, some of which are multinucleated.
   b. The fibroblastic component of these lesions is arranged in fascicles with interlacing bundles dispersed among the histiocytes.

2. These lesions are found most often in the dermis, although they also may occur in deeper tissues. Some lesions demonstrate a prominent vascularity.

3. Fibrous histiocytomas are subdivided into groups depending upon their most prominent histologic feature.
   a. Fibrous **xanthoma** is characterized by numerous foam cells.
   b. **Giant cell tumor of tendon sheaths** has many giant cells and is found characteristically in the hands and fingers.
   c. **Sclerosing hemangioma** has prominent vascularity.

D. HEMANGIOMA is common in children and is frequently red or blue in color.

1. Various forms occur, including capillary, cavernous, and venous types, depending on the size of the vessels comprising the lesion.

2. Bleeding is occasionally a problem clinically. Those lesions that reach large size may produce thrombocytopenia (**Kasabach-Merritt syndrome**).

E. KELOID is a strictly **dermal** post-traumatic lesion.

F. NEURAL SHEATH TUMORS (SCHWANNOMAS) are usually subcutaneous or dermal tumors, which may be pedunculated. Rarely, they can occur in deeper soft tissues.

1. **Neurofibroma**, one of two common histologic subtypes, may or may not be circumscribed. It consists of spindle- to comma-shaped cells in a myxoid background, with the arrangement of cells giving a wavy appearance to the lesion. Multiple neurofibromas in association with café

au lait spots on the skin are known as **von Recklinghausen's neurofibromatosis** (a familial disorder).

    2. Neurilemoma, the other common subtype, is encapsulated, often has alternating myxoid and cellular areas (Antoni A and Antoni B patterns), and contains prominent thick-walled blood vessels.

    3. The **granular cell tumor** (formerly called the granular cell myoblastoma) is a relatively common lesion believed by many authors to be related histogenetically to Schwann cells.

        a. The lesion is composed of distinctive, large plate-like cells with finely granular cytoplasm and is found chiefly in the dermis and submucosal areas (tongue and larynx).

        b. Characteristically, the overlying squamous epithelium is thickened, and it may proliferate to such an extent as to simulate a squamous cell carcinoma (a condition termed **pseudoepitheliomatous hyperplasia**).

G. LEIOMYOMA is a benign neoplasm that recapitulates smooth muscle and that may arise anywhere in the soft tissue, often in or near vascular walls.

    1. The lesion is usually a small, circumscribed nodule that microscopically is composed of bundles of elongated pink cells with fibrillar cytoplasm, resembling nonskeletal muscle.

    2. Mitoses are rare and cellularity is usually even throughout the tumor.

H. RHABDOMYOMA is a very rare lesion that resembles skeletal muscle and usually arises in the tongue.

V. MALIGNANT NEOPLASMS (SARCOMAS)

A. GENERAL CONSIDERATIONS

    1. Sarcoma is a general term for malignant soft tissue lesions. The lesions usually infiltrate and invade surrounding tissues and have the capacity to metastasize, characteristically via the bloodstream. Prognosis depends upon the histologic subtype and the degree of differentiation. Survival rates are usually poor.

    2. Although sarcomas can arise in viscera and hollow organs (e.g., the uterus or stomach), this discussion will be limited to sarcomas that arise in extravisceral, extraskeletal mesenchymal tissues. Criteria for determining malignancy, and hence prognosis, may vary for those tumors that arise in soft tissues and those lesions that appear identical but arise in viscera. (For uterine smooth muscle tumors to be considered sarcomas, average mitotic rates of 10/10 high-power fields should be seen; similar smooth muscle tumors in the leg should be considered sarcomas, however, with mitotic rates of 3 to 5/50 high-power fields.) These different diagnostic criteria are based on careful clinicopathologic correlative and follow-up studies, which have shown that histology is not the only predictive factor but that the site of origin also is important.

    3. Sarcomas are named after the adult tissue that they most closely resemble. This principle was based on an old assumption that adult tissue gave rise to sarcomas (e.g., that skeletal muscle cells transformed into rhabdomyosarcoma). It is reasonable to assume, however, that this is not the case, and many pathologists now believe that sarcomas are derived from **uncommitted pluripotential cells**, which during neoplastic change acquire the capacity to recapitulate adult mesenchymal tissue. Most pathologists still refer, however, to sarcomas as tumors derived from mature adult mesenchymal tissues.

    4. Clinical Correlates of Sarcomas.

        a. Most sarcomas appear as solitary, deep-seated masses. (Benign and reactive lumps, in contrast, generally affect tissue that is more superficial and tend to be smaller.)

        b. Sarcomas appear fleshy and often bulge on cut surfaces.

        c. The most common sites affected are the extremities and the retroperitoneum.

        d. Sarcomas comprise most pediatric solid tumors but account for fewer than 5 percent of adult malignancies.

        e. As a group, sarcomas typically metastasize hematogenously, most commonly to the lungs and liver. They can extend directly or metastasize by embolic means, however, to regional nodes. (The most common sarcomas to metastasize by lymphatic embolic means are synovial sarcoma and malignant fibrous histiocytoma.)

        f. Histology cannot be the sole diagnostic criterion for sarcomas. Clinically benign lesions may resemble sarcomas microscopically. Misdiagnosis can be avoided only by adequate knowledge of the site of origin of a specimen.

    g. Sarcomas are classified according to the following.

       (1) Activity.

          (a) Locally aggressive, recurring tumors can cause death because of the sites where they occur (e.g., fibromatosis of the upper arm can invade the thorax and pleural cavity).

          (b) Metastasizing neoplasms usually kill by replacing vital organs.

       (2) Grade. The grade of a sarcoma is determined by the degree of differentiation (how closely it resembles adult mesenchymal tissue). Low-grade (better differentiated) lesions tend to follow a more indolent course than high-grade tumors.

       (3) Stage. The three stages are localized, regional, and metastatic (systemic).

    h. Of the sarcomas listed in Table 21-1, rhabdomyosarcoma, synovial sarcoma, and angiosarcoma are always considered grade III because they have a uniformly poor prognosis, despite the degree of differentiation.

    i. Therapy for soft tissue sarcomas is divided into three categories.

       (1) Surgical excision is indicated for localized lesions. Often, radical surgery is necessary since these tumors are seen to be large and more extensive microscopically than grossly.

       (2) Radiation therapy is indicated for lesions of regional extension to sterilize the local tumor bed and to treat inadequately removed tumors (those extending to the margins).

       (3) Systemic chemotherapy is indicated to control recognized or subclinical hematogenous metastases. Chemotherapy is often administered after surgery and sometimes after surgery and radiation therapy.

5. Classification. Malignant neoplasms can be divided into eight groups.

    a. Liposarcoma

    b. Malignant fibrous histiocytoma

    c. Fibrosarcoma

    d. Rhabdomyosarcoma

    e. Malignant schwannoma

    f. Synovial sarcoma

    g. Angiosarcoma

    h. Leiomyosarcoma

B. LIPOSARCOMA

1. Clinical Data.

    a. Liposarcoma is the most frequently encountered sarcoma. Affected patients usually present with a large, bulky, myxoid mass that is most commonly located in the thigh or retroperitoneum. The tumor is extremely rare in children.

    b. Well-differentiated variants tend to recur but do not metastasize, although they can cause death by involvement of vital retroperitoneal structures (e.g., the aorta or ureters).

    c. Less-differentiated and pleomorphic liposarcomas may give rise to distant metastases.

2. The **histologic varieties** of liposarcoma can be grouped as either **myxoid** or **nonmyxoid**. Generally, patients who have nonmyxoid types develop metastases more commonly than those with myxoid varieties. The more common myxoid type is characterized by proliferating lipoblasts in different stages of differentiation, prominent vascularity with a plexiform arrangement of capillaries, and a matrix rich in mucopolysaccharides.

3. Among the factors that are important in the **treatment** of liposarcomas are the histologic type and the extent of the tumor.

    a. Myxoid tumors infiltrate locally, and wide surgical excision is the treatment of choice. Many of these tumors are deceptively circumscribed, and if they are simply excised (shelled out), the chances of recurrence are very high.

    b. Amputation is not necessary in all cases of liposarcoma occurring in the extremities but should be considered in recurring lesions or when local excision is not feasible.

    c. Radiation has not been advocated as a standard method of treatment in liposarcoma, but it is occasionally employed for inoperable cases or for those who have developed metastatic disease.

C. MALIGNANT FIBROUS HISTIOCYTOMA ranks second to liposarcoma in frequency, occurs more often in males than in females, and may be seen in any age group, although it occurs most commonly in adults.

1. Clinical Data. The tumor may be found on an extremity, the head or neck, or in the retroperitoneum. It may infiltrate widely and metastasize.

2. Histologically, the tumor contains a mixture of "facultative" fibroblasts (sometimes disposed in storiform or pinwheel patterns) and histiocytes. Cytologic evidence for malignancy includes pleomorphism, hyperchromatism of nuclei, abnormal mitoses, and the presence of tumor giant cells.

D. FIBROSARCOMA is a highly cellular, spindle-cell tumor, with a moderate to high mitotic rate. It also is capable of bloodborne metastases and should be distinguished from fibromatosis (see VI B).

E. RHABDOMYOSARCOMA recapitulates embryonic myogenesis in a disorganized and haphazard pattern.

1. **Clinical Data.** The most common complaint is the presence of a mass that is neither painful nor tender despite its rapid growth. Other symptoms relate to the site of the tumor.

2. Two main varieties of rhabdomyosarcoma are recognized: the juvenile and the adult forms.
   a. **Juvenile Rhabdomyosarcoma.**
      (1) **Embryonal rhabdomyosarcoma** closely resembles the developing muscle of the 7- to 10-week fetus and occurs most commonly in children who are less than 6 years old.
         (a) The tumor usually is located in the head and neck regions, particularly in the orbit, nasopharynx, and middle ear. It also may occur in the retroperitoneum and urogenital tract.
         (b) This neoplasm must be differentiated from other small cell tumors of childhood, such as malignant lymphoma, leukemia, Ewing's sarcoma, and neuroblastoma.
         (c) **Sarcoma botryoides** is a form of embryonal rhabdomyosarcoma.
            (i) It tends to occur in the genitourinary, biliary, or upper respiratory tract of very young children.
            (ii) Botryoides refers to the grape-like gross appearance of the lesion, which is assumed when the lesion grows beneath a mucous membrane. The tumor is polypoid, soft, and jelly-like in appearance.
            (iii) Usually the lining epithelium of the mucosa is preserved, and a dense zone of undifferentiated rhabdomyoblasts is seen immediately beneath the epithelium (cambium layer). Mitoses are numerous.
      (2) **Alveolar rhabdomyosarcoma** recapitulates a later stage of fetal muscle development than the embryonal form and is found in a slightly older age group (10 to 25 years).
         (a) The common **sites of origin** are the extremities, particularly the flexor areas of the forearms and hands and the hypothenar eminences.
         (b) **Histologically**, aggregates of loosely arranged, small undifferentiated cells are separated into nests by dense fibrous septa. Because of the loss of cohesiveness, only a single layer of tumor cells remains firmly attached to the fibrous trabeculae, resulting in an alveolar or pseudoglandular appearance.
   b. **Pleomorphic rhabdomyosarcoma** occurs almost exclusively in adults, generally in the fourth to seventh decades of life.
      (1) About 70 percent of these tumors arise from the muscles of the lower extremities, particularly the thigh.
      (2) **Grossly**, the tumor is characteristically deep-seated within the musculature and varies from a relatively small to a large bulky mass. The consistency is usually soft and fleshy.
      (3) **Microscopically**, the tumors vary greatly in appearance and differentiation but are characterized by the **rhabdomyoblast**, a large, bizarre cell with eosinophilic cytoplasm and demonstrable cross striations.

3. The **prognosis** of all rhabdomyosarcomas is dismal, with local recurrence and metastases to lungs common in adult forms despite various forms of therapy. For the juvenile types, the **treatment** includes radical surgery, followed by irradiation and chemotherapy. Encouraging results from using such regimens for the treatment of embryonal rhabdomyosarcoma have occurred; this is not true for the treatment of the other forms.

F. MALIGNANT SCHWANNOMAS usually arise in or near a nerve trunk or in association with neurofibroma. Hence, such lesions may occur anywhere.

1. Rapid growth of a lesion in a patient who has von Recklinghausen's disease usually means that malignant schwannoma has arisen.

2. Generally, these neoplasms are highly malignant tumors composed of very cellular spindle cells arranged in a wavy pattern; many mitoses and foci of necrosis are common.

3. The prognosis is quite poor.

G. **SYNOVIAL SARCOMA** may affect patients of all ages, but it is most frequently found in young adults. In most series, the tumor has a slight preponderance in males.

1. **Clinical Data**. Synovial sarcoma commonly occurs in the lower limbs, specifically in the region of the knee. The tumor may develop, however, in any site where there are tendons, joints, or bursae. The sarcoma may be small or large, is often well circumscribed and painless, and usually is slow in enlarging.

2. **Histologically**, the tumor does not arise from synovial membranes but is classified as being of synovial origin because it is **biphasic**, that is, having a spindle cell fibrosarcoma-like element and a pseudoglandular (epithelioid) one, resembling normal synovial membrane. Calcification is often noted both radiologically and microscopically.

3. The **prognosis** is generally poor. Nodal metastases occur in up to 30 percent of cases, and bloodborne spread, especially to the lungs, is common.

4. Wide excision, including amputation, is the **treatment** of choice. Surgical intervention usually is performed late in the course of the disease and often is inadequate because the tumor appears encapsulated. The incidence of local recurrence is high, reflecting this failure.

5. A recently recognized and probably related lesion is the **epithelioid sarcoma**, which arises in distal portions of the extremities, frequently producing multiple nodules along the length of the tendon.
   a. **Histologically**, this lesion shows granulomatous features with large histiocytic or epithelioid cells surrounding zones of necrosis. This latter feature has led to misdiagnosis of the lesion as a rheumatoid nodule.
   b. The natural history is one of multiple recurrences and eventual distant metastasis. The course of the disease may extend over many years.

H. **ANGIOSARCOMA** (hemangiosarcoma) is an uncommon tumor that typically occurs in the skin or breast but rarely may arise in soft tissues.

1. **Clinical Data**. The tumor is grossly hemorrhagic and often necrotic. It may attain a large size rapidly and metastasizes readily to the lungs and liver.

2. **Histologically**, the appearance of this tumor may range from differentiated, (i.e., showing easily recognizable blood vessels) to a solid anaplastic neoplasm.

3. The **prognosis** is almost uniformly fatal within 2 years, death often being caused by exsanguinating hemorrhage.

I. **LEIOMYOSARCOMA**, a malignancy resembling smooth muscle, usually arises in the uterus or gastrointestinal tract. The tumor also may occur in the retroperitoneum or extremities, occasionally originating from large veins. It ranges in size from small to very large and has no characteristic gross appearance.

1. **Histologically**, the leiomyosarcoma is composed of elongated smooth muscle cells with pink fibrillary cytoplasm. Mitoses are present but may range from as few as 3/50 high power fields to many mitoses/1 high power-field. Not infrequently, large bizarre cells are present.

2. The **prognosis** for a leiomyosarcoma is poor, with bloodborne metastases common. Lesions in the retroperitoneum or the extremities usually have a worse prognosis than those in the uterus or gastrointestinal tract.

VI. LOCALLY AGGRESSIVE LESIONS

A. **GENERAL CONSIDERATIONS**

1. This group consists of nonencapsulated neoplasms that invade surrounding tissues and structures. Frequently, extension of the lesion is greater than can be appreciated grossly, and thus the tumors often are excised inadequately. The tendency to recur locally is very high. These tumors **do not metastasize** but may cause death by local extension and involvement of vital structures.

2. **Classification**. Locally aggressive lesions can be classified into three groups.
   a. Fibromatosis
   b. Dermatofibrosarcoma protuberans
   c. Well-differentiated myxoid liposarcoma

B. **FIBROMATOSIS**, also known as desmoid tumor, typically occurs in the shoulder area, pelvic girdle area, the neck, or the anterior abdominal wall. Although comprised chiefly of bland collagenous tissue and fibrocytes with rare mitoses, the lesion infiltrates surrounding muscle and soft tissue, often beyond apparent gross limits. Thus, inadequate excisions often are performed, and recurrences are quite common.

C. **DERMATOFIBROSARCOMA PROTUBERANS**, a type of fibrous histiocytoma that may become quite large, is a slowly growing protuberant tumor involving the skin and subcutis (see V C). The tumor is typified by radial whorls of fibroblasts, producing a characteristic storiform pattern. The tumor often recurs locally, may be difficult to control, and on rare occasions metastasizes.

D. **WELL-DIFFERENTIATED MYXOID LIPOSARCOMA** tends to pursue a locally aggressive course and rarely metastasizes (see V B).

STUDY QUESTIONS

Directions: Each question below contains five suggested answers. Choose the **one best** response to each question.

1. A 56-year-old woman has a recurrent myxoid liposarcoma of the upper thigh and inguinal region. The most successful curative therapy for this patient would be

(A) local excision

(B) local excision and regional lymphadenectomy

(C) hemipelvectomy

(D) localized radiation

(E) systemic chemotherapy including adriamycin

2. A 32-year-old woman noted a 3-cm, painless mass, which she attributed to an athletic injury, lateral to her left popliteal fossa. Three months later, the mass was biopsied, and a diagnosis of synovial sarcoma was made. Which of the following statements concerning the prognosis for this patient is true?

(A) Following radical local excision, the tumor is unlikely to recur

(B) Following radical local excision, the tumor may recur but is unlikely to metastasize

(C) Prophylactic lymph node dissection combined with radical local excision will decrease the chance of tumor recurrence

(D) If the tumor does not recur within 5 years of adequate treatment, it is unlikely ever to recur

(E) None of the above

3. Which of the following patients is most likely to have nodular fasciitis?

(A) A 52-year-old man who has had a painful 3-cm nodule on his chest for 6 months

(B) A 72-year-old woman who has had a tender 5-cm nodule on her back for 1 year

(C) A 24-year-old woman who has had a tender 2-cm nodule on her right arm for 2 weeks

(D) A 19-year-old man who has had a painless 5-cm nodule on his left leg for 2 months

(E) A 7-year-old boy who has had a painless 1-cm nodule on his left knee as a result of a fall occurring 1 month ago

Directions: The group of questions below consists of lettered choices followed by several numbered items. For each numbered item select the **one** lettered choice with which it is **most** closely associated. Each lettered choice may be used once, more than once, or not at all.

Questions 4–8

For each type of sarcoma that follows, select its "supposed" tissue of origin.

(A) Endothelium

(B) Adipose tissue

(C) Connective tissue

(D) Skeletal muscle

(E) Schwann cell

4. Rhabdomyosarcoma

5. Neurofibrosarcoma

6. Angiosarcoma

7. Liposarcoma

8. Fibrosarcoma

ANSWERS AND EXPLANATIONS

1. The answer is C. (*V B 3 b–c*) Myxoid liposarcoma infiltrates locally and demands wide surgical excision. Although amputation is not necessary in all cases of liposarcoma occurring in an extremity, hemipelvectomy is the treatment of choice in the patient presented who has a recurring lesion. Radiation would be ineffective as would be local excision. Systemic chemotherapy would not be useful because a myxoid liposarcoma is unlikely to have distant metastases. Lymphadenectomy would not be needed because liposarcomas rarely, if ever, spread to nodes.

2. The answer is E. (*V G*) Synovial sarcomas usually are slow growing and thus may have a prolonged natural history, but they metastasize given enough time. Because of a lack of early signs or symptoms, surgical intervention often is performed late in the course of these tumors and often is inadequate because the tumors appear encapsulated. Local recurrences thus are frequent. Recently, the addition of new therapeutic modalities to treatment by wide surgical excision (and amputation when possible) has improved the prognosis.

3. The answer is C. (*II F 2 a–d*) Nodular (pseudosarcomatous) fasciitis typically affects the upper extremities or trunk of young adults, is discovered soon after onset, and follows a history of trauma in one-third to one-half of cases. The nodule produced characteristically is tender and less than 3 cm.

4–8. The answers are: 4-D, 5-E, 6-A, 7-B, 8-C. (*V A 2; Table 1*) Although modern theory suggests that most, if not all, sarcomas arise from totipotential mesenchymal stem cells, because the histologic pattern of most sarcomas recapitulates a particular type of mesenchymal tissue, the tumors traditionally have been named for such tissues. Thus, rhabdomyosarcoma recapitulates striated (skeletal) muscle; neurofibrosarcoma, nerve (Schwann) cells; angiosarcoma, blood vessels (endothelium); liposarcoma, fat cells (adipose tissue); and fibrosarcoma, fibrocytes (connective tissue).

Post-test

STUDY QUESTIONS

Directions: Each question below contains five suggested answers. Choose the **one best** response to each question.

1. An exuberant hypertrophic collagenous reaction occurs in some individuals following an injury. The term that best describes this condition is

(A) cicatrix
(B) keloid
(C) callus
(D) granulation tissue
(E) wound

2. Lymphedema of an extremity can be the result of infestation by which of the following parasites?

(A) *Plasmodium vivax*
(B) *Entamoeba histolytica*
(C) *Strongyloides stercoralis*
(D) *Schistosoma mansoni*
(E) *Filaria bancrofti*

3. What are the two types of small cell carcinomas?

(A) Oat cell and anaplastic cell
(B) Oat cell and intermediate cell
(C) Carcinoid cell and intermediate cell
(D) Carcinoid cell and anaplastic cell
(E) Anaplastic cell and intermediate cell

4. Cystic changes that consist of microscopic tubular malformations lined by cuboidal epithelium admixed with bands of smooth muscle cause a congenital lung malformation called

(A) cystic fibrosis
(B) pulmonary sequestration
(C) bronchogenic cysts
(D) congenital lobar emphysema
(E) congenital adenomatoid malformation

5. Which of the following types of esophagitis is the most common?

(A) Reflux
(B) Viral
(C) Fungal
(D) Acute corrosive
(E) Chronic granulomatous

6. Barrett's epithelium is found in what part of the gastrointestinal tract?

(A) Esophagus
(B) Stomach
(C) Small intestine
(D) Large intestine
(E) Rectum

7. What is the most common benign tumor of the stomach?

(A) Polypoid adenoma
(B) Leiomyoma
(C) Glomus tumor
(D) Lipoma
(E) Schwannoma

8. What name is given to metastatic gastric carcinoma of the ovary?

(A) Brenner tumor
(B) Erdheim tumor
(C) Rokitansky's tumor
(D) Krukenberg's tumor
(E) Grawitz's tumor

9. What parasite is the most common cause of appendicitis in the United States?

(A) *Giardia lamblia*
(B) *Oxyuris vermicularis*
(C) *Schistosoma mansoni*
(D) *Schistosoma japonicum*
(E) *Cryptosporidium*

10. Which inflammatory condition of the intestine is characterized by segmental involvement, which usually includes the terminal ileum and cecum, transmural inflammation with lymphoid aggregates scattered throughout all histologic layers, and the development of epithelioid granulomas?

(A) Diverticulitis
(B) Colitis cystica profunda
(C) Cryptosporidiosis
(D) Crohn's disease
(E) Ulcerative colitis

11. A 16-year-old female with gallstones is most likely to

(A) be obese and diabetic
(B) be taking birth control pills
(C) be jaundiced
(D) have congenital spherocytosis
(E) have a history of drug abuse

12. A 10-year-old boy enters the hospital with lethargy, anorexia, and hypoglycemia. He quickly develops seizures and metabolic acidosis and lapses into a coma. A liver biopsy shows small fatty droplets. What is the most likely diagnosis?

(A) Hepatitis A infection
(B) Reye's syndrome
(C) Obstructive biliary cirrhosis
(D) Schistosomiasis
(E) Cystic fibrosis

13. What is the most common renal tumor in children?

(A) Angiomyolipoma
(B) Renal cell carcinoma
(C) Wilms' tumor
(D) Mesoblastic nephroma
(E) Neuroblastoma

14. Which of the following lesions of the penis is virus-induced?

(A) Erythroplasia of Queyrat
(B) Squamous cell carcinoma
(C) Condyloma acuminatum
(D) Bowen's disease
(E) Prurigo

15. Psammoma bodies are most often found in which type of ovarian cancer?

(A) Brenner tumor
(B) Germ cell tumor
(C) Serous cystadenocarcinoma
(D) Mucinous cystadenoma
(E) Mucinous cystadenocarcinoma

16. The most common cause of death in women beyond the fifth decade of life in the United States is now

(A) leukemia
(B) myocardial infarction
(C) breast carcinoma
(D) lung carcinoma
(E) cervical carcinoma

17. A 60-year-old woman with a history of breast carcinoma that had been treated with surgical excision, radiation, and chemotherapy 2 years ago is undergoing routine follow-up. Although she is asymptomatic, her hemoglobin concentration is 8.7 g/dl and the hematocrit is 27 percent. The most likely explanation is

(A) iron deficiency anemia

(B) chemotherapy-induced marrow injury

(C) acute leukemia

(D) metastatic breast cancer

(E) inadequate data is given for a conclusion

fluctuates in palpation *characteristic of* *WARthin tumor*

18. A 68-year-old man presents with a fluctuant parotid mass, which he says has been present for about 10 years. He denies any recent growth of this mass, has no pain, no nerve paralysis in the area, and no lymphadenopathy. What is the most likely diagnosis?

(A) Malignant lymphoma

(B) Pleomorphic adenoma

(C) Mucoepidermoid carcinoma

(D) Papillary cystadenoma lymphomatosum

(E) Adenoid cystic carcinoma

19. Although gout may produce arthritis, its primary pathologic abnormalities are

(A) autoimmune

(B) neoplastic

(C) metabolic

(D) inflammatory

(E) infectious

Directions: Each question below contains four suggested answers of which **one or more** is correct. Choose the answer

    A   if **1, 2, and 3** are correct
    B   if **1 and 3** are correct
    C   if **2 and 4** are correct
    D   if **4** is correct
    E   if **1, 2, 3, and 4** are correct

20. True statements describing the phenomenon of white cell emigration from vessels in areas of inflammation include

(1) cell emigration occurs through gaps between the endothelial cells

(2) the accompanying loss of fluid blood elements is passive

(3) cell emigration is independent of endothelial cell motion

(4) polymorphonuclear neutrophils are the first cells to emigrate

21. The classic signs and symptoms of inflammation include

(1) dolor

(2) calor

(3) rubor

(4) tumor

22. The modified Jones criteria are clinical manifestations of which of the following diseases?

(1) Syphilis

(2) Secondary hypertension

(3) Cyanotic heart disease

(4) Rheumatic fever

SUMMARY OF DIRECTIONS

A	B	C	D	E
1,2,3 only	1,3 only	2,4 only	4 only	All are correct

---

23. Congenital heart lesions that usually cause cyanosis include

(1) patent ductus arteriosus
(2) Eisenmenger's complex
(3) atrial septal defect
(4) tetralogy of Fallot

24. Common lesions that can be demonstrated in atherosclerotic patients include

(1) fatty streaks
(2) atheromas
(3) intimal plaques
(4) medial granulomas

25. Colonic polyps that are considered to be pre-cancerous include

(1) adenomatous polyps
(2) villous adenomas
(3) familial multiple polyposis
(4) hyperplastic polyps

26. The major types of stomach carcinoma include which of the following?

(1) Ulcerated
(2) Diffuse (linitis plastica)
(3) Superficial
(4) Fungating

27. Factors known to predispose to peptic ulcers include

(1) hyperacidity
(2) familial history
(3) excessive gastrin production
(4) heavy cigarette smoking

28. Characteristic histopathologic features found in chronic active hepatitis include

(1) lymphocytic infiltrates
(2) fibrous tissue septa
(3) bridging necrosis
(4) piecemeal necrosis

29. Transitional cell carcinomas of the urinary bladder have been associated with which of the following conditions?

(1) Beta-naphthylamine exposure
(2) Schistosomiasis
(3) Heavy cigarette smoking
(4) Exstrophy of the bladder

30. True statements concerning renal cell carcinoma include

(1) patients may present with hematuria
(2) lungs and brain are common sites of metastases
(3) metastatic spread is primarily via the bloodstream
(4) peak incidence is in the fourth decade of life

31. Of the following statements concerning carcinoma of the prostate, those generally accepted as true include

(1) serum acid phosphatase levels can be elevated
(2) it is linked to environmental exposure to certain compounds
(3) metastatic bone disease is a common outcome
(4) it most often originates in the posterior lobe of the gland

32. Factors affecting the prognosis for a patient with an ovarian carcinoma include

(1) stage of the tumor
(2) grade of the tumor
(3) histologic type of the tumor
(4) amount of tumor necrosis

33. The characteristics by which adenocarcinoma of the endocervical glands resembles endometrial carcinoma more closely than squamous cell carcinoma of the cervix include

(1) age of the patient
(2) pattern of metastatic spread
(3) occurrence in obese, diabetic women
(4) association with skin papillomas

34. Important prognostic factors for patients with breast carcinoma include the

(1) age of the patient
(2) histologic tumor type
(3) presence of estrogen receptors in the tumor
(4) presence of metastases

35. Currently accepted modes of therapy for breast carcinoma include

(1) simple mastectomy
(2) lumpectomy and radiation therapy
(3) modified radical mastectomy
(4) mastectomy, radiation therapy, and chemotherapy

36. True statements concerning carcinoma of the mouth include

(1) it can be multifocal
(2) it is more common in smokers and alcoholics
(3) it is most often a squamous cell type
(4) it can metastasize to the cervical lymph nodes

37. Patients under long-term Dilantin therapy may develop which of the following complications?

(1) Leukoplakia
(2) Moniliasis
(3) Dental caries
(4) Gingival hyperplasia

38. The functions of osteoclasts include

(1) secretion of immunoglobulins
(2) resorption of bone mineral crystal
(3) synthesis of new collagen
(4) lysis of bone matrix

39. In general, true statements concerning chondrosarcomas include

(1) they can begin in benign cartilage tumors
(2) they have a tendency to recur
(3) they are common in the pelvic bones
(4) they are very sensitive to radiation therapy

40. Which of the following conditions can be classified as a bullous disease?

(1) Pemphigus
(2) Dermatitis herpetiformis
(3) Erythema multiforme
(4) Herpes simplex

Directions: The groups of questions below consist of lettered choices followed by several numbered items. For each numbered item select the **one** lettered choice with which it is **most** closely associated. Each lettered choice may be used once, more than once, or not at all.

Questions 41–45

Match each statement below with the mediastinal compartment that it describes.

(A) Superior mediastinum
(B) Anterior mediastinum
(C) Middle mediastinum
(D) Posterior mediastinum
(E) Entire mediastinum

41. This is the most likely mediastinal compartment to contain a bronchogenic cyst.

42. The heart lies within the pericardial sac in this mediastinal compartment.

43. Rupture of the lower esophagus can cause an inflammation of this mediastinal compartment, resulting in acute mediastinitis.

44. The great vessels originate from the aortic arch in this compartment of the mediastinum.

45. Granulomatous disease such as tuberculosis and histoplasmosis can produce chronic mediastinitis of this compartment.

Questions 46–50

For each of the following disorders of the central nervous system, match the area that is dominantly affected.

(A) Peripheral sensory neurons
(B) Cerebellum
(C) Substantia nigra
(D) Cerebral cortex
(E) Anterior horn cells of the spinal cord

46. Huntington's chorea
47. Charcot-Marie-Tooth disease
48. Amyotrophic lateral sclerosis
49. Parkinson's disease
50. Pick's disease

Questions 51–55

For each disease process listed below, select the lymph node histologic characteristic with which it is associated.

(A) Fibrosis
(B) Histiocytic proliferation
(C) Serpiginous necrosis
(D) Inclusion bodies
(E) Melanin

51. Toxoplasmosis
52. Herpesvirus
53. Syphilis
54. Dermatopathia
55. Cat-scratch fever

Questions 56–60

Match each description of a skin lesion below with the name of the lesion.

(A) Macule
(B) Papule
(C) Nodule
(D) Wheal
(E) Vesicle

56. A circumscribed, flat area of skin distinguished by color from the surrounding skin

57. A palpable, solid, round or ellipsoid lesion situated deep in the skin or in the subcutaneous tissue

58. A well-circumscribed solid elevation of the skin

59. A small, circumscribed elevation of the skin containing serum or other fluid

60. A short-lived, circumscribed area of elevated skin produced by focal edema of the upper dermis

ANSWERS AND EXPLANATIONS

1. The answer is B. (*Chapter 1 III B 3*) A keloid is the term given to excessive collagen formation in the connective tissues of certain individuals. Keloid formation can be a problem in both primary and secondary forms of healing in individuals with an apparent genetic predisposition to it. When keloids form in exposed skin areas, considerable cosmetic problems can occur since repeated excision of keloids may result in a cycle of subsequent keloid formation in the incisions.

2. The answer is E. (*Chapter 5 IV C 5*) Filariasis is the common name for Bancroftian filariasis, which is caused by infestation of the parasite *Wuchereria (Filaria) bancrofti.* The larvae enter the dermal lymphatics when an individual is bitten by a carrier mosquito. The adult worms often take up residence in the regional lymphatics and nodes of the lower extremities. The inflammatory and fibrotic reaction to the dead worms causes lymphatic obstruction with lymphedema sometimes so gross as to cause elephantiasis.

3. The answer is B. (*Chapter 6 VIII B 3 b*) Small cell carcinoma of the lung is a distinct tumor type with two general subgroups—the oat cell or lymphocyte-like form, which accounts for about 42 percent of cases, and the intermediate cell form, which includes fusiform and polygonal cell types, accounting for 58 percent of cases. Small cell carcinomas represent nearly 10 percent of all lung cancers. Almost all the victims are men, more than 75 percent of whom have a history of smoking.

4. The answer is E. (*Chapter 6 III B*) Congenital adenomatoid malformation is associated with poly-hydramnios, hydrops fetalis, and respiratory distress syndrome in the newborn. In older children this malformation leads to recurrent pulmonary infections.

5. The answer is A. (*Chapter 8 I C 1 b*) Inflammation of the esophagus is most often the result of an incompetent lower esophageal sphincter, which permits reflux of gastric contents into the lower esophagus, causing chemical irritation. Viral and fungal esophagitis occur primarily in patients with diminished immune responses. Corrosive esophagitis results from ingestion of corrosive chemicals, which are usually in the form of cleaning agents. Granulomatous esophagitis is a relatively uncommon condition, occurring in individuals with one of the granulomatous diseases (e.g., tuberculosis).

6. The answer is A. (*Chapter 8 I C 2*) Barrett's epithelium is columnar, mucous-type epithelium located in the distal esophagus. The cells are believed to be the result of metaplastic change of the normal squamous epithelium of the esophagus. Ulcerations of this altered esophageal epithelium closely resemble peptic ulcers of the stomach. There is nearly a 10 percent incidence of adenocarcinoma of Barrett's epithelium in the affected population.

7. The answer is B. (*Chapter 8 II D 1*) Leiomyoma is a benign smooth muscle tumor and is the most common benign gastric neoplasm. Leiomyomas can be multiple. The tumor originates from the smooth muscle cells of the muscularis mucosa or the longitudinal or circular smooth muscle layers of the stomach. A small leiomyoma may not produce symptoms until ulceration of the mucosa leads to hemorrhage, with signs of blood loss in the gastrointestinal tract.

8. The answer is D. (*Chapter 8 II E 1 e*) Krukenberg's tumor is the term given to metastatic carcinoma of the ovary secondary to mucinous carcinoma of the stomach. The metastases, which are often bilateral, result from the lymphatic spread of the primary gastric carcinoma. The metastatic tumor in the ovaries often contains signet ring cells distended with mucin, which displaces the nucleus toward the periphery of the cell. The presence of these signet ring cells indicates that the tumor is not a primary ovarian cancer.

9. The answer is B. (*Chapter 8 IV B 1*) *Oxyuris vermicularis* is a pinworm that is the cause of approximately 3 percent of the cases of appendicitis in the United States. This infestation usually affects children, but the parasite is often only identified during histologic examination of the appendix. *Schistosoma mansoni* can also infest the appendix, although not to the extent of *Oxyuris vermicularis* infestation.

10. The answer is D. (*Chapter 8 V D 4*) Crohn's disease is a chronic inflammatory disorder of the gastrointestinal tract. It has a typically segmental pattern of involvement, hence its alternate name, regional enteritis. The terminal ileum is involved in nearly two-thirds of the patients, and about one-half have concurrent involvement of the colon. The histologic pattern of inflammation in Crohn's disease includes ulceration of the mucosa, submucosal inflammation and fibrosis, and pronounced subserosal inflammation and fibrosis. Granulomas are found in approximately three-fourths of cases of Crohn's disease.

11. The answer is D. (*Chapter 9 II D 2*) Age is a major clue. The patient probably has bilirubinate stones resulting from hemolysis, which leads to excess bilirubin and its subsequent precipitation as stones.

12. The answer is B. (*Chapter 10 IV A 2*) Symptoms of Reye's syndrome include acute encephalopathy with fatty infiltration of the liver. The liver in Reye's syndrome is unique because of the microvesicular accumulation of fat in the hepatocyte cytoplasm and the cytoplasm's uniform foamy appearance. Brain tissue from Reye's victims has edematous myelin sheaths and changes in the neuronal mitochondria that are similar to those seen in the liver mitochondria: matrix rarefaction, pleomorphism, swelling, loss of dense bodies, and glycogen depletion.

13. The answer is C. (*Chapter 11 VIII A*) Wilms' tumor (nephroblastoma) is the second most common visceral tumor of early childhood—the most common is neuroblastoma. Wilms' tumor occurs with equal frequency in both sexes. Nearly two-thirds of the tumors present in children under 3 years of age.

14. The answer is C. (*Chapter 12 V C, D*) Benign condyloma acuminatum is a papillary excrescence of the penis, which is caused by viral infection. Erythroplasia of Queyrat, squamous cell carcinoma, Bowen's disease, and prurigo have not been proven to be of viral etiology.

15. The answer is C. [*Chapter 13 VI A 3 a (2) (c)*] Serous cystadenocarcinoma is the most common of all malignant ovarian tumors, accounting for nearly 40 percent of ovarian malignancies. Grossly, the tumor is composed of cysts and papillary structures, sometimes with zones of hemorrhage and necrosis. The surface of the tumor is covered with diffuse papillary excrescences, which are formed by pluristratified epithelium with abundant psammoma bodies. Psammoma bodies are small calcified concentrically laminated structures, which are believed to form from degenerated epithelial cells in the papillae.

16. The answer is C. (*Chapter 14 VIII A 1*) Carcinoma of the breast is now the leading cause of death in the United States in women over the age of 40 years. Although the incidence of lung carcinoma is rapidly increasing in the female population, still 1 in 13 women will develop breast carcinoma. Thus far, there has been no screening test developed to detect breast carcinoma comparable to Papanicolaou's (Pap) test for early identification of cervical neoplasias.

17. The answer is E. [*Chapter 17 II A 3 b (1) (a); II A 3 b (2); IV B 2 b; II A 3 b (3)*] Although iron deficiency anemia, chemotherapy-induced marrow injury, acute leukemia, and metastatic breast cancer are all possible explanations of the symptoms, without detailed peripheral smear morphology and further laboratory data, the diagnosis cannot be determined definitively. Elderly individuals may have nutritional deficiencies from poor or inadequate diet; another possibility is gastrointestinal blood loss from an undefined condition (e.g., a cancer). Chemotherapy can depress and injure marrow, producing anemia, and in some cases, the marrow injury may be prolonged. Cases of postchemotherapy acute leukemia also occur. Finally, metastatic tumors of the bone marrow can produce a marrow-replacement type of anemia.

18. The answer is D. (*Chapter 18 VI B 1 b*) The history given by the patient suggests a benign lesion. The fluctuation on palpation is characteristic of papillary cystadenoma lymphomatosum (Warthin's tumor). These tumors account for about 10 percent of benign salivary tumors. Although there is a male predominance of nearly 10:1 in incidence of Warthin's tumor, the reason is unknown.

19. The answer is C. (*Chapter 19 II B 2 b*) Gout produces both acute and chronic arthritis because of the deposition of urates in the joints. The acute form of gout is characterized only by nonspecific acute inflammation of the synovial tissue, which is provoked by the deposition of microcrystals of urate. Chronic gout is distinguished by larger amounts of urate crystals on articular joint surfaces and by tophi formation in the capsular connective tissues around the joints.

20. The answer is E (all). (*Chapter 1 I D 2*) Emigration of motile white cells from the blood vessels into the perivascular tissues is a vital component of the inflammatory response. The mobile cells insert pseudopodia into endothelial cell junctions and show active, purposeful movement through the endothelial gaps without evidence of phagocytic-like phenomena by the endothelial cells. The first or immediate wave of migration is that of predominantly polymorphonuclear leukocytes, closely followed by monocytes.

21. The answer is E (all). (*Chapter 1 I A 2*) Dolor, calor, rubor, and tumor are the Latin terms for the four classic signs and symptoms of inflammation: pain, warmth or fever, redness, and swelling. These four cardinal signs were recognized by a Roman writer of the first century, A.D., Celsus. Galen, a second-century Greek physician, later added a fifth sign, functio laesa, which means loss of function.

22. The answer is D (4). (*Chapter 4 II C 1*) The modified Jones criteria are major and minor manifestations of rheumatic fever upon which the clinical diagnosis can be made. Patients with two major manifestations or one of the major and two minor manifestations are thought to have high probability of rheumatic fever if there is historic evidence of streptococcal infection.

23. The answer is C (2, 4). (*Chapter 4 II D 1, 2*) Cyanosis depends in large part on the amount of incompletely oxygenated blood that reaches the systemic circulation because of anomalous development of the circulatory system. Tetralogy of Fallot is one of the most common congenital anomalies producing the condition. Eisenmenger's complex produces cyanosis when pulmonary resistance is greater than systemic resistance so that a right-to-left shunt occurs. Patent ductus arteriosus or atrial septal defect alone does not typically produce cyanosis.

24. The answer is A (1, 2, 3). (*Chapter 5 II B 1*) Fatty streaks, intimal plaques, and atheromas are the classic lesions of atherosclerosis. When atheromas are complicated by ulceration, calcification, thrombosis, and intraplaque hemorrhage, the lesions are referred to as "complicated plaques." The fatty streaks have been found in children, leading to the speculation that atherosclerosis may begin at a very early age.

25. The answer is A (1, 2, 3). (*Chapter 8 V F*) Polyps in the colon are proliferations of mucosal epithelium—both glandular and surface epithelium, which protrude into the intestinal lumen. Hyperplastic polyps are benign and are not considered to be precancerous. Adenomatous polyps occur in three main forms: tubular, tubulovillous, and villous; while adenomatous polyps represent benign neoplastic growths, the prevalent opinion is that it is from these growths that most cancers of the colon arise. It is very likely in the familial polyposis syndromes that the patient will develop one or more carcinomas of the colon unless all of the polyps are removed or a total colectomy is performed.

26. The answer is E (all). (*Chapter 8 II E 1*) Of the major stomach carcinomas, the ulcerated, fungating, and diffuse (linitis plastica) types account for nearly two-thirds. The superficial form is thought to represent an "early" carcinoma, with tumor cells growing extensively in the mucosal layer before invasion of the deeper layers or lymph node metastases occur. The nodular form is the fifth type of gastric carcinoma.

27. The answer is E (all). (*Chapter 8 II C 1 d*) Peptic ulcers are chronic ulcerations of the gastrointestinal mucosa at any site exposed to acid-pepsin secretions; however, nearly all peptic ulcers occur in the duodenum or in the stomach. Individuals with peptic ulcers have much higher acid secretion levels than normal individuals. Increased gastrin secretion, particularly in patients with gastrin-secreting tumors, leads to hyperacidity with the consequent development of more peptic ulcers. There is a strong familial tendency to duodenal ulcers but less so to gastric ulcers. While there is no one simple etiology for peptic ulcers, there are definite associations. For example, heavy cigarette smokers have nearly twice the incidence of peptic ulcers in comparison to nonsmokers.

28. The answer is E (all). [*Chapter 10 III B 4 a (2) (a)*] The diagnosis of chronic active hepatitis can be confusing because of the implication that a precise duration of disease must have occurred before this diagnosis can be rendered. Two subdivisions of the disease are recognized: chronic persistent hepatitis, which is generally a mild nonprogressive illness, and chronic active or aggressive hepatitis, in which the severity of the illness may fluctuate. Piecemeal necrosis, a histologic pattern observed in chronic active hepatitis, is the severe necrosis of hepatocytes that is seen predominately at the edges of the hepatic parenchymal limiting plates, portal zones, and along tracts of previous hepatocyte necrosis and fibrosis.

29. The answer is E (all). (*Chapter 11 IX C 1*) A large amount of data suggests a link between the development of bladder carcinoma and exposure to chemical carcinogens, such as beta-naphthylamine and tobacco tars, high urinary levels of metabolites of tryptophan, and irritations from various sources, such as schistosomiasis of the bladder. The development of bladder carcinomas is also associated with congenital conditions, including bladder exstrophy.

30. The answer is A (1, 2, 3). (*Chapter 11 VIII B*) The peak incidence of renal cell carcinoma occurs near the sixth decade of life. The classical symptoms of the neoplasm include hematuria, pain, and a flank mass. Metastases occur primarily through the bloodstream, commonly to the lungs and brain.

31. The answer is E (all). (*Chapter 12 IV E 1*) Prostate carcinoma is the most common malignancy in the male population beyond the fifth decade of life. An endocrine cause as well as various viral and environmental causes (e.g., cadmium exposure) have been postulated as etiologic explanations. Sensitive assays for the elevation of serum acid phosphatase levels of prostatic origin have helped in early diagnosis, but unfortunately, bone metastases as well as metastases to the lymph nodes, lungs, liver, and brain still account for significant morbidity. Nearly 75 percent of prostate carcinomas are thought to originate in the posterior lobe of the gland.

32. The answer is A (1, 2, 3). [*Chapter 13 VI A 3 a (2) (c) (iii)*] The overall 5-year survival rate for patients with ovarian cancers depends greatly upon the stage or extent of spread of the tumor at the time of diagnosis. The grade of the individual neoplasm also affects the prognosis: the higher the grade, the worse the prognosis. Certainly, the type of tumor is also an important determinant of prognosis. For example, variants such as endometrioid tumors have a better prognosis than serous carcinomas. The amount of necrosis does not correlate with prognosis for patients with ovarian cancers.

33. The answer is B (1, 3). (*Chapter 13 V B, C*) Endocervical adenocarcinoma is comparable to cervical squamous cell carcinoma in its pattern of metastatic spread; both cancers metastasize via lymphatics. However, endocervical adenocarcinoma is like endometrial carcinoma in that it affects postmenopausal women who are obese, diabetic, and hypertensive; these patients are also often multiparous. Squamous cell cervical carcinoma accounts for nearly 95 percent of cervical cancers, and adenocarcinoma of the endocervical glands accounts for the other 5 percent.

34. The answer is E (all). (*Chapter 14 IX*) Although long-term survival for patients with breast carcinoma is difficult to predict precisely, a large number of studies have shown that there are several important prognostic factors. These include the rapidity of diagnosis, the histologic features of the tumor, the age of the patient at time of diagnosis, stage of spread of the cancer, host immunologic response to the tumor, presence or absence of estrogen receptors in the tumor cells, and the presence or absence of distant organ metastases.

35. The answer is E (all). (*Chapter 14 X*) Simple mastectomy, lumpectomy followed by radiation therapy, modified radical mastectomy, and mastectomy, radiation therapy, and chemotherapy are all presently used to treat patients with breast carcinoma. The therapy for an individual patient is decided upon according to the stage of spread of the cancer, the estrogen-receptor status of the tumor tissue, the histologic type of the tumor, and the patient's wishes.

36. The answer is E (all). (*Chapter 18 II E*) The most common malignant lesion of the oral mucous membranes is squamous cell carcinoma. This lesion, particularly of the tongue and larynx, occurs most often in smokers, especially heavy smokers who also drink alcohol excessively. When multiple sites of tumor are present, the patient's prognosis is worse. Some primary squamous cell carcinomas metastasize via lymphatics to the cervical lymph nodes.

37. The answer is D (4). (*Chapter 18 II C 1*) Gingival hyperplasia occurs predominately in patients receiving long-term Dilantin therapy. Lobulated masses of gingival tissue enlarge due to proliferation of collagen and new vessel formation. The hyperplasia usually recedes following discontinuation of the drug therapy.

38. The answer is C (2, 4). (*Chapter 19 I A 2 c*) Three types of cells compose bone, excluding the bone marrow elements and vascular endothelium. Osteoclasts are the cells that dissolve the mineral crystalline bone structure and lyse the remaining bone matrix elements. The cells may be multinucleated. Osteoblasts are actively engaged in synthesizing new collagen. The third cell type, osteocytes, are osteoblasts that become embedded and are incorporated into an osteoid matrix.

39. The answer is A (1, 2, 3). (*Chapter 19 I H 3 b*) Chondrosarcoma is not a particularly radiosensitive tumor; thus, it is treated surgically. However, an unfortunate tendency of the tumor is local recurrence, with more aggressive growth and likelihood of metastases if the surgical excision is not complete. The most common sites of origin are reported to be the spine, pelvis, and ends of the femur and humerus.

40. The answer is E (all). (*Chapter 20 III C 3, 5, 6, 7*) Pemphigus, dermatitis herpetiformis, erythema multiforme, and herpes simplex all are classified as bullous diseases by virtue of producing blisters, vesicles, or bullae. The lesions are formed by the destruction of individual cells or the intracellular connections. Trauma to the epidermis can also disrupt the keratinocyte connections. Blisters, vesicles, and bullae can contain serum or blood, depending upon the disease.

41–45. The answers are: 41-C, 42-C, 43-D, 44-A, 45-B. (*Chapter 7 III B; I C; II A; I A; II B*) The midsection of the thorax, which is the extrapleural space between the lungs, has been divided arbitrarily by anatomists and surgeons into subdivisions. The division of the mediastinum into superior, anterior, middle, and posterior is generally accepted; however, differences in terminology and referencing do exist. There are separate mediastinal compartments containing specific organs and tissues, and thus disease arising in these particular spaces can be better diagnosed with an appreciation of the mediastinal anatomy. For example, although rare, bronchogenic cysts can produce serious infections in the middle mediastinum, with the possible formation of lung abscesses if an infected bronchogenic cyst should rupture into the airways. Similarly, acute mediastinitis can be a life-threatening condition requiring surgical attention when there is traumatic perforation of the esophagus with its contents spilling into the posterior mediastinum.

46–50. The answers are: 46-B, 47-A, 48-E, 49-C, 50-D. (*Chapter 16 II F 2 a; II I 4; II I 7*) Huntington's disease, which consists of abnormal, involuntary movements (chorea) and mental deterioration, affects the cerebellum. Charcot-Marie-Tooth disease involves the peripheral sensory nerves, which show degenerated axons, loss of myelin, and fibrosis. Atrophy of the anterior horns of the spinal cord (especially of the cervical and lumbar areas) is associated with massive loss of neurons and gliosis and is characteristic of amyotrophic lateral sclerosis. Clinically, there is corresponding muscle weakness and spasticity. Loss of pigmented nuclei of the brainstem is characteristic of Parkinson's disease; usually, this includes depigmentation of the substantia nigra. Pick's disease is a presenile dementia characterized by degeneration (loss of neurons) of the frontal and temporal lobes of the cerebral cortex.

51–55. The answers are: 51-B, 52-D, 53-A, 54-E, 55-C. (*Chapter 17 VI A; VI B 2; VII A*) Small collections of histiocytes are seen in the sinusoids and nodal substance of nodes affected by toxoplasmosis. Histologically, the lymph nodes show prominent capsular fibrosis in syphilitic lymphadenitis. Sinus histiocytes containing melanin are characteristic of excoriative dermatopathia. The mature lesion of cat-scratch fever is an abscess with central necrosis. Characteristic of changes seen in some viral infections (including those of herpesvirus) is the formation of inclusion bodies in the cells.

56–60. The answers are: 56-A, 57-C, 58-B, 59-E, 60-D. (*Chapter 20 II A*) Macule, papule, nodule, wheal, and vesicle are all terms that describe the lesions that are produced by various diseases of the skin. For example, tender red nodules, which are found in the pretibial skin surfaces, are the classic findings in erythema nodosum, an inflammatory disease of the skin and subcutaneous tissue. Molluscum contagiosum is a poxvirus infection characterized by flesh-colored, smooth papules of the skin. Macules varying from white to brown in color are seen in tinea versicolor—a yeast infection caused by *Pityrosporon orbiculare*. Wheals and vesicles characterize the various eruptions that may follow oral and parenteral administration of a drug.

Index

Page numbers in *italics* refer to illustrations; those followed by a (t) denote tables.

nague Herman
879-8272

mr Jesus Pengson Hernandez
One Davis Drive
P.O. Box 6662
Saginaw, MI 48608

pg 227